Cochrane Handbook for
Systematic Reviews of
Diagnostic Test Accuracy

Cochrane Handbook for Systematic Reviews of Diagnostic Test Accuracy

Edited by

Senior Editors
Jonathan J. Deeks
Patrick M. Bossuyt

Associate Editors
Mariska M. Leeflang
Yemisi Takwoingi

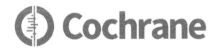

Registered Offices
John Wiley & Sons, Inc., 111 River Street, Hoboken, NJ 07030, USA
John Wiley & Sons Ltd, The Atrium, Southern Gate, Chichester, West Sussex, PO19 8SQ, UK

For details of our global editorial offices, customer services, and more information about Wiley products visit us at www.wiley.com.

Wiley also publishes its books in a variety of electronic formats and by print-on-demand. Some content that appears in standard print versions of this book may not be available in other formats.

Library of Congress Cataloging-in-Publication Data
Names: Deeks, Jonathan J., editor. | Bossuyt, Patrick, editor. | Leeflang,
    Mariska M., editor. | Takwoingi, Yemisi, editor. | Cochrane
    Collaboration, publisher.
Title: Cochrane handbook for systematic reviews of diagnostic test accuracy
    / edited by senior editors, Jonathan J. Deeks, Patrick M. Bossuyt ;
    associate editors, Mariska M. Leeflang, Yemisi Takwoingi.
Other titles: Handbook for systematic reviews of diagnostic test accuracy
Description: Hoboken, NJ : Wiley-Blackwell ; [London] : The Cochrane
    Collaboration, 2023. | Includes bibliographical references and index.
Identifiers: LCCN 2022052835 (print) | LCCN 2022052836 (ebook) | ISBN
    9781119756163 (cloth) | ISBN 9781119756170 (adobe pdf) | ISBN
    9781119756187 (epub)
Subjects: MESH: Systematic Reviews as Topic | Diagnostic Techniques and
    Procedures | Validation Studies as Topic
Classification: LCC RC71.5 (print) | LCC RC71.5 (ebook) | NLM W 20.5 |
    DDC 616.07/5–dc23/eng/20230119
LC record available at https://lccn.loc.gov/2022052835
LC ebook record available at https://lccn.loc.gov/2022052836

Cover Design: Wiley
Cover Images: © thanmano/Adobe Stock Photos; NVB Stocker/Adobe stock Photos; Kitreel/Adobe Stock Photos; angellodeco/Adobe Stock Photos; only4denn/Adobe Stock Photos; Tasha/Adobe Stock Photos; JarekKilian/Adobe Stock Photos; Nomad_Soul/Adobe Stock Photos; igorkol_ter/Adobe Stock Photos; utah51/Adobe Stock Photos; Marjan Apostolovic/Shutterstock

Set in 10/12pt SourceSansPro by Straive, Pondicherry, India
SKY10048700_060123

Contents

Contributors *xv*

Preface *xix*

Part One About Cochrane Reviews of diagnostic test accuracy *1*

1 Planning a Cochrane Review of diagnostic test accuracy *3*
1.1 Introduction *4*
1.2 Why do a systematic review of test accuracy? *4*
1.3 Undertaking a Cochrane Review of diagnostic test accuracy *5*
    1.3.1 The role of the Diagnostic Test Accuracy Editorial Team *5*
    1.3.2 Expectations for the conduct and reporting of Cochrane Reviews of diagnostic test accuracy *5*
    1.3.3 Data management and quality assurance *6*
    1.3.4 Keeping the Review up to date *6*
1.4 Proposing a new Cochrane Review of diagnostic test accuracy *6*
1.5 Cochrane Protocols *7*
1.6 The author team *11*
    1.6.1 The importance of the team *11*
    1.6.2 Criteria for authorship *12*
    1.6.3 Incorporating relevant perspectives and stakeholder involvement *12*
1.7 Resources and support *13*
    1.7.1 Identifying resources and support *13*
    1.7.2 Funding and conflicts of interest *14*
    1.7.3 Training *14*
    1.7.4 Software *15*
1.8 Chapter information *15*
1.9 References *16*

Part Two Introducing test accuracy *19*

2 Evaluating medical tests *21*
2.1 Introduction *21*
2.2 Types of medical tests *22*
2.3 Test accuracy *23*
2.4 How do diagnostic tests affect patient outcomes? *24*

2.4.1   Direct test effects   *25*
2.4.2   Altering clinical decisions and actions   *25*
2.4.3   Changes to time frames and populations   *25*
2.4.4   Influencing patient and clinician perceptions   *26*
2.5   Evaluations of test accuracy during test development   *26*
2.5.1   Evaluations of accuracy during biomarker discovery   *26*
2.5.2   Early evaluations of test accuracy   *27*
2.5.3   Clinical evaluations of test accuracy   *28*
2.6   Other purposes of medical testing   *28*
2.6.1   Predisposition   *29*
2.6.2   Risk stratification   *29*
2.6.3   Screening   *29*
2.6.4   Staging   *29*
2.6.5   Prognosis   *30*
2.6.6   Treatment selection   *30*
2.6.7   Treatment efficacy   *31*
2.6.8   Therapeutic monitoring   *31*
2.6.9   Surveillance for progression or recurrence   *31*
2.7   Chapter information   *32*
2.8   References   *32*

3   Understanding the design of test accuracy studies   *35*
3.1   Introduction   *35*
3.2   The basic design for a test accuracy study   *36*
3.3   Multiple groups of participants   *39*
3.4   Multiple reference standards   *42*
3.5   More on reference standards   *44*
3.5.1   Delayed verification   *44*
3.5.2   Composite reference standard   *44*
3.5.3   Panel-based reference   *44*
3.5.4   Latent class analysis   *45*
3.5.5   Gold standard   *45*
3.5.6   Clinical reference standard   *45*
3.6   Comparative test accuracy studies   *45*
3.6.1   Paired comparative accuracy study   *46*
3.6.2   Randomized comparative accuracy study   *46*
3.6.3   Non-randomized comparative accuracy study   *47*
3.7   Additional aspects of study designs   *47*
3.7.1   Prospective versus retrospective   *48*
3.7.2   Pragmatic versus explanatory   *48*
3.8   Concluding remarks   *49*
3.9   Chapter information   *49*
3.10   References   *50*

4   Understanding test accuracy measures   *53*
4.1   Introduction   *53*
4.2   Types of test data   *54*

4.3   Inconclusive index test results   *55*
4.4   Target condition   *56*
4.5   Analysis of a primary test accuracy study   *56*
       4.5.1   Sensitivity and specificity   *57*
       4.5.2   Predictive values   *58*
       4.5.3   Proportion with the target condition   *58*
       4.5.4   Pre-test and post-test probabilities   *59*
       4.5.5   Interpretation of sensitivity, specificity and predictive values   *59*
       4.5.6   Confidence intervals   *60*
       4.5.7   Other test accuracy measures   *61*
4.6   Positivity thresholds   *64*
4.7   Receiver operating characteristic curves   *66*
4.8   Analysis of a comparative accuracy study   *68*
4.9   Chapter information   *71*
4.10   References   *72*

Part Three   Methods and presentation of systematic reviews of test accuracy   *73*

5   **Defining the review question   *75***
5.1   Introduction   *75*
5.2   Aims of systematic reviews of test accuracy   *76*
       5.2.1   Investigations of heterogeneity   *77*
5.3   Identifying the clinical problem   *77*
       5.3.1   Role of a new test   *77*
       5.3.2   Defining the clinical pathway   *80*
       5.3.3   Unclear and multiple clinical pathways   *83*
5.4   Defining the review question   *84*
       5.4.1   Population   *84*
       5.4.2   Index test(s)   *85*
       5.4.3   Target condition   *85*
       5.4.4   The review question: PIT   *86*
       5.4.5   From review question to objectives   *86*
       5.4.6   Broad versus narrow questions   *87*
5.5   Defining eligibility criteria   *88*
       5.5.1   Types of studies   *88*
       5.5.2   Participants   *89*
       5.5.3   Index test(s)   *90*
       5.5.4   Target condition   *91*
       5.5.5   Reference standard   *92*
5.6   Chapter information   *93*
5.7   References   *93*

6   **Searching for and selecting studies   *97***
6.1   Introduction   *98*
6.2   Searching for studies   *98*
       6.2.1   Working in partnership   *100*
       6.2.2   Advice for review teams that do not include an information specialist   *101*

6.3   Sources to search   *101*
    6.3.1   Bibliographic databases   *101*
        6.3.1.1   MEDLINE, PubMed and Embase   *102*
        6.3.1.2   National and regional databases   *103*
        6.3.1.3   Subject-specific databases   *103*
        6.3.1.4   Dissertations and theses databases   *104*
    6.3.2   Additional sources to search   *104*
        6.3.2.1   Related reviews, guidelines and reference lists as sources
                  of studies   *105*
        6.3.2.2   Handsearching   *105*
        6.3.2.3   Forward citation searching and co-citation searching   *105*
        6.3.2.4   Web searching   *106*
        6.3.2.5   Grey literature databases   *107*
        6.3.2.6   Trial registries   *107*
        6.3.2.7   Contacting colleagues, study authors and
                  manufacturers   *108*
6.4   Designing search strategies   *108*
    6.4.1   Structuring the search strategy   *109*
    6.4.2   Controlled vocabulary and text words   *110*
    6.4.3   Text word or keyword searching   *112*
    6.4.4   Search filters   *113*
    6.4.5   Language, date and type of document restrictions   *113*
    6.4.6   Identifying fraudulent studies, other retracted publications, errata
            and comments   *114*
    6.4.7   Minimizing the risk of bias through search methods   *114*
6.5   Documenting and reporting the search process   *115*
    6.5.1   Documenting the search process   *116*
    6.5.2   Reporting the search process   *116*
        6.5.2.1   Reporting the search process in the protocol   *116*
        6.5.2.2   Reporting the search process in the review   *117*
6.6   Selecting relevant studies   *119*
    6.6.1   Examine full-text reports for compliance of studies with eligibility
            criteria   *120*
6.7   Future developments in literature searching and selection   *121*
6.8   Chapter information   *121*
6.9   References   *122*

7   Collecting data   *131*
7.1   Introduction   *132*
7.2   Sources of data   *132*
    7.2.1   Studies (not reports) as the unit of interest   *133*
    7.2.2   Correspondence with investigators   *134*
7.3   What data to collect   *135*
    7.3.1   What are data?   *135*
    7.3.2   Study methods (participant recruitment and sampling)   *137*
    7.3.3   Participant characteristics and setting   *138*

7.3.4   Index test(s)   *139*
7.3.5   Target condition and reference standard   *140*
7.3.6   Flow and timing   *140*
7.3.7   Extracting study results and converting to the desired format   *141*
            7.3.7.1   Obtaining 2×2 data from accuracy measures   *141*
            7.3.7.2   Using global measures   *144*
            7.3.7.3   Challenges defining reference standard positive and
                         negative: strategies when there are more than
                         two categories   *145*
            7.3.7.4   Challenges defining index test positive and negative:
                         inconclusive results   *145*
            7.3.7.5   Challenges defining index test positive and negative:
                         test failures   *147*
            7.3.7.6   Challenges defining index test positive and negative: dealing
                         with multiple thresholds and extracting data from ROC curves
                         or other graphics   *147*
            7.3.7.7   Extracting data from figures with software   *148*
            7.3.7.8   Corrections for missing data: adjusting for partial verification
                         bias   *148*
            7.3.7.9   Multiple index tests from the same study   *148*
            7.3.7.10   Subgroups of patients   *150*
            7.3.7.11   Individual patient data   *150*
            7.3.7.12   Extracting covariates   *151*
7.3.8   Other information to collect   *151*
7.4   Data collection tools   *152*
7.4.1   Rationale for data collection forms   *152*
7.4.2   Considerations in selecting data collection tools   *152*
7.4.3   Design of a data collection form   *154*
7.5   Extracting data from reports   *157*
7.5.1   Introduction   *157*
7.5.2   Who should extract data?   *157*
7.5.3   Training data extractors   *158*
7.5.4   Extracting data from multiple reports of the same study   *158*
7.5.5   Reliability and reaching consensus   *159*
7.5.6   Suspicions of scientific misconduct   *159*
7.5.7   Key points in planning and reporting data extraction   *160*
7.6   Managing and sharing data and tools   *160*
7.7   Chapter information   *163*
7.8   References   *164*

8   **Assessing risk of bias and applicability**   *169*
8.1   Introduction   *170*
8.2   Understanding bias and applicability   *171*
8.2.1   Bias and imprecision   *171*
8.2.2   Bias versus applicability   *171*
8.2.3   Biases in test accuracy studies: empirical evidence   *172*

8.3   QUADAS-2   *173*
    8.3.1   Background   *173*
    8.3.2   Risk-of-bias assessment   *173*
    8.3.3   Applicability assessment   *174*
    8.3.4   Using and tailoring QUADAS-2   *174*
    8.3.5   Flow diagram   *174*
    8.3.6   Performing the QUADAS-2 assessment   *175*
8.4   Domain 1: Participant selection   *176*
    8.4.1   Participant selection: risk-of-bias signalling questions (QUADAS-2)   *176*
    8.4.2   Participant selection: additional signalling questions for comparative accuracy studies (QUADAS-C)   *178*
    8.4.3   Participant selection: concerns regarding applicability   *181*
8.5   Domain 2: Index test   *182*
    8.5.1   Index test: risk-of-bias signalling questions (QUADAS-2)   *182*
    8.5.2   Index test: additional signalling questions for comparative accuracy studies (QUADAS-C)   *183*
    8.5.3   Index test: concerns regarding applicability   *186*
8.6   Domain 3: Reference standard   *187*
    8.6.1   Reference standard: risk-of-bias signalling questions (QUADAS-2)   *187*
    8.6.2   Reference standard: additional signalling questions for comparative accuracy studies (QUADAS-C)   *188*
    8.6.3   Reference standard: concerns regarding applicability   *189*
8.7   Domain 4: Flow and timing   *191*
    8.7.1   Flow and timing: risk-of-bias signalling questions (QUADAS-2)   *191*
    8.7.2   Flow and timing: additional signalling questions for comparative accuracy studies (QUADAS-C)   *193*
8.8   Presentation of risk-of-bias and applicability assessments   *196*
8.9   Narrative summary of risk-of-bias and applicability assessments   *197*
8.10   Chapter information   *197*
8.11   References   *198*

9   **Understanding meta-analysis**   *203*
9.1   Introduction   *203*
    9.1.1   Aims of meta-analysis for systematic reviews of test accuracy   *204*
    9.1.2   When not to use a meta-analysis in a review   *204*
    9.1.3   How does meta-analysis of diagnostic test accuracy differ from meta-analysis of interventions?   *205*
    9.1.4   Questions that can be addressed in test accuracy analyses   *206*
        9.1.4.1   What is the accuracy of a test?   *206*
        9.1.4.2   How does the accuracy vary with clinical and methodological characteristics?   *206*
        9.1.4.3   How does the accuracy of two or more tests compare?   *206*
    9.1.5   Planning the analysis   *207*
9.2   Graphical and tabular presentation   *208*
    9.2.1   Coupled forest plots   *208*
    9.2.2   Summary ROC plots   *208*

9.2.3   Linked SROC plots   *210*
    9.2.3.1   Example 1: Anti-CCP for the diagnosis of rheumatoid arthritis –
        descriptive plots   *210*
9.2.4   Tables of results   *211*
9.3   Meta-analytical summaries   *211*
9.3.1   Should I estimate an SROC curve or a summary point?   *212*
9.3.2   Heterogeneity   *214*
9.4   Fitting hierarchical models   *215*
9.4.1   Bivariate model   *216*
9.4.2   Example 1 continued: anti-CCP for the diagnosis of rheumatoid
    arthritis   *217*
9.4.3   The Rutter and Gatsonis HSROC model   *219*
9.4.4   Example 2: Rheumatoid factor as a marker for rheumatoid
    arthritis   *220*
9.4.5   Data reported at multiple thresholds per study   *221*
9.4.6   Investigating heterogeneity   *222*
    9.4.6.1   Criteria for model selection   *223*
    9.4.6.2   Heterogeneity and regression analysis using the bivariate
        model   *223*
    9.4.6.3   Example 1 continued: Investigation of heterogeneity in
        diagnostic performance of anti-CCP   *224*
    9.4.6.4   Heterogeneity and regression analysis using the Rutter
        and Gatsonis HSROC model   *227*
    9.4.6.5   Example 2 continued: Investigating heterogeneity in diagnostic
        accuracy of rheumatoid factor (RF)   *228*
9.4.7   Comparing index tests   *230*
    9.4.7.1   Test comparisons based on all available studies   *230*
    9.4.7.2   Test comparisons using the bivariate model   *231*
    9.4.7.3   Example 3: CT versus MRI for the diagnosis of coronary artery
        disease   *232*
    9.4.7.4   Test comparisons using the Rutter and Gatsonis HSROC
        model   *234*
    9.4.7.5   Test comparison based on studies that directly compare
        tests   *235*
    9.4.7.6   Example 3 continued: CT versus MRI for the diagnosis of
        coronary artery disease   *236*
9.4.8   Approaches to analysis with small numbers of studies   *238*
9.4.9   Sensitivity analysis   *239*
9.5   Special topics   *241*
9.5.1   Imperfect reference standard   *241*
9.5.2   Investigating and handling verification bias   *241*
9.5.3   Investigating and handling publication bias   *242*
9.5.4   Developments in meta-analysis for systematic reviews of test
    accuracy   *243*
9.6   Chapter information   *243*
9.7   References   *244*

10   Undertaking meta-analysis   *249*
10.1   Introduction   *249*
10.2   Estimation of a summary point   *251*
        10.2.1 Fitting the bivariate model using SAS   *251*
        10.2.2 Fitting the bivariate model using Stata   *253*
        10.2.3 Fitting the bivariate model using R   *256*
        10.2.4 Bayesian estimation of the bivariate model   *261*
                10.2.4.1   Specification of the bivariate model in rjags   *261*
                10.2.4.2   Monitoring convergence   *263*
                10.2.4.3   Summary statistics   *264*
                10.2.4.4   Generating an SROC plot   *265*
                10.2.4.5   Sensitivity analyses   *266*
10.3   Estimation of a summary curve   *266*
        10.3.1 Fitting the HSROC model using SAS   *268*
        10.3.2 Bayesian estimation of the HSROC model   *268*
                10.3.2.1   Specification of the HSROC model in rjags   *268*
                10.3.2.2   Monitoring convergence   *270*
                10.3.2.3   Summary statistics and SROC plot   *271*
                10.3.2.4   Sensitivity analyses   *272*
10.4   Comparison of summary points   *272*
        10.4.1 Fitting the bivariate model in SAS to compare summary points   *274*
        10.4.2 Fitting the bivariate model in Stata to compare summary points   *280*
        10.4.3 Fitting the bivariate model in R to compare summary points   *284*
        10.4.4 Bayesian inference for comparing summary points   *287*
                10.4.4.1   Summary statistics   *289*
10.5   Comparison of summary curves   *291*
        10.5.1 Fitting the HSROC model in SAS to compare summary curves   *292*
        10.5.2 Bayesian estimation of the HSROC model for comparing summary curves   *294*
                10.5.2.1   Monitoring convergence   *295*
                10.5.2.2   Summary statistics   *295*
10.6   Meta-analysis of sparse data and a typical data sets   *296*
        10.6.1 Facilitating convergence   *297*
        10.6.2 Simplifying hierarchical models   *301*
10.7   Meta-analysis with multiple thresholds per study   *305*
        10.7.1 Meta-analysis of multiple thresholds with R   *306*
        10.7.2 Meta-analysis of multiple thresholds with rjags   *311*
10.8   Meta-analysis with imperfect reference standard: latent class meta-analysis   *316*
        10.8.1 Specification of the latent class bivariate meta-analysis model in rjags   *316*
        10.8.2 Monitoring convergence   *317*
        10.8.3 Summary statistics and summary ROC plot   *317*
        10.8.4 Sensitivity analyses   *320*
10.9   Concluding remarks   *321*
10.10   Chapter information   *321*
10.11   References   *322*

11   **Presenting findings**   *327*
11.1   Introduction   *327*
11.2   Results of the search   *328*
11.3   Description of included studies   *328*
11.4   Methodological quality of included studies   *329*
11.5   Individual and summary estimates of test accuracy   *329*
    11.5.1   Presenting results from included studies   *330*
    11.5.2   Presenting summary estimates of sensitivity and specificity   *330*
    11.5.3   Presenting SROC curves   *330*
    11.5.4   Describing uncertainty in summary statistics   *332*
    11.5.5   Describing heterogeneity in summary statistics   *333*
11.6   Comparisons of test accuracy   *333*
    11.6.1   Comparing tests using summary points   *333*
    11.6.2   Comparing tests using SROC curves   *334*
    11.6.3   Interpretation of confidence intervals for differences in test accuracy   *336*
11.7   Investigations of sources of heterogeneity   *336*
11.8   Re-expressing summary estimates numerically   *340*
    11.8.1   Frequencies   *340*
    11.8.2   Predictive values   *341*
    11.8.3   Likelihood ratios   *344*
11.9   Presenting findings when meta-analysis cannot be performed   *344*
11.10   Chapter information   *346*
11.11   References   *347*

12   **Drawing conclusions**   *349*
12.1   Introduction   *349*
12.2   'Summary of findings' tables   *350*
12.3   Assessing the strength of the evidence   *352*
    12.3.1   Key issues to consider when assessing the strength of the evidence   *352*
        12.3.1.1   How valid are the summary estimates?   *359*
        12.3.1.2   How applicable are the summary estimates?   *359*
        12.3.1.3   How heterogeneous are the individual study estimates?   *359*
        12.3.1.4   How precise are the summary estimates?   *360*
        12.3.1.5   How complete is the body of evidence?   *361*
        12.3.1.6   Were index test comparisons made between or *within* primary studies?   *362*
12.4   GRADE approach for assessing the certainty of evidence   *362*
    12.4.1   GRADE domains for assessing certainty of evidence for test accuracy   *363*
        12.4.1.1   Risk of bias   *363*
        12.4.1.2   Indirectness (applicability)   *363*
        12.4.1.3   Inconsistency (heterogeneity)   *364*
        12.4.1.4   Imprecision   *365*
        12.4.1.5   Publication bias   *365*

12.5	Summary of main results in the Discussion section	*365*
12.6	Strengths and weaknesses of the review	*366*
	12.6.1 Strengths and weaknesses of included studies	*366*
	12.6.2 Strengths and weaknesses of the review	*367*
	12.6.2.1 Strengths and weaknesses due to the search and selection process	*367*
	12.6.2.2 Strengths and weaknesses due to methodological quality assessment and data extraction	*367*
	12.6.2.3 Weaknesses due to the review analyses	*368*
	12.6.2.4 Direct and indirect comparisons	*368*
	12.6.3 Comparisons with previous research	*369*
12.7	Applicability of findings to the review question	*369*
12.8	Drawing conclusions	*369*
	12.8.1 Implications for practice	*370*
	12.8.2 Implications for research	*373*
12.9	Chapter information	*374*
12.10	References	*374*
13	Writing a plain language summary	*377*
13.1	Introduction	*377*
13.2	Audience and writing style	*378*
13.3	Contents and structure of a plain language summary	*379*
	13.3.1 Title	*380*
	13.3.2 Key messages	*380*
	13.3.3 'Why is improving [. . .] diagnosis important?'	*381*
	13.3.4 'What is the [. . .] test?'	*382*
	13.3.5 What did we want to find out?	*382*
	13.3.6 What did we do?	*383*
	13.3.7 What did we find?	*383*
	13.3.7.1 Describing the included studies	*383*
	13.3.7.2 Presenting information on test accuracy	*384*
	13.3.7.3 Presenting single estimates of accuracy	*385*
	13.3.7.4 Presenting multiple estimates of accuracy: two index tests	*386*
	13.3.7.5 Presenting multiple estimates of accuracy: more than two index tests	*387*
	13.3.7.6 When presenting a numerical summary of test accuracy is not appropriate	*387*
	13.3.7.7 Graphical illustration of test accuracy results	*388*
	13.3.8 What are the limitations of the evidence?	*391*
	13.3.9 How up to date is this evidence?	*392*
13.4	Chapter information	*392*
13.5	References	*393*
13.6	Appendix: Additional example plain language summary	*394*
	Index	*399*

Contributors

Arevalo-Rodriguez, Ingrid
Hospital Universitario Ramón y Cajal
(IRYCIS)
CIBER Epidemiology and Public Health
(CIBERESP)
Madrid
Spain

Bossuyt, Patrick M
Department of Epidemiology and Data
Science
Amsterdam UMC
University of Amsterdam
Amsterdam
The Netherlands

Chandler, Jacqueline
Wessex Academic Health Science Network
Southampton
UK

Cumpston, Miranda S
School of Public Health and Preventive
Medicine
Monash University
Melbourne;
Cochrane Public Health
School of Medicine and Public Health
University of Newcastle
Newcastle
Australia

Davenport, Clare
Institute of Applied Health Research
University of Birmingham
Birmingham
UK

Deeks, Jonathan J
Institute of Applied Health Research
University of Birmingham
Birmingham
UK

Dendukuri, Nandini
McGill University
Montreal
Canada

Dinnes, Jacqueline
Institute of Applied Health Research
University of Birmingham
Birmingham
UK

Eisinga, Anne
Cochrane UK
Oxford University Hospitals NHS Foundation
Trust
Oxford
UK

Flemyng, Ella
Cochrane
London
UK

Gatsonis, Constantine
School of Public Health
Brown University
Providence, RI
USA

Glanville, Julie
glanville.info
York
UK

Jones, Hayley E
Population Health Sciences
Bristol Medical School
University of Bristol
Bristol
UK

Leeflang, Mariska M
Department of Epidemiology and Data
Science
Amsterdam UMC
University of Amsterdam
Amsterdam
The Netherlands

Li, Tianjing
Department of Ophthalmology
School of Medicine
University of Colorado Anschutz Medical
Campus
Aurora, CO
USA

Macaskill, Petra
Sydney School of Public Health
Faculty of Medicine and Health
University of Sydney
Sydney
Australia

Partlett, Christopher
Nottingham Clinical Trials Unit
University of Nottingham
Nottingham
UK

Reitsma, Johannes B
Julius Center for Health Sciences and
Primary Care
University Medical Center Utrecht
Utrecht University
Utrecht
The Netherlands

Rücker, Gerta
Institute of Medical Biometry and Statistics
Faculty of Medicine and Medical Center
University of Freiburg
Freiburg
Germany

Rutjes, Anne W
Department of Medical and Surgical
Sciences SMECHIMAI
University of Modena and Reggio Emilia
Modena
Italy

Schiller, Ian
Centre for Outcomes Research
McGill University Health Centre – Research
Institute
Montreal
Canada

Scholten, Rob J
Cochrane Netherlands
Julius Center for Health Sciences and
Primary Care
University Medical Center Utrecht
Utrecht University
Utrecht
The Netherlands

Spijker, René
Cochrane Netherlands
Julius Center for Health Sciences and
Primary Care
University Medical Center Utrecht
Utrecht University
Utrecht;
Medical Library
Amsterdam UMC
University of Amsterdam
Amsterdam
The Netherlands

Steingart, Karen R
Department of Clinical Sciences
Liverpool School of Tropical Medicine
Liverpool
UK

Takwoingi, Yemisi
Institute of Applied Health Research
University of Birmingham
Birmingham
UK

Whiting, Penny
Population Health Sciences
Bristol Medical School
University of Bristol
Bristol
UK

Yang, Bada
Julius Center for Health Sciences and
Primary Care
University Medical Center Utrecht
Utrecht University
Utrecht
The Netherlands

Preface

Patrick M. Bossuyt, Jonathan J. Deeks, Mariska M. Leeflang, Yemisi Takwoingi and Ella Flemyng

Medical tests are an indispensable element of modern-day health care. Clinicians rely on medical tests to find the likely cause of a patient's signs and symptoms, to evaluate the extent of disease, to predict the future course of the condition, to screen for asymptomatic disease and in many other situations.

Like any other intervention in health care, a medical test should be properly evaluated before its use can be recommended. Tests must make little error in measuring chemical, biological or physical quantities, or in detecting features, whether a clinical doctor assessing symptoms, a pathologist seeing a biopsy or a radiologist identifying an image. However, as well as being accurate, tests must also provide the right information to guide clinical actions. For this reason, a medical test must be evaluated for its clinical performance.

For diagnostic tests, this clinical performance is referred to as diagnostic accuracy: the ability of a test to correctly identify people who have or do not have the target condition. A diagnostic accuracy study assesses the results of an index test (test of interest) against a reference standard and provides estimates of the test's performance. Such evaluations of clinical performance should be done in a real-world setting within the context of a clinical pathway taking into account the intended use and target population.

For many tests a range of diagnostic accuracy studies have been reported in the medical literature. As in other areas of science, systematic reviews of such studies can provide informative syntheses of the available evidence. A systematic review can provide decision makers and other stakeholders with an overview of the currently available evidence about a test's diagnostic accuracy. We expect such reviews to include a well-defined review question, systematic searches of all relevant studies, evaluations of

This chapter should be cited as: Bossuyt PM, Deeks JJ, Leeflang, MM, Takwoingi Y, Flemyng E. Preface. In: Deeks JJ, Bossuyt PM, Leeflang MM, Takwoingi Y, editors. *Cochrane Handbook for Systematic Reviews of Diagnostic Test Accuracy*. 1st edition. Chichester (UK): John Wiley & Sons, 2023: xix–xxiv.

the risk of bias and applicability of identified studies and, if possible, meta-analyses that statistically combine the results of multiple studies.

The methods for systematic reviews of diagnostic accuracy studies were slow to develop, compared to methods for systematic reviews of randomized controlled trials of interventions. This difference parallels a difference in rigour in the primary studies and an understanding of sources of bias. Other explanations can be found as well: the wide differences in study objectives and designs of test accuracy studies, ranging from bio-marker discovery studies to large-scale clinical applications in the intended use setting. This variation and complexity of study designs can lead to results that are either not rel-evant or not valid for answering a test accuracy review question. This is further com-pounded by the fact that measures of test accuracy are not automatically transferable across different populations and settings. Unlike randomized controlled trials, test accu-racy studies typically provide paired proportions to indicate how well the test performs in those who have and those who do not have the target condition, i.e. the test's sensitiv-ity and specificity. This poses specific challenges for meta-analysis. Furthermore, sensi-tivity and specificity vary considerably more across studies than estimates of relative risk from clinical trials because they are proportions, not relative or absolute differences.

"Another challenge is in addressing clinically important comparative questions when there are competing tests that can be used at the same point in the clinical path-way. Systematic reviews of test accuracy can evaluate and compare the accuracy of two or more tests. While many studies evaluate the accuracy of a single index test, far fewer compare the accuracy of two or more index tests. Such comparative test accuracy stud-ies, which can provide robust evidence to inform test selection, deserve greater appre-ciation from clinical investigators, researchers, grant-awarding organizations funding test research, and those developing test use recommendations."

"Evidence on how the results of primary studies differ according to methodological features may be provided by meta-epidemiological studies. These meta-epidemiologi-cal studies often use data collected from systematic reviews. For example, the earliest meta-epidemiological studies based on Cochrane reviews strengthened the impor-tance of allocation concealment in randomised trials. Similar empirical studies using systematic reviews of diagnostic accuracy have confirmed essential elements of valid test accuracy studies, from avoiding the unnecessary inclusion of healthy controls to the need for appropriate statistical methods."

"This *Handbook* is informed by currently available empirical evidence and theoretical understanding of primary diagnostic accurarcy studies, review methods, and tech-niques for meta-analysis. The ongoing creation of Cochrane reviews will provide data for future studies that will shape our knowledge of how primary test accuracy studies and systematic reviews could be better performed."

This *Handbook* has a long history. Its development started around 2002, when a num-ber of us felt that the methodology for systematic reviews of test accuracy studies had sufficiently advanced to guide researchers. Since then, an incredible number of col-leagues have contributed to its gestation. Many of these have become authors of chap-ters in this *Handbook*. Others are explicitly acknowledged in various chapters for their contribution. Yet many more have contributed, through various discussions in methods groups sessions, conferences and other meetings. While we worked on this *Handbook* progress did not halt and in several steps of the review process more methodological advances were made, while best practices emerged in other areas.

Considerable progress has been made in searching, in evaluating risk of bias and applicability and in meta-analysis. The continuing development of software programs and user-written macros has made meta-analysis methods more accessible. A challenging area remains the communication of findings from reviews to decision makers and other stakeholders. Systematic reviews typically reveal substantial variability across studies and this variability makes it challenging to appreciate the true diagnostic accuracy of medical tests.

The authors of this *Handbook* have aimed to develop guidance based on the best current knowledge. We expect that several of the methods and practices will be advanced even further in the coming years, necessitating an update of this *Handbook* in the future. We are confident that the guidance in this *Handbook* will enable researchers in Cochrane and beyond to prepare informative reviews of the available literature to benefit patients and clinicians. In short: to all of us.

About Cochrane

Cochrane is an international network of health practitioners, researchers, methodologists, patients and carers, and others, with a vision of a world of better health for all people where decisions about health and care are informed by high-quality evidence (www.cochrane.org). Founded as The Cochrane Collaboration in 1993, it is a not-for-profit organization whose members aim to produce credible, accessible health information that is free from commercial sponsorship and other conflicts of interest.

Cochrane works collaboratively with health professionals, policy makers and international organizations, such as the World Health Organization (WHO), to support the development of evidence-informed guidelines and policy. WHO guidelines on critical public health issues such as the consolidated guidelines on systematic screening for tuberculosis disease (2021) and rapid diagnostics for tuberculosis detection (2021), and the WHO Essential Diagnostics List (2021), are underpinned by Cochrane Reviews.

There are examples of the impact of Cochrane Reviews on health and health care. Globally in 2020, a WHO-recommended rapid molecular test was used as the initial diagnostic test for 1.9 million (33%) of the 5.8 million people newly diagnosed with tuberculosis in 2020 (Global Tuberculosis Report 2021). Several rapid diagnostic tests (RDTs) for tuberculosis have been endorsed by the WHO since 2010 based on evidence from many Cochrane Reviews. A Cochrane Special Collection on diagnosing tuberculosis, first published in 2019 and last updated in March 2022 to celebrate World Tuberculosis Day (www.cochranelibrary.com/collections/doi/SC000034/full), highlighted the influential Cochrane reviews that have informed the two WHO consolidated guidelines on systematic screening and rapid diagnostics for tuberculosis. The use of RDTs for tuberculosis has contributed to the decentralization of testing and allowed patients to be diagnosed quickly with earlier initiation of appropriate treatment in many low- and middle-income countries. Rapid and reliable testing has also facilitated earlier detection of drug resistance and reduced mortality from tuberculosis among persons living with HIV.

Cochrane Reviews are published in full online in the *Cochrane Database of Systematic Reviews*, which is a core component of the Cochrane Library (www.cochranelibrary.com). The Cochrane Library was first published in 1996, and is now an online collection of multiple databases. The first Cochrane Review of diagnostic test accuracy was published in 2008.

About this *Handbook*

Work on a handbook to support authors of Cochrane Reviews of diagnostic test accuracy began in 2002, with draft chapters shared with the community online. It has evolved and grown into this second version since 2020, which is also the first print edition of the *Cochrane Handbook for Systematic Reviews of Diagnostic Test Accuracy*.

This *Handbook* is the official guide that describes in detail the process of preparing and maintaining systematic reviews of test accuracy for Cochrane. The *Handbook* has been produced by the Cochrane Screening and Diagnostic Tests Methods Group (www.methods.cochrane.org/sdt). It is a step-by-step guide for those conducting systematic reviews of test accuracy and a reference for more experienced authors.

The *Handbook* is divided into three parts. Part 1 covers information specific to Cochrane Reviews of diagnostic test accuracy. Part 2 introduces test accuracy studies and discusses when it might be appropriate to conduct them. Part 3 covers the methods used in systematic reviews of test accuracy and how to present the findings, including collecting data, assessing risk of bias in the included studies, and undertaking meta-analysis. It is applicable to all systematic reviews of test accuracy, though it is specifically relevant to Cochrane Reviews.

The *Handbook* is updated regularly to reflect advances in systematic review methodology and in response to feedback from users. Please refer to training.cochrane.org/handbook-diagnostic-test-accuracy for the most recent online version, for interim updates to the guidance and for details of previous versions of the *Handbook*. Feedback and corrections to the *Handbook* are also welcome via the contact details on the website.

Key details about this edition

This edition is the first complete version of this *Handbook*. The *Handbook* has been restructured, with reorganization or splitting of existing chapters and the addition of several new chapters. The *Handbook* covers:

- Updated guidance on understanding test accuracy measures (Chapter 4), searching for and selecting studies (Chapter 6), assessing the risk of bias and applicability in included studies (Chapter 8), understanding meta-analysis (Chapter 9), presenting findings (Chapter 11) and drawing conclusions (Chapter 12).
- New guidance on planning a Cochrane Review of diagnostic test accuracy (Chapter 1).
- New guidance on evaluating medical tests (Chapter 2).
- New guidance on the design of test accuracy studies (Chapter 3).
- New guidance on defining the review question (Chapter 5).
- New guidance on data extraction (Chapter 7).
- New guidance on undertaking meta-analysis (Chapter 10).
- New guidance on writing a plain language summary (Chapter 13).

How to cite this book

Deeks JJ, Bossuyt PM, Leeflang MM, Takwoingi Y, editors. *Cochrane Handbook for Systematic Reviews of Diagnostic Test Accuracy*. 1st edition. Chichester (UK): John Wiley & Sons, 2023.

Acknowledgements

We thank all of our contributing authors and chapter editors for their patience and responsiveness in preparing this *Handbook*. We are also indebted to all those who have contributed to previous versions of the *Handbook*, and particularly to past editor Rob J. Scholten.

Many people contributed constructive and timely peer review for this edition. We thank Alex Sutton, Anna Noel-Storr, April Coombe, Bada Yang, Bella Harris, Brian Duncan, Chris Hyde, Cochrane Information Specialist Executive, Daniël Korevaar, Danielle van der Windt, Denise Mitchell, Dimitrinka Nikolova, Eleanor Ochodo, Gianni Virgili, Ingrid Arevalo-Rodriguez, Jean-Paul Salameh, Jacqueline Dinnes, Jenny Doust, Jenny Negus, Jérémie Cohen, Karen R. Steingart, Kayleigh Kew, Kurinchi Gurusamy, Marta Roque, Matthew McInnes, Mia Schmidt-Hansen, Miranda Langendam, Sarah Berhane, Stephanie Boughton, Sophie Beese and Trevor McGrath.

Specific administrative support and copyediting for this version of the *Handbook* were provided by Laura Mellor, and we are deeply indebted to Laura for her many contributions. We would also like to thank staff at Wiley for their patience, support and advice, including Priyanka Gibbons (Commissioning Editor), Jennifer Seward (Senior Project Editor) and Samras Johnson Vanathaiya (Content Refinement Specialist). Finally, we thank Sally Osborn for copyediting the whole volume.

This *Handbook* would not have been possible without the generous support provided to the editors by colleagues at the University of Birmingham, the University of Amsterdam, and the Cochrane Evidence Production and Methods Directorate at Cochrane Central Executive. We particularly thank Karla Soares-Weiser (Editor in Chief, Cochrane) and acknowledge Ella Elliot (Wiley), Ingrid Arevalo-Rodriguez and other people from Wiley involved in the cover design.

Finally, the Editors would like to thank the thousands of Cochrane authors who volunteer their time to collate evidence for people making decisions about health care, and the methodologists, editors and trainers who support them.

Additional sources of support the editors would like to declare include that Jonathan J. Deeks is a UK National Institute for Health Research (NIHR) Senior Investigator Emeritus. Yemisi Takwoingi is funded by a UK National Institute for Health Research (NIHR) Postdoctoral Fellowship. Jonathan J. Deeks and Yemisi Takwoingi are supported by the NIHR Birmingham Biomedical Research Centre at the University Hospitals Birmingham NHS Foundation Trust and the University of Birmingham. The views expressed are those of the authors and not necessarily those of the NHS, the NIHR or the Department of Health and Social Care.

The *Handbook* editorial team

Jonathan J. Deeks (Senior Editor) is Professor at the Institute of Applied Health Research, University of Birmingham, UK, as well as a member of Cochrane's Diagnostic Test Accuracy Editorial Team.

Patrick M. Bossuyt (Senior Editor) is Professor at the Amsterdam UMC, University of Amsterdam, Department of Epidemiology and Data Science, The Netherlands; and a member of Amsterdam Public Health, Methodology, The Netherlands.

Mariska M. Leeflang (Associate Editor) is Associate Professor at the Amsterdam UMC, University of Amsterdam, Department of Epidemiology and Data Science, The Netherlands; a member of Amsterdam Public Health, Methodology, The Netherlands; as well as a Convenor of Cochrane's Screening and Diagnostic Tests Methods Group and member of Cochrane's Diagnostic Test Accuracy Editorial Team.

Yemisi Takwoingi (Associate Editor) is Professor at the Institute of Applied Health Research, University of Birmingham, UK, as well as a Convenor of Cochrane's Screening and Diagnostic Tests Methods Group and a member of Cochrane's Diagnostic Test Accuracy Editorial Team.

Ella Flemyng (Managing Editor) is Editorial Product Lead in Cochrane's Evidence Production and Methods Directorate, part of Cochrane's Central Executive Team, UK.

Part One

About Cochrane Reviews of diagnostic test accuracy

1

Planning a Cochrane Review of diagnostic test accuracy

Ella Flemyng, Miranda S. Cumpston, Ingrid Arevalo-Rodriguez, Jacqueline Chandler and Jonathan J. Deeks

---

KEY POINTS

- Systematic reviews of test accuracy (i.e. systematic reviews of studies of the accuracy of one or more medical tests) aim to address a need for health decision makers to have access to high-quality, relevant and up-to-date information regarding the use of a test in a specific healthcare setting.
- Systematic reviews of test accuracy, like all systematic reviews produced within Cochrane, aim to minimize bias through the use of pre-specified research questions and methods that are documented in protocols, and by basing their findings on reliable research.
- Author teams of systematic reviews of test accuracy should include members with appropriate methodological expertise in diagnostic test accuracy research.
- Proposals for new Cochrane Reviews of diagnostic test accuracy are generally submitted by author teams to Cochrane for approval before they are started.
- The Diagnostic Test Accuracy Editorial Team provides input into the editorial process for Cochrane Reviews of diagnostic test accuracy, by advising from the title stage to the final publication, offering methodological feedback on protocols and reviews.
- Review authors should be familiar with, and follow, the guidance developed by Cochrane for the conduct and reporting of their systematic reviews of test accuracy, as well as Cochrane's editorial policies such as avoiding and declaring potential conflicts of interest.

This chapter should be cited as: Flemyng E, Cumpston M S, Arevalo-Rodriguez I, Chandler J, Deeks JJ. Chapter 1: Planning a Cochrane Review of diagnostic test accuracy. In: Deeks JJ, Bossuyt PM, Leeflang MM, Takwoingi Y, editors. *Cochrane Handbook for Systematic Reviews of Diagnostic Test Accuracy*. 1st edition. Chichester (UK): John Wiley & Sons, 2023: 3–18.

This chapter re-uses and builds on material included in the following chapters of the *Cochrane Handbook for Systematic Reviews of Interventions* to ensure consistency in guidance for authors of Cochrane Reviews.

Cumpston M, Chandler J. Chapter II: Planning a Cochrane Review. In: Higgins JPT, Thomas J, Chandler J, Cumpston M, Li T, Page MJ, Welch VA, editors. *Cochrane Handbook for Systematic Reviews of Interventions* Version 6.1 (updated September 2020). Cochrane, 2020. Available from training.cochrane.org/handbook.

Lasserson TJ, Thomas J, Higgins JPT. Chapter 1: Starting a review. In: Higgins JPT, Thomas J, Chandler J, Cumpston M, Li T, Page MJ, Welch VA, editors. *Cochrane Handbook for Systematic Reviews of Interventions* Version 6.1 (updated September 2020). Cochrane, 2020. Available from training.cochrane.org/handbook.

1.1 Introduction

This chapter describes the general process for considering, planning and organizing a Cochrane Review of diagnostic test accuracy.

The process of preparing and publishing a Cochrane Review is different from that for other journals. This chapter builds on the information detailed in Chapter II (Planning a Cochrane Review) of the *Cochrane Handbook for Systematic Reviews of Interventions* with specific details on planning and preparing a Cochrane Review of diagnostic test accuracy (Lasserson 2020).

1.2 Why do a systematic review of test accuracy?

In general, systematic reviews were developed out of a need to ensure that decisions affecting people's lives can be informed by an up-to-date and complete understanding of the relevant research evidence. A systematic review attempts to collate all the empirical evidence that fits pre-specified eligibility criteria in order to answer a specific research question. It uses explicit, systematic methods that are selected with a view to minimizing bias, thus providing more reliable findings from which conclusions can be drawn and decisions made (Antman 1992, Oxman 1993).

Systematic review methodology, pioneered and developed by Cochrane, sets out a highly structured, transparent and reproducible methodology (Chandler and Hopewell 2013). This involves specifying a research question a priori; clarity on the scope of the review and which studies are eligible for inclusion; making every effort to find all relevant research and to ensure that issues of bias in included studies are accounted for; and analysing the included studies in order to draw conclusions based on all the identified research in an impartial and objective way (Lasserson 2020).

Cochrane Reviews can be categorized by the type of question they seek to address. Cochrane's first *Handbook* was dedicated to systematic reviews that seek to assess the benefits and harms of interventions, commonly referred to as Cochrane Reviews of interventions, which is the most common type of Cochrane Review. The *Cochrane Handbook for Systematic Reviews of Diagnostic Test Accuracy* focuses on the second most common type of Cochrane Review, which aims for the formal evaluation, including assessments of the methodological quality, of the available evidence on the performance of one or more medical tests, in a specific population and healthcare setting, for a specific testing purpose (Leeflang 2013, McInnes 2018, Schünemann 2020a).

The methods used are different for systematic reviews of test accuracy compared to systematic reviews of interventions, and this *Handbook* focuses on the methods recommended by Cochrane to plan, conduct and report the former to a high standard.

1.3   Undertaking a Cochrane Review of diagnostic test accuracy

Cochrane Reviews of diagnostic test accuracy have specific features that set them apart from reviews for other journals.

1.3.1   The role of the Diagnostic Test Accuracy Editorial Team

The Cochrane Diagnostic Test Accuracy Editorial Team currently supports the editorial process for Cochrane Reviews of diagnostic test accuracy. In 2023, Cochrane moves to a centralised editorial process for all evidence syntheses published on the Cochrane Library in 2023 and so this role may change. The Diagnostic Test Accuracy Editorial team consists of methodologists and clinicians with expertise in test accuracy research. They provide advice during all stages of the process, including the review of new titles, if requested, as well as methodological peer review and editorial assessment of all Cochrane Protocols and Reviews of diagnostic test accuracy. If improvements are needed, the Diagnostic Test Accuracy Editorial Team provides comprehensive guidance to be shared with the review authors, detailing the changes required to meet Cochrane's publication standards. The most up to date information about the Diagnostic Test Accuracy Editorial Team is available via the Screening and Diagnostic Tests Methods Group website (www.methods.cochrane.org/sdt).

1.3.2   Expectations for the conduct and reporting of Cochrane Reviews of diagnostic test accuracy

For Cochrane Reviews of diagnostic test accuracy, authors should follow the methodo-logical expectations detailed in this *Handbook*. Some specific expectations for plain language summaries of Cochrane Reviews of diagnostic test accuracy are detailed in Chapter 13. These expectations, informed by Cochrane editors and review authors, draw on experience of publishing systematic reviews of test accuracy since 2009.

Authors of Cochrane Reviews of diagnostic test accuracy should follow the Preferred Reporting Items for Systematic reviews and Meta-Analyses extension for Diagnostic Test Accuracy (PRISMA-DTA) Statement, as ensuring compliance with these reporting standards facilitates a full assessment of the methods and findings of the review (McInnes 2018).

Finally, as with all medical writing, it is important to consider the readers when deciding on the writing style, language, detail and level of assumed knowledge. In general, Cochrane Protocols and Reviews are read by informed patients as well as by clinicians, other healthcare professionals and policy makers. They are widely read by people whose first language is not English. It is thus important that the content and writing style, as far as possible, ensure that these reviews are accessible to this wide audience. Full details are available in the Cochrane Style Manual (www.community.cochrane.org/style-manual).

1.3.3 Data management and quality assurance

Cochrane Reviews of diagnostic test accuracy should be recorded and reported in sufficient detail for them to be replicable. Retaining a record of inclusion decisions, data collection and any transformations or adjustment to the extracted data will help to establish a secure and retrievable audit trail (Stegeman 2020).

Systematic reviews of test accuracy can be operationally complex projects, often involving large research teams working from different sites across the world. Good data management processes are essential to ensure that data and decisions are not inadvertently lost, facilitating the identification and correction of errors and supporting future efforts to update and maintain the review. Transparent reporting of review decisions enables readers to assess the reliability of the review for themselves (Lasserson 2020).

Further details about data management and quality assurance are available in Chapter 1 (Starting a review) of the *Cochrane Handbook for Systematic Reviews of Interventions* (Lasserson 2020).

1.3.4 Keeping the Review up to date

Cochrane Reviews should be updated if new, relevant evidence becomes available, especially when it would have an impact on the authors' conclusions. When proposing a new review, author teams should be committed both to completing the review and to maintaining it once it is published. However, there can be flexibility in this. Further details on updating are available in Chapter IV (Updating a review) of the *Cochrane Handbook for Systematic Reviews of Interventions* (Cumpston 2020b).

A 'living' systematic review is a systematic review that is continually updated, with new (or newly identified) evidence incorporated as soon as it becomes available (Elliott 2014a, Elliott 2017). Cochrane Reviews of diagnostic test accuracy can be conducted in living mode in situations where the evidence base is growing or evolving rapidly, to ensure that policy and practice are underpinned by the most up-to-date research. Any Cochrane Review in living mode should have approval from Cochrane, meet certain criteria (community.cochrane.org/review-production/production-resources/living-systematic-reviews) and follow specific guidance for the production and publication of living systematic reviews.

1.4 Proposing a new Cochrane Review of diagnostic test accuracy

Cochrane Reviews of diagnostic test accuracy go through a proposal process to check that the scope of the proposed review is appropriate and avoids duplication with existing and ongoing Cochrane Reviews, and that the author team have the skills, experience and resources to conduct the review (see Section 1.6). The proposal process also allows Cochrane staff to provide early editorial support and signposting to methods resources. Information about how to propose a Cochrane Review of diagnostic test accuracy is available online (www.methods.cochrane.org/sdt).

A proposal for a Cochrane Review of diagnostic test accuracy is checked for the suitability of the review question, approach and methods. As explained in Chapter 2 and Chapter 5, some test evaluation issues are not suitable for evaluation in test accuracy studies, including the reliability of a test, the agreement among different users when the test is applied, and the consequences for patient-important outcomes when the test is used (Lord 2006, Schünemann 2019, Schünemann 2020a, Schünemann 2020b).

Once a title is registered, the review authors will be required to develop and submit a formal protocol (see Section 1.5) incorporating feedback provided on the review proposal. Following peer review and approval, the protocol will be published in the *Cochrane Database of Systematic Reviews (CDSR)*. Author teams can then proceed to complete the full review. Both protocols and reviews should meet Cochrane's standards and adhere to Cochrane's editorial policies (www.community.cochrane.org/review-production/production-resources/cochrane-editorial-and-publishing-policy-resource). Cochrane may reject manuscripts that are not of a sufficient standard for publication following Cochrane's rejection policy (www.cochranelibrary.com/cdsr/editorial-policies#rejection-appeals).

The review title should succinctly reflect the review's objective. Typically, the key components of the title are:

- the population (stating what symptoms they present with, the healthcare setting, and what tests they have received before);
- the target condition or health status to be diagnosed (including the stage or subtype of disease that, for example, may determine eligibility for subsequent treatment);
- the diagnostic test or tests being evaluated (including their intended role and place in the current clinical diagnostic pathway).

An overview of test accuracy and test evaluation is available in Chapter 2 and details on designs for test accuracy studies are available in Chapter 3.

Four title formats are possible (Table 1.4.a) depending on the number of tests being evaluated (options 1 and 3 are for two or more tests, options 2 and 4 work for either a single test or a single group of tests) and whether the patient description is required (options 1 and 2) or can be omitted (options 3 and 4). Options 3 and 4, which do not include a patient description, should only be used where the target condition clearly implies a particular patient group.

1.5 Cochrane Protocols

Protocols for systematic reviews of test accuracy provide clear statements of the objectives of the research, including a focus on the comparisons that will be made, if needed, as well as the methods to conduct the review. They communicate important background information to provide a clinical context and define key clinical issues regarding the index test under assessment. The protocol also justifies the rationale and need for the review in the context of the existing scientific literature and current diagnostic

Table 1.4.a Structure for titles of Cochrane Reviews of diagnostic test accuracy

Option	Scenario	Structure	Examples
1	The full structure for a review title can include a comparison of two or more named index tests, a target condition and a population	\<Index test(s) 1\> *versus*/or \<index test(s) 2†\> *versus*/or . . . *for* \<target condition(s)\> *in* \<population\> († if the comparison is with current diagnostic practice, the second index test will be the comparator test – for instance, the test intended to be replaced)	Computed tomography angiography or magnetic resonance angiography for detection of intracranial vascular malformations in people with intracerebral haemorrhage Ultrasound, CT, MRI or PET-CT for staging and re-staging of adults with cutaneous melanoma
2	The second index test can be dropped when only a single test is considered, or when there is a name that describes the group of tests being compared	\<Index test(s)\> *for* \<target condition(s)\> *in* \< population\>	Optical coherence tomography (OCT) for detection of macular oedema in patients with diabetic retinopathy Rapid diagnostic tests for diagnosing uncomplicated P. falciparum malaria in endemic countries Plasma interleukin-6 concentration for the diagnosis of sepsis in critically ill adults
3	The population or setting can also occasionally be dropped where these will be obvious from the tests or the target condition	\<Index test(s) 1\> *versus*/or \<index test(s) 2†\> *versus*/or . . . *for* \<target condition(s)\> († if the comparison is with current diagnostic practice, the second index test will be the comparator test)	Human papillomavirus testing versus repeat cytology for triage of minor cytological cervical lesions Transabdominal ultrasound or endoscopic ultrasound for diagnosis of gallbladder polyps
4	The simplest option drops both the second test group and the population	\<Index test(s)\> *for* \<target condition(s)\>	Second trimester serum tests for Down's Syndrome screening Rapid diagnostic tests for plague

pathways to detect the target condition. Crucially, the protocol defines the methods by which the review will be undertaken, stating study eligibility criteria; search strategies, selection and quality assessment methods; and a statistical analysis plan.

Given the complexity of preparing Cochrane Reviews, a protocol should be written prospectively. There are a number of reasons that Cochrane Reviews should have a published protocol, including but not limited to the following: to reduce the risk of introducing bias in the review process; to improve the quality of the review as protocols undergo editorial, clinical and methodological peer review to ensure the methods are appropriate for the review question before the review is started; and to reduce the risk of duplicating efforts if other similar reviews are already underway. More details on the rationale for protocols is available in Chapter 1 (Starting a review) of the *Cochrane Handbook of Systematic Reviews of Interventions* (Lasserson 2020).

Cochrane Protocols and Reviews of diagnostic test accuracy follow a standard structure that facilitates review reporting and peer review. Most headings are common between the protocol and the review, including the Background and Methods sections, so only minor changes will be required between stages, such as a change in writing tense (from future to past). The exception will be where there are declared differences between a published protocol and a review, which should be described in the 'Differences between protocol and review' section of the completed review.

The full structure of a Cochrane Review of diagnostic test accuracy is seen in Box 1.5.a, along with which sections are found in the protocol. A full reporting template for

---

Box 1.5.a Sections of a Cochrane Review of diagnostic test accuracy

Title
Abstract*
Plain language summary*
Summary of findings*
Background

- Target condition being diagnosed
- Index test(s)
- Clinical pathway
  - Prior test(s)
  - Role of index test(s)
  - Alternative test(s)
- Rationale

Objectives
Methods

- Criteria for considering studies for this review
  - Types of studies
  - Participants
  - Index tests
  - Target conditions
  - Reference standards

- Search methods for identification of studies
  - Electronic searches
  - Searching other resources
- Data collection and analysis
  - Selection of studies
  - Data extraction and management
  - Assessment of methodological quality
  - Statistical analysis and data synthesis
  - Investigations of heterogeneity
  - Sensitivity analyses
  - Assessment of reporting bias

Results*

- Results of search
- Methodological quality of included studies
- Findings

Discussion*

- Summary of main results
- Strengths and weaknesses of review
- Applicability of findings to review question

Authors' conclusions*

- Implications for practice
- Implications for research

Appendices

- Search strategy
- Review-specific tailoring of QUADAS2

Information

- Authors
- Contribution of authors
- Sources of support
- Declarations of interest
- Acknowledgements
- Version history
- Differences between protocol and review*

References
Characteristics of studies*
Data and analyses*
Figures and tables

*Sections of a completed Review, not required in a Protocol.

Cochrane Protocols of diagnostic test accuracy is available as online supplementary material (1.S1 Writing a Cochrane Protocol of diagnostic test accuracy) and more details about protocol development in Cochrane more generally are available in Chapter 1 (Starting the review) in the *Cochrane Handbook for Systematic Reviews of Interventions* (Lasserson 2020).

1.6   The author team

1.6.1   The importance of the team

Synthesizing research about tests is more complex than synthesizing intervention studies (Naaktgeboren 2014, Beese 2018). In addition, the quality of systematic reviews of test accuracy published in the medical literature is currently poor (Mallett 2006, Willis 2011, Arevalo-Rodriguez 2014, Spencer-Bonilla 2017). It is imperative that the team planning the development of a systematic review of test accuracy includes individuals with the multidisciplinary skills needed to successfully complete the task from the beginning of the process.

In all cases Cochrane Reviews should be undertaken by more than one person and often require more than two. Review teams should include clinical and methodological expertise in the topic area being reviewed, as well as the perspectives of stakeholders (see Section 1.6.3 on which stakeholders are recommended for systematic reviews of test accuracy). For systematic reviews of test accuracy, it is often helpful to include both health professionals who use the index test in daily practice for the purpose specified in the review, and experts who are familiar with the relevant technical details related to its implementation. This will ensure that the team includes both those who face the clinical problem and those able to fully understand the study reports at a technical level.

Given the technical nature and complexity of test accuracy study reports and the clinical nuances that should be considered in making diagnoses in real-world settings, it is important to include on the team people with both topic and methodological expertise. This should help to ensure a balanced approach and a good mix of skills and knowledge, as well as a comprehensive assessment of the evidence regarding the accuracy of the index test.

For systematic reviews of test accuracy, author teams should include members with expertise in literature searching, completing systematic reviews, test research methods and statistics. The information specialists and statistical experts should be aware of the particular methodology for searching and data analysis for systematic reviews of test accuracy, as detailed in this *Handbook* in Chapter 6, Chapter 9 and Chapter 10.

When a proposal for a new review is under consideration, Cochrane's editorial teams will consider not only the clarity of the review question, but also the skills and experience of the team proposing the new review. All review authors are encouraged to make use of Cochrane training and guidance resources to ensure they have the skills required to conduct the review (see Section 1.7). First-time review authors are also encouraged to work with others who are experienced in the process of conducting systematic reviews of test accuracy.

1.6.2 Criteria for authorship

Authorship of all scientific publications (including Cochrane Protocols and Reviews) establishes accountability, responsibility and credit. Cochrane follows the International Committee of Medical Journal Editors (ICMJE) criteria for authorship (ICMJE 2018). When deciding who should appear in the byline of a Cochrane Review, it is important to distinguish individuals who have made a substantial contribution to the review (and who should be listed) from those who have helped in other ways (who should be mentioned in the Acknowledgements section). More information about authorship and contributorship is available in the Cochrane Editorial and Publishing Policy Resource (community.cochrane.org/review-production/production-resources/cochrane-editorial-and-publishing-policy-resource).

Methodological specialists such as statisticians and information specialists should be included as review authors where they meet the ICMJE authorship criteria, particularly where they have been substantively involved in the design and execution of the review's methods.

1.6.3 Incorporating relevant perspectives and stakeholder involvement

Engaging consumers and other stakeholders, such as policy makers, research funders and healthcare professionals, increases relevance, promotes mutual learning, improves uptake and decreases research waste. Review author teams are therefore encouraged to seek and incorporate the views of a variety of stakeholders and users during the review process.

As a review author, mapping out all potential stakeholders specific to the review question is a helpful first step to considering who might be invited to be involved in the review's development. Stakeholders typically include patients and consumers; consumer advocates; policy makers and other public officials; guideline developers; professional organizations; researchers; funders of health services and research; healthcare practitioners; and, on occasion, journalists and other media professionals. Balancing seniority, credibility within the given field and diversity should be considered. Review authors should also take account of the needs of low- and middle-income countries and regions, as well as vulnerable and marginalized people and societies, in the review process and invite appropriate input on the scope of the review and the questions it will address (Lasserson 2020).

Some author teams decide to form an Advisory Group with representation from multiple stakeholders. The Effective Public Health Practice Project, Canada, found that six members is generally large enough to cover all issues and is manageable for public health reviews (Effective Public Health Practice Project 2007). However, the broader the review, the broader the experience required of Advisory Group members. Terms of reference, job descriptions or person specifications for an Advisory Group may be developed to ensure clarity about the task(s) required.

More ways of working with consumers and other stakeholders are detailed in Chapter 1 (Starting a review) of the *Cochrane Handbook for Systematic Review of Interventions* (Lasserson 2020).

It is established good practice to ensure that consumers are involved and engaged in health research, including systematic reviews. Cochrane uses the term 'consumers' to refer to a wide range of people, including patients or people with personal experience of a healthcare condition, carers and family members, representatives of patients and carers, service users and members of the public.

Cochrane believes that consumer involvement is important because it (i) promotes transparency, accountability and trust in the way that research is produced; (ii) results in evidence that addresses consumers' needs, reduces waste in research, improves the translation of research into policy and practice, and ultimately leads to improved bene-fits for health systems and outcomes for patients; and (iii) is consistent with current health research approaches and is expected or mandated by some funders, partners and consumers. The benefits of consumer involvement are best realized when consumers contribute throughout the process of production and dissemination of research (see the Statement of Principles for Consumer Involvement in Cochrane, www.consumers.cochrane.org/news/statement-principles-consumer-involvement-cochrane).

Whenever consumers (or others) contribute during the development of a protocol or review, their contribution should be acknowledged in the Acknowledgements section or as an author if they meet the criteria for authorship (see Section 1.6.2).

1.7   Resources and support

1.7.1   Identifying resources and support

The main resource required by review authors is their own time. Most review authors will contribute their time free of charge because it will be viewed as part of their existing research or efforts to keep up to date in their areas of interest. However, Cochrane can facilitate author training opportunities and methodological support, among other support services.

The amount of time required to conduct a systematic review of test accuracy will vary, depending on the review question, the number of studies identified by the search strat-egies, the methods used, the experience of the review authors and the types of support available (Beese 2018). The workload associated with undertaking a review is thus very variable. However, early consideration of the tasks involved and the time required for each of these might help review authors to estimate the total amount of time that will be required during the entire review process. These tasks include training, meetings, protocol development, searching for studies, assessing citations and full-text reports of studies for eligibility, assessing the risk of bias and applicability of included studies, collecting data, pursuing missing data and unpublished studies, analysing the data, interpreting the results, and writing the review.

A time chart with target dates for accomplishing key tasks can help with scheduling the time needed to complete a review. Such targets may vary widely from review to review. Review authors, together with Cochrane, should determine an appropriate time frame for a specific review.

Resources that might be required for these tasks, in addition to the review authors' time, include:

- study-searching expertise;
- additional library resources, including access to electronic databases for searching and interlibrary loans;

- statistical support for synthesizing (if appropriate) the results of the included studies;
- equipment (e.g. computing hardware and software);
- supplies and services (internet connection, printing, telephone charges);
- office space for staff; and
- travel funds to attend review team meetings or present the results of the review.

1.7.2   Funding and conflicts of interest

Many organizations currently provide funding for high-priority systematic reviews. These include research-funding agencies, organizations that provide or fund healthcare services, those responsible for health technology assessment and those involved in the development of clinical practice guidelines. Author teams may wish to identify and seek funding from such organizations operating in their region or field of health care.

Conflict of interest in the funding and authorship of research gives rise to significant issues, which Cochrane takes very seriously (Bero 2018, Soares-Weiser 2019). Under Cochrane's policy on conflict of interest (www.cochranelibrary.com/cdsr/editorial-policies), a Cochrane Review cannot be funded or conducted by commercial sponsors or commercial sources with a financial interest in the topic of a specific review.

All prospective review authors should complete a declaration of interests form when proposing a review, and update this annually thereafter until publication, and just before publication of the protocol and the completed review. Individuals who are employed by, or own, a company that has a financial interest in the topic of the Cochrane Review (including, but not limited to, drug companies or medical device manufacturers), or who hold or have applied for a patent related to the topic of the Cochrane Review, are prohibited from being Cochrane Review authors. Additional restrictions apply for other financial interests. If any interests change over time, review authors should alert Cochrane and determine whether they affect the author's involvement in the review.

Restrictions also apply to any authors of the review who were involved in the conduct of one or more of the review's included studies. Review authors should not determine the eligibility of these studies, extract data from them or assess the methodological quality of these studies. Neither should they be involved in assessing the strength of the evidence involving studies they have (co-)authored. These tasks must be undertaken by other members of the team.

Full details on conflicts of interest and Cochrane Reviews, including all of the implications for review authors, are available in the Conflict of Interest Policy for Cochrane content (www.cochranelibrary.com/cdsr/editorial-policies).

Further discussion of the issues around conflicts of interest in research, and in particular how they apply to the studies included within a review, is outlined in Boutron et al (2020).

1.7.3   Training

Review authors new to Cochrane Reviews of diagnostic test accuracy may have previous training and experience in conducting Cochrane Reviews of interventions and other systematic reviews, but may benefit from additional guidance in the specialized methods required for systematic reviews of test accuracy. Cochrane provides a range of support services to facilitate learning of the specific methodology related to these reviews to assist those contributing to Cochrane Reviews of diagnostic test accuracy in gaining the knowledge and skills they need.

Cochrane also provides a range of online training resources, as well as face-to-face events in locations around the world. Details of current resources and events are available on the Cochrane Training website (training.cochrane.org) and via the Screening and Diagnostic Tests Methods Group website (methods.cochrane.org/sdt).

1.7.4   Software

Cochrane Reviews are supported by an ecosystem of software tools to assist with different aspects of the review process (Elliott et al 2014b). The primary piece of software is the review authoring tool Review Manager (RevMan; training.cochrane.org/online-learning/core-software/revman). It provides structured text drafting, standard tables and reference formats, meta-analysis, online help and error-checking mechanisms.

RevMan does not contain the statistical functionality required for meta-analysis of systematic reviews of test accuracy. Review teams therefore need to use RevMan in conjunction with a statistical package capable of fitting hierarchical models, such as Stata, SAS, R or WinBUGS. Study data entered into RevMan can be exported in a format suitable for import into these packages, and parameter estimates obtained from analyses in these packages can be entered back into RevMan to create the final meta-analytical summary receiver operating characteristic (SROC) plots and forest plots for inclusion in the review. Chapter 10 of this *Handbook* provides guidance on using these software packages for test accuracy meta-analysis. Tutorial documents and a resource of helpful computer macros are available on the Screening and Diagnostic Tests Methods Group website (methods.cochrane.org/sdt/).

Review authors may wish to consider other software resources (community.cochrane. org/help/tools-and-software) that might assist them with managing the review process (e.g. the selection of references to be included in the review). The choice of software tools may depend on the review authors' preference, the availability of a stable internet connection, the cost and other considerations. A register of tools designed for use in systematic reviews is maintained in the Systematic Review Toolbox (www. systematicreviewtools.com). Authors are advised to check with Cochrane and seek methodological advice before incorporating new technologies into their reviews.

For editorial stages, Cochrane uses the editorial management system Editorial Manager (training.cochrane.org/online-learning/em-training).

1.8   Chapter information

Authors: Ella Flemyng (*Cochrane, London, UK*), Miranda S. Cumpston (*School of Public Health and Preventive Medicine, Monash University, Cochrane Public Health, University of Newcastle, Australia*), Ingrid Arevalo-Rodriguez (*Hospital Universitario Ramón y Cajal (IRYCIS); CIBER Epidemiology and Public Health (CIBERESP), Madrid, Spain*), Jacqueline Chandler (*Wessex Academic Health Science Network, Southampton, UK*), Jonathan J. Deeks (*Institute of Applied Health Research, University of Birmingham, UK*).

Sources of support: Ella Flemyng is employed by and receives a salary from Cochrane. Ingrid Arevalo-Rodriguez is funded by the Instituto de Salud Carlos III through the "Acción Estrategica en Salud 2017-2020 / Contratos Miguel Servet 2020/CD20/00152". Jonathan J. Deeks is a UK National Institute for Health Research (NIHR) Senior Investigator Emeritus. Jonathan J. Deeks is supported by the NIHR Birmingham Biomedical Research Centre at the University Hospitals Birmingham NHS Foundation Trust and the University of Birmingham. The views expressed are those of the authors and not necessarily those of the NHS, the NIHR or the Department of Health and Social Care. No other authors declare sources of support for writing this chapter.

Declarations of interest: Ella Flemyng works in Cochrane's Evidence Production and Methods Directorate, part of Cochrane's Central Executive Team. Miranda S. Cumpston is an Editor with Cochrane Public Health. Ingrid Arevalo-Rodriguez and Jonathan J. Deeks are members of Cochrane's Diagnostic Test Accuracy Editorial Team. The authors declare no other potential conflicts of interest relevant to the topic of this chapter.

Acknowledgements: This chapter re-uses and builds on material included in the following chapters of the *Cochrane Handbook for Systematic Reviews of Interventions* to ensure consistency in guidance for authors of Cochrane Reviews: (1) Cumpston M, Chandler J. Chapter II: Planning a Cochrane Review. In: Higgins JPT, Thomas J, Chandler J, Cumpston M, Li T, Page MJ, Welch VA, editors. *Cochrane Handbook for Systematic Reviews of Interventions* Version 6.1 (updated September 2020). Cochrane, 2020. Available from training.cochrane.org/handbook. (2) Lasserson TJ, Thomas J, Higgins JPT. Chapter 1: Starting a review. In: Higgins JPT, Thomas J, Chandler J, Cumpston M, Li T, Page MJ, Welch VA, editors. *Cochrane Handbook for Systematic Reviews of Interventions* Version 6.1 (updated September 2020). Cochrane, 2020. Available from training. cochrane.org/handbook.

The authors thank Ginny Brunton, Clare Davenport, Sally Green, Julian Higgins, Nicki Jackson, Monica Kjeldstrøm, Toby Lasserson, Sandy Oliver and Susanna Wisniewski for contributions to previous versions of this chapter. The authors also thank Liz Wager for her assistance in preparing the text for the chapter previously titled 'Guide to the contents of a Cochrane Diagnostic Test Accuracy Protocol', which was incorporated into this chapter, and Nynke Smidt and Theresa Moore for their contributions to the previous version of that chapter.

The authors would like to thank Sophie Beese, Stephanie Boughton, Isobel Harris, Kayleigh Kew and Dimitrinka Nikolova for helpful peer review comments.

1.9 References

Antman EM, Lau J, Kupelnick B, Mosteller F, Chalmers TC. A comparison of results of meta-analyses of randomized control trials and recommendations of clinical experts. Treatments for myocardial infarction. *JAMA* 1992; **268**: 240–248.

Arevalo-Rodriguez I, Segura O, Solà I, Bonfill X, Sanchez E, Alonso-Coello P. Diagnostic tools for alzheimer's disease dementia and other dementias: an overview of diagnostic test accuracy (DTA) systematic reviews. *BMC Neurology* 2014; **14**: 183.

Beese S, Harris B, Davenport C, Mallet S, Takwoingi Y, Deeks J. The first ten years of Cochrane DTA reviews: progress and common methodological challenges. *Abstracts of the 25th Cochrane Colloquium*. Edinburgh (UK): Cochrane Database of Systematic Reviews, 2018.

Bero L. More journals should have conflict of interest policies as strict as Cochrane. *BMJ Opinion*; 2018. Available at blogs.bmj.com/bmj/2018/11/12/lisa-bero-more-journals-should-have-conflict-of-interest-policies-as-strict-as-cochrane/.

Boutron I, Page M, Higgins J, Altman D, Lundh A, Hróbjartsson A. Chapter 7: Considering bias and conflicts of interest among the included studies. In: Higgins J, Thomas J, Chandler J, Cumpston M, Li T, Page M, Welch V, editors. *Cochrane Handbook for Systematic Reviews of Interventions* Version 6.1 (updated September 2020). Cochrane, 2020. Available from training.cochrane.org/handbook.

Chandler J, Hopewell S. Cochrane methods—twenty years experience in developing systematic review methods. *Systematic Reviews* 2013; **2**: 76.

Cumpston M, Chandler J. Chapter II: Planning a Cochrane Review. In: Higgins J, Thomas J, Chandler J, Cumpston M, Li T, Page M, Welch V, editors. *Cochrane Handbook for Systematic Reviews of Interventions* Version 6.1 (updated September 2020). Cochrane, 2020a. Available from training.cochrane.org/handbook.

Cumpston M, Chandler J. Chapter IV: Updating a review. In: Higgins J, Thomas J, Chandler J, Cumpston M, Li T, Page M, Welch V, editors. *Cochrane Handbook for Systematic Reviews of Interventions* Version 6.1 (updated September 2020). Cochrane, 2020b. Available from training.cochrane.org/handbook.

Effective Public Health Practice Project. Effective Public Health Practice Project 2007. Available at www.city.hamilton.on.ca/PHCS/EPHPP.

Elliott JH, Turner T, Clavisi O, Thomas J, Higgins JP, Mavergames C, Gruen RL. Living systematic reviews: an emerging opportunity to narrow the evidence-practice gap. *PLoS Medicine* 2014a; **11**: e1001603.

Elliott JH, Sim I, Thomas J, Owens N, Dooley G, Riis J, Wallace B, Thomas J, Noel-Storr A, Rada G, Struthers C, Howe T, MacLehose H, Brandt L, Kunnamo I, Mavergames C. #CochraneTech: technology and the future of systematic reviews. *Cochrane Database of Systematic Reviews* 2014b, **9**: ED000091.

Elliott JH, Synnot A, Turner T, Simmonds M, Akl EA, McDonald S, Salanti G, Meerpohl J, MacLehose H, Hilton J, Tovey D, Shemilt I, Thomas J. Living systematic review: 1. Introduction—the why, what, when, and how. *Journal of Clinical Epidemiology* 2017; **91**: 23–30.

ICMJE. Recommendations for the Conduct, Reporting, Editing, and Publication of Scholarly Work in Medical Journals. International Committee of Medical Journal Editors, 2018. Available at www.icmje.org/recommendations.

Lasserson T, Thomas J, Higgins J. Chapter 1: Starting a review. In: Higgins J, Thomas J, Chandler J, Cumpston M, Li T, Page M, Welch V, editors. *Cochrane Handbook for Systematic Reviews of Interventions* Version 6.1 (updated September 2020). Cochrane, 2020. Available from training.cochrane.org/handbook.

Leeflang MM, Deeks JJ, Takwoingi Y, Macaskill P. Cochrane diagnostic test accuracy reviews. *Systematic Reviews* 2013; **2**: 82.

Lord SJ, Irwig L, Simes RJ. When is measuring sensitivity and specificity sufficient to evaluate a diagnostic test, and when do we need randomized trials? *Annals of Internal Medicine* 2006; **144**: 850–855.

Mallett S, Deeks JJ, Halligan S, Hopewell S, Cornelius V, Altman DG. Systematic reviews of diagnostic tests in cancer: review of methods and reporting. *BMJ* 2006; **333**: 413.

McInnes MDF, Moher D, Thombs BD, McGrath TA, Bossuyt PM, Clifford T, Cohen JF, Deeks JJ, Gatsonis C, Hooft L, Hunt HA, Hyde CJ, Korevaar DA, Leeflang MMG, Macaskill P, Reitsma JB, Rodin R, Rutjes AWS, Salameh JP, Stevens A, Takwoingi Y, Tonelli M, Weeks L, Whiting P, Willis BH. Preferred Reporting Items for a Systematic Review and Meta-analysis of Diagnostic Test Accuracy Studies: The PRISMA-DTA Statement. *JAMA* 2018; **319**: 388–396.

Naaktgeboren CA, van Enst WA, Ochodo EA, de Groot JA, Hooft L, Leeflang MM, Bossuyt PM, Moons KG, Reitsma JB. Systematic overview finds variation in approaches to investigating and reporting on sources of heterogeneity in systematic reviews of diagnostic studies. *Journal of Clinical Epidemiology* 2014; **67**: 1200–1209.

Oxman AD, Guyatt GH. The science of reviewing research. *Annals of the New York Academy of Sciences* 1993; **703**: 125–133; discussion 133-124.

Schünemann HJ, Mustafa RA, Brozek J, Santesso N, Bossuyt PM, Steingart KR, Leeflang M, Lange S, Trenti T, Langendam M, Scholten R, Hooft L, Murad MH, Jaeschke R, Rutjes A, Singh J, Helfand M, Glasziou P, Arevalo-Rodriguez I, Akl EA, Deeks JJ, Guyatt GH. GRADE guidelines: 22. The GRADE approach for tests and strategies—from test accuracy to patient-important outcomes and recommendations. *Journal of Clinical Epidemiology* 2019; **111**: 69–82.

Schünemann HJ, Mustafa RA, Brozek J, Steingart KR, Leeflang M, Murad MH, Bossuyt P, Glasziou P, Jaeschke R, Lange S, Meerpohl J, Langendam M, Hultcrantz M, Vist GE, Akl EA, Helfand M, Santesso N, Hooft L, Scholten R, Rosen M, Rutjes A, Crowther M, Muti P, Raatz H, Ansari MT, Williams J, Kunz R, Harris J, Rodriguez IA, Kohli M, Guyatt GH. GRADE guidelines: 21 part 1. Study design, risk of bias, and indirectness in rating the certainty across a body of evidence for test accuracy. *Journal of Clinical Epidemiology* 2020a; **122**: 129–141.

Schünemann HJ, Mustafa RA, Brozek J, Steingart KR, Leeflang M, Murad MH, Bossuyt P, Glasziou P, Jaeschke R, Lange S, Meerpohl J, Langendam M, Hultcrantz M, Vist GE, Akl EA, Helfand M, Santesso N, Hooft L, Scholten R, Rosen M, Rutjes A, Crowther M, Muti P, Raatz H, Ansari MT, Williams J, Kunz R, Harris J, Rodriguez IA, Kohli M, Guyatt GH. GRADE guidelines: 21 part 2. Test accuracy: inconsistency, imprecision, publication bias, and other domains for rating the certainty of evidence and presenting it in evidence profiles and summary of findings tables. *Journal of Clinical Epidemiology* 2020b; **122**: 142–152.

Soares-Weiser K. A more rigorous conflict of interest policy is coming for Cochrane; 2019. Available at www.cochrane.org/news/more-rigorous-conflict-interest-policy-coming-cochrane.

Spencer-Bonilla G, Singh Ospina N, Rodriguez-Gutierrez R, Brito JP, Iñiguez-Ariza N, Tamhane S, Erwin PJ, Murad MH, Montori VM. Systematic reviews of diagnostic tests in endocrinology: an audit of methods, reporting, and performance. *Endocrine* 2017; **57**: 18–34.

Stegeman I, Leeflang MMG. Meta-analyses of diagnostic test accuracy could not be reproduced. *Journal of Clinical Epidemiology* 2020; **127**: 161–166.

Willis BH, Quigley M. The assessment of the quality of reporting of meta-analyses in diagnostic research: a systematic review. *BMC Medical Research Methodology* 2011; **11**: 163.

Part Two

Introducing test accuracy

2

Evaluating medical tests

Jonathan J. Deeks and Patrick M. Bossuyt

KEY POINTS

- Medical tests are procedures to assess an individual's current health state or predict their future health state.
- Commonly used tests include clinical history taking and physical examination, questionnaire-based measurement tools, physiological measurements, in vitro tests of many different forms, radiological imaging, endoscopic and other optical examinations, and risk scores that combine test results of different types.
- Medical tests that provide evidence for diagnosis, staging, screening, monitoring and surveillance of disease are often evaluated using test accuracy studies. However, assessing the ability to determine disease predisposition, prognosis or treatment response requires longitudinal rather than cross-sectional test accuracy studies.
- Improving test accuracy can improve patient outcomes if more accurate tests lead to more effective interventions being given to the right patients.
- Evaluating test accuracy is necessary but not sufficient to assess whether tests benefit patients, as tests may also affect patients in other ways.

2.1 Introduction

In this chapter we consider various sorts of medical tests, and briefly introduce the types of test technology most commonly encountered in medical care and the research literature. We then review the multiple purposes for which medical tests are used and identify those that can be evaluated using the test accuracy paradigm and that therefore can be included in Cochrane Reviews of diagnostic test accuracy. For several of these purposes we explain the need for evidence in addition to test accuracy to fully understand a test's impact on patients. We describe the types of research that may be

This chapter should be cited as: Deeks JJ, Bossuyt PM. Chapter 2: Evaluating medical tests. In: Deeks JJ, Bossuyt PM, Leeflang MM, Takwoingi Y, editors. *Cochrane Handbook for Systematic Reviews of Diagnostic Test Accuracy*. 1st edition. Chichester (UK): John Wiley & Sons, 2023: 21–34.

Cochrane Handbook for Systematic Reviews of Diagnostic Test Accuracy, First Edition. Edited by Jonathan J. Deeks, Patrick M. Bossuyt, Mariska M. Leeflang and Yemisi Takwoingi.
© 2023 The Cochrane Collaboration. Published 2023 by John Wiley & Sons Ltd.

undertaken when evaluating medical tests, and identify the place that test accuracy has in the evaluation pathway. Finally, we review the impact of tests on patients, consider the role that test accuracy has in predicting the effect of testing and treatment on patients, and discuss the additional evidence that may be required to decide whether using a test is likely to do more good than harm.

2.2 Types of medical tests

A medical test refers to any procedure performed on a person's fluids, cells, tissue or on the person themself, to detect, diagnose or monitor a condition or the course of a condition. Medical tests come in many different forms, from patient history and physical and visual examination to lab tests and imaging, as well as risk scores that combine multiple pieces of information from different sources.

Diagnostic tests are medical tests undertaken in patients who present to health services with signs or symptoms. They are typically used to identify the likely cause of these symptoms, by identifying an underlying disease, and to decide whether treatment is required.

Cochrane places no restrictions on types of tests for inclusion as review topics, and defines testing as anything that records a characteristic, measurement or observation from an individual, regardless of the technology used to obtain it. The defining feature is that the observation, resulting from the test or procedure, is made to infer something about the health state of the individual at that point in time. Table 2.2.a lists the types

Table 2.2.a Major types of tests

Test type	Example Cochrane Review of diagnostic test accuracy
Taking a medical history	First rank symptoms of schizophrenia
Clinical examination	Clinical assessment to screen for the detection of oral cavity cancer and potentially malignant disorders in apparently healthy adults
Questionnaires	Informant Questionnaire on Cognitive Decline in the Elderly (IQCODE) for the diagnosis of dementia within a general practice (primary care) setting
Physiological measurements	Ankle brachial index for the diagnosis of symptomatic peripheral arterial disease
In vitro diagnostics	Procalcitonin, C-reactive protein, and erythrocyte sedimentation rate for the diagnosis of acute pyelonephritis in children
Radiological imaging	Magnetic resonance imaging versus computed tomography to detect acute vascular lesions in patients presenting with stroke symptoms
Optical imaging	Capsule endoscopy for the diagnosis of oesophageal varices in people with chronic liver disease or portal vein thrombosis
Risk scores	Second trimester serum tests for Down syndrome screening

of tests and technologies most commonly used for diagnosis with examples from Cochrane Reviews.

2.3 Test accuracy

This *Handbook* provides guidance for performing systematic reviews of test accuracy studies. Test accuracy studies evaluate the ability of a test to correctly classify study participants, based on the test results, as having the target condition or not. In most cases, that information will be relevant when the test is considered for diagnostic reasons: to identify the condition that most likely is responsible for the signs and symptoms of the patient. Chapter 3 describes the study designs for such studies.

Because the purpose of testing may not be strictly the detection of disease, we are, more generally, referring to the detection of a condition. The target condition is the condition that the test aims to detect. In test evaluation, the target condition may be a specific disease, such as chronic kidney disease. It may also be a syndrome (e.g. Down syndrome, acute coronary syndrome) or a disease stage (e.g. end-stage kidney disease, also known as renal failure).

The results from a medical test may be qualitative (expressed in a report) or quantitative (expressed in numbers). Essential for evaluations of test accuracy is that the test result can be classified as pointing to the target condition, or not. The first situation – test result points to the presence of the target condition – is usually called a positive test result; the second situation – test result does not point to the presence of the target condition – is correspondingly called a negative test result. This means that all test results are classified as either positive test results or negative test results.

In evaluations of the accuracy of medical tests, this classification into positive and negative test results is compared with a similar classification, but made by using the results from the reference standard. The reference standard is usually the best available method for finding out whether people have the target condition (see Chapter 3).

When we evaluate test accuracy, we compare two classifications: the one made based on the test results (positive versus negative) and the one made based on the reference standard (target condition present or not). Test positives – those with a positive test result – can then be found out to have a true positive test result (the reference standard confirms the presence of the target condition) or a false positive test result (the reference standard shows that the target condition is not present. Similarly, test negatives can be further classified as true negatives or false negatives. Test accuracy measures, such as sensitivity and specificity, are statistical summaries of such comparisons. Chapter 4 discusses the various ways in which the results of this comparison of classifications can be summarized.

When the test is aimed to assist in making a diagnosis, the accuracy of that test can be referred to as its diagnostic accuracy. The question about the diagnostic accuracy of a test is a cross-sectional question: it addresses the extent to which a classification, based on the test results, corresponds to a classification of the same people, had they been evaluated by the reference standard, at that specific point in time.

Test accuracy is sometimes referred to in other terms. It is also known as the discriminatory performance or discrimination. Accuracy is but one of the possible ways to evaluate the clinical performance of a medical test. Clinical performance is a more general term, referring to the ability of a test to yield results that are correlated with a particular clinical condition or a physiological or pathological process or state (Horvath 2014, European Parliament and Council of the European Union 2017).

2.4   How do diagnostic tests affect patient outcomes?

It is now recognized that recommendations about the use of medical tests should be based on the ability of tests or testing strategies to improve outcomes: to improve or preserve the health of those being tested, or to make health care more efficient without detrimental health effects (Lord 2006, Schünemann 2008).

The impact of a test on patient outcomes is best assessed in randomized trials that allocate participants to diagnostic pathways that do and do not contain the new test and compare patient outcomes once all consequent interventions have been undertaken (Bossuyt 2000). Systematic reviews of these studies are included in the Cochrane Library as systematic reviews of interventions, not of test accuracy. An alternative approach is a decision analysis that compares different diagnostic strategies using different sources of information for test accuracy and treatment efficacy, presuming particular models of clinician diagnostic and management behaviour (National Institute for Health and Clinical Excellence 2011, Chang 2012).

Randomized trials of testing strategies have advantages since they can also assess how other differences in the testing pathway affect patient outcomes (as described in Section 2.4.2). However, they are challenging to mount, needing large sample sizes and require clinicians to adhere to diagnostic and treatment protocols (or at least to record them) (Ferrante di Ruffano 2017a).

While these randomized trials are often proposed as the ideal method for judging the value of a diagnostic test, few such trials have been undertaken in diagnostic settings (Ferrante di Ruffano 2012a) and many have been underpowered or methodologically lacking (Ferrante di Ruffano 2017b). In some fields, such as infectious diseases, trials of tests are used (Odaga 2014). More success has been achieved in undertaking randomized trials of screening interventions, several of which have been evaluated in Cochrane Reviews of interventions (e.g. screening for prostate cancer, colorectal cancer and lung cancer) (Hewitson 2007, Gøtzsche 2013, Ilic 2013, Manser 2013).

Evidence of improved test accuracy may not necessarily be sufficient for a test to lead to improved patient outcomes (Lord 2006). In fact, as there are other ways in which tests affect patients that can lead to changes in outcomes, it is not even necessary for a new test to be as accurate as an existing test to benefit patients overall. It is important to be aware of the possible ways in which each new test can act, and to assess the evidence for each effect (Ferrante di Ruffano 2012b).

Cochrane Reviews of diagnostic test accuracy can provide evidence of the accuracy of a test, but often need to be used alongside other evidence to make a holistic judgement of the likely impact on patients. There may even be some circumstances where trade-offs between harms (e.g. reduced accuracy) over benefits (e.g. less use of risky invasive testing) may need to be assessed. This section outlines the main issues that should be considered. These considerations should be mentioned in both the Background and Discussion sections of a Cochrane Review.

Ferrante di Ruffano and colleagues (Ferrante di Ruffano 2012b) proposed using a checklist to compare testing strategies to identify the key differences that might affect patient outcomes. The key aspects in this framework are described below.

2.4.1   Direct test effects

Tests may directly harm patients if they are invasive. It is important to be aware of what these harms may be and how frequently they are encountered. While some tests may involve passing discomfort, others may have long-term sequelae, or put patients at risk of serious and sometimes life-threatening complications. Undergoing testing may also have psychological harms and benefits. Regardless of the test results, testing may cause anxiety through raising the possibility of discovering life-changing health states, but may also provide reassurance by reducing the uncertainty afforded by a diagnosis.

2.4.2   Altering clinical decisions and actions

More accurate tests will improve patient outcomes if the reductions in false positive or false negative results lead to more people receiving appropriate diagnoses and appropriate treatment. The degree to which appropriate treatment can improve patient outcomes depends on its efficacy. However, it is also important to be wary of the harms associated with false positive and false negative diagnoses. People who receive false positive diagnoses may undergo additional unnecessary testing and interventions, which may have adverse effects. They may also suffer unnecessary anxiety. Those who get false negative results from testing may be denied, or experience delays in receiving, effective treatment.

Although diagnostic yield generally increases with accuracy, it is also affected by a doctor's confidence in the diagnostic test. Tests inducing greater confidence could benefit patients by reducing the need for further investigations and shortening the time to treatment. Doctors' confidence can also influence the actual treatment delivered, particularly in surgery.

Tests will not affect clinical decisions if they are prone to technical failure or if they deliver results that are difficult to interpret. Either problem could require additional investigations, increasing the time to diagnosis, incorrect decision-making or poor diagnostic confidence. It is thus important to assess failure rates and non-diagnostic results, both of which are commonly reported in test accuracy studies.

2.4.3   Changes to time frames and populations

In some clinical problems the speed with which the correct treatment is identified and given can be critical to a patient's disease course. Thus, tests that can be undertaken earlier or produce results more quickly can improve health outcomes. However, quicker results are beneficial only if they produce earlier diagnosis and treatment, which may depend on factors other than the speed of the test.

Earlier diagnosis can also provide psychological benefit by dispelling anxiety or providing earlier reassurance, but can also cause psychological harm, particularly if effective treatments are unavailable.

The value of a test within a health system will also increase with the number of patients who are able to access it. This may depend on the mode by which it is delivered, which may improve access, but also on any contraindications to its use, which may exclude particular patient groups.

2.4.4 Influencing patient and clinician perceptions

Predicting and measuring patients' and clinicians' perceptions of testing and their impact on health outcomes may be difficult, and many of these aspects may vary between patients, clinicians and health systems, and have the potential to be modifiable.

Patients' perceptions of testing, their experience of the testing process and their understanding of the test result can all affect their health. Many studies show social, emotional, cognitive and behavioural effects of testing across various clinical conditions. Evaluation of the acceptability of a test is important to assess whether patients are willing to undergo a procedure. This is especially important if multiple testing is required; an unpleasant first test can adversely influence patients' willingness to attend follow-up testing or treatment. The experience of undergoing tests can also influence illness beliefs. Diagnostic placebo effects might occur if the impression of a thorough investigation improves perceptions of health status. Receiving a diagnosis can have behavioural and health consequences – for example, by confirming patients' negative health beliefs.

Patients' experiences and perceptions of testing will also affect subsequent health behaviours, such as the willingness or motivation to adhere to medical advice. Negative perceptions or experiences of testing and clinical diagnosis could cause patients to lose confidence in the diagnosis or management plan, making them reluctant to have subsequent testing or treatment.

Doctors' emotional, cognitive, social or behavioural perspectives, although external to objective medical concerns, are nevertheless important in decision-making. Referring doctors might modify management to reassure and satisfy patients or to prevent perceived threats of malpractice, often by requesting additional diagnostic information. This defensive medicine tends to raise the diagnostic threshold needed to trigger a change in management, and if additional tests are less accurate, harmful or lead to treatment delays, patients will be adversely affected.

2.5 Evaluations of test accuracy during test development

Evaluations of the accuracy of a medical test or procedure can be performed during various stages of the development of a medical test. To appreciate the validity and applicability of these evaluations in Cochrane Reviews, we should understand the differences.

2.5.1 Evaluations of accuracy during biomarker discovery

Many medical tests are assays that measure a specific biomarker. A biomarker is a characteristic that serves as an indicator of normal biological or pathogenic processes, or pharmacological responses to a therapeutic intervention (FDA-NIH Biomarker Working Group 2016). Assays on the other hand are analytical procedures for detecting or measuring the presence, amount, state or functional activity of a biomarker (Horvath 2014). In vitro medical tests often use laboratory assays of one or more biomarkers, in a specific clinical context and for a specific clinical purpose, in a specific patient population.

Biomarkers may be discovered in different ways, including scientific reasoning and experimentation, and targeted technological development. In most circumstances no formal medical test exists at this point. However, some forms of modern biomarker development generate data on the ability of biomarker measurement to correctly identify patients with a known condition, and express the results in accuracy terms, for example as the sensitivity and specificity of the biomarker. Very often, several putative biomarkers are evaluated in parallel in marker discovery studies.

These evaluations during biomarker discovery are regularly done in very specific groups, not representative of any clinical population, and often without a specific intended use. It is therefore not always known whether the biomarker will be used for a screening test or for a diagnostic test, for example. As a consequence, such evaluations are not very informative for actual decision-making in clinical practice. They are primarily done to evaluate the hypothesis that a biomarker holds promise, and biomarkers with encouraging findings may eventually lead to useful medical tests.

2.5.2 Early evaluations of test accuracy

Assays, particularly in vitro diagnostics, undergo studies of analytical performance before their accuracy is evaluated. Their ability to detect conditions in artificial laboratory conditions is investigated and their measurement properties established. Occasionally such studies are described as studies of analytical accuracy, and report estimates of analytical sensitivity (the assay's ability to detect very low concentrations of a given substance in a biological specimen) and analytical specificity (the assay's ability to detect the intended target, without concerns about cross-reactivity or interference). Such studies are not appropriate to be considered in a systematic review of test accuracy, as they evaluate measurement properties, not the ability of a test to correctly classify patients in clinical practice.

Early studies of accuracy may be proof-of-concept studies that challenge the biomarker to discriminate between people with established disease and those who are healthy. Should a biomarker fail to meet this artificial but easy challenge, it will not be evaluated further.

Further challenges may then be set to investigate whether the biomarker can discriminate between those with the target condition and others with similar conditions, and can detect the condition at different points in its natural history. Such studies may be undertaken using easily available samples stored in biobanks. Often the health status of the study participants will already be known and reference standards need not be undertaken.

As discussed in Chapter 3 and Chapter 8, the estimates of sensitivity and specificity from these studies are unlikely to be representative of the performance of the test in practice, but these studies will identify whether the test has the potential to be clinically useful.

2.5.3   Clinical evaluations of test accuracy

The test accuracy studies most appropriate for inclusion in Cochrane Reviews are those that are undertaken in the population where the test would normally be implemented, for the intended use, and at the point in the clinical pathway where it would actually be used. Such studies require evaluation with a reference standard in all participants. These studies are most likely to provide estimates of test accuracy that will be applicable to patient care, as discussed in Chapter 3 and Chapter 4.

A further step is to undertake test accuracy studies that allow the accuracy of the new test to be compared with the accuracy of alternative tests, particularly against current testing practice. Comparative test accuracy studies will be useful in assessing whether new tests improve the accuracy of diagnoses and they provide the strongest type of evidence for selecting tests based on test accuracy. The Cochrane process pays particular attention to studies of this nature as they have the greatest ability to inform management decisions.

2.6   Other purposes of medical testing

Test accuracy studies can also be performed when the test is used for other purposes than arriving at a diagnosis. This section provides a more extensive overview of the reasons to consider medical testing, and to what extent test accuracy can be used to express the clinical performance of the test. Depending on the circumstances, the same procedure can be used as a medical test for more than one purpose.

While a single application of a test may provide information for multiple purposes for an individual patient, the evaluation of the ability of a test to perform each of the roles is likely to need a separate research study, as explained in Table 2.6.a.

Table 2.6.a Purposes of medical testing

Test use	Clinical question
Predisposition	Is this healthy person at risk of developing the condition in the future?
Risk stratification	How likely is this person to develop a condition in the future?
Screening	Does this asymptomatic person have early disease or a precursor of disease?
Diagnosis	What condition is causing the symptoms in this person?
Staging	How severe is the condition in this person?
Prognosis	What is likely to be the outcome of the condition in this person?
Treatment selection	Is this person likely to benefit from the treatment considered?
Treatment monitoring	Is the condition changing under treatment?
Monitoring	Is this chronic condition under control?
Surveillance	Has the condition progressed or recurred?

2.6.1 Predisposition

Tests of predisposition are undertaken in healthy individuals to identify those at increased risk of developing a particular disease. Knowledge of being at high risk may prompt individuals to modify health-related behaviours, to undergo enhanced surveillance for developing disease or to undergo prophylactic interventions.

Tests for predisposition are based on how a person's fixed characteristics, such as their family or medical history or genetic make-up, relate to the incidence of a disease. Such tests require information from longitudinal studies that compare disease incidence in people with and without each characteristic. Studies may be done either prospectively or retrospectively, but due to their longitudinal nature they are not suited for evaluation within the test accuracy framework.

2.6.2 Risk stratification

Tests can be used to calculate the chances of developing an event or a condition in the future, based on a combination of fixed and variable characteristics. Well-known examples are the cardiovascular risk scores, such as QRISK3, which are based on sex, age, total cholesterol, systolic blood pressure, smoking status and other risk factors.

Like tests for predisposition, the development and validation of tools for risk stratification require longitudinal cohort studies and, as such, they are not suited for evaluation within the test accuracy framework.

2.6.3 Screening

Screening involves looking for early-stage disease, precursors of disease or emerging risk factors in people who are asymptomatic and apparently healthy. It aims to identify disease at an early stage when it can successfully be treated, rather than to wait until it becomes symptomatic and less amenable to treatment.

It may be desirable to evaluate the accuracy of a screening test in detecting the early-stage disease by comparing the screening test results against the reference standard. This would fit the test accuracy framework, even though screening tests are performed in asymptomatic people, in contrast with diagnostic tests. Systematic reviews of the accuracy of screening tests may be undertaken. Systematic reviews of test accuracy may also be useful to compare the accuracy of a new screening test with an existing one.

However, assessing whether a screening programme creates more benefit than harm requires consideration of the outcomes of the consequent interventions, which is best undertaken in randomized trials. Cochrane Reviews of these trials are published as reviews of interventions and not of test accuracy.

2.6.4 Staging

Tests may be used to stage disease, to find out how advanced or severe it is. Staging tests are undertaken only in patients found to have the disease, and may help identify the most appropriate choice of intervention depending on the severity of the disease. Staging thus classifies patients with a known condition into subcategories.

Evaluating the accuracy of a staging test is similar to evaluating a diagnostic test, in that results of the new test are compared with results of a reference standard. However, staging tests often classify patients into more than two categories, which makes the application of accuracy measures such as sensitivity and specificity difficult, as these are designed for binary classifications of data.

Staging tests also frequently function as tests of prognosis, in that patients with severe disease often have poorer outcomes. However, longitudinal studies are required to evaluate the relationship between disease stage and future likely outcomes (the prognostic value of the test) and to assess the accuracy of a staging test.

2.6.5 Prognosis

Prognostic tests are used to predict what the future state of a disease is likely to be. Knowledge of likely future health states may lead to modification of a patient's treatment, or enable the patient to make appropriate plans.

Tests for prognosis are similar to those for predisposition, in that they aim to predict what the future holds for a patient and their evaluation requires longitudinal follow-up. Unlike predisposition studies, prognosis studies examine the relationship between test results and a health outcome, such as death or recovery, rather than the onset of disease. Prognosis may be investigated in a sample of all those who have the disease, while predisposition is investigated in healthy people who do not yet have the disease.

Prognosis studies may be done either prospectively or retrospectively, but due to their longitudinal nature they are not immediately suited for evaluation within the test accuracy framework. However, some clinical scenarios where outcomes are observed over a standard time period, such as predicting pregnancy within a year or the outcome of pregnancy, have strong commonalities with test accuracy studies.

2.6.6 Treatment selection

Stratified or precision medicine focuses on identifying subgroups of patients who will benefit from particular interventions, often through pairing a new test or biomarker with an intervention. The greatest advances are being made where the molecular understanding of a disease leads to development of both a biomarker to detect the molecular target and a targeted therapy. Typically, this involves the use of molecular pathology tests such as genomics, proteomics and metabolomics, which have had their greatest successes in cancer.

Benefit from treatment is defined as a difference in outcomes: a better outcome after treatment compared with the counterfactual outcome when not being treated. Such a difference in outcome can never be directly observed, and a reference standard for benefit may be difficult to define. Hence, the evaluation of treatment selection tests rarely fits the test accuracy paradigm.

Evaluation of test–treatment combinations is best achieved through randomized trials. Ideally, randomized trials randomly allocate participants to treatment or a comparator, and investigate whether the observed treatment effect differs between patients who are biomarker positive and those who are biomarker negative, via a test of the interaction. Such evaluations are more suited to the format of Cochrane Reviews of interventions than those of test accuracy.

2.6.7   Treatment efficacy

Medical tests may be used in both clinical practice and research to predict whether a treatment has worked or not, particularly to get an early indication of a response to a new treatment when long-term follow-up would otherwise be required. In oncology, such tests are called predictive tests, to distinguish them from prognostic tests, which would predict the future health state under no or under conventional treatment.

Such trials often evaluate the presence or absence of a response after treatment in studies in which all participants receive treatment and compare the proportion of responders between biomarker positives and biomarker negatives. Though the results can be expressed in terms of accuracy, the longitudinal nature of such treatment studies makes them unfit for the test accuracy paradigm.

2.6.8   Therapeutic monitoring

Therapeutic monitoring involves using a test repeatedly in a group of patients to see whether their disease is being appropriately controlled by a therapy. For example, patients who are prescribed anti-hypertensive drugs will have their blood pressure regularly measured to assess whether the drug and its dosage are appropriate. If their blood pressure remains high, the dose may be increased, or further anti-hypertensive agents may be added. If their blood pressure is too low, the drug dosage may be reduced.

To inform treatment decisions reliably, monitoring tests need to have good test accuracy to correctly classify individuals. However, monitoring tests must also respond to changes in patients' health state quickly, and their clinical value will also depend on how often they are used and whether the associated changes in management actually improve patient health. Evaluation of whether using a monitoring strategy leads to patient benefit is also best assessed using a randomized trial, as for screening interventions, and is amenable to systematic review using the Cochrane methods for reviewing intervention studies.

2.6.9   Surveillance for progression or recurrence

Tests are also used repeatedly in patients who have a progressive disease or have recently undergone an intervention to check for disease progression or recurrence, which may prompt changes in patient management. This is sometimes called surveillance, a form of monitoring.

Surveillance has many similarities to screening, but screening is performed in asymptomatic people while surveillance is planned in individuals known to have a disease or known to have undergone an intervention.

Surveillance, like monitoring, requires tests that are accurate but also respond to changes in patient status. Thus, systematic reviews of the accuracy of tests for surveillance are informative, but whether or not surveillance testing benefits patients is also best assessed in randomized trials.

2.7   Chapter information

Authors: Jonathan J. Deeks (*Institute of Applied Health Research, University of Birmingham, UK*); Patrick M. Bossuyt *(Department of Epidemiology and Data Science, University of Amsterdam, The Netherlands)*.

Sources of support: Jonathan J. Deeks is a UK National Institute for Health Research (NIHR) Senior Investigator Emeritus. Jonathan J. Deeks is supported by the NIHR Birmingham Biomedical Research Centre at the University Hospitals Birmingham NHS Foundation Trust and the University of Birmingham. The views expressed are those of the authors and not necessarily those of the NHS, the NIHR or the Department of Health and Social Care. The authors declare no other sources of support for writing this chapter.

Declarations of interest: Jonathan J. Deeks is a member of Cochrane's Diagnostic Test Accuracy Editorial Team. The authors declare no other potential conflicts of interest relevant to the topic of this chapter.

Acknowledgements: The authors would like to thank Jenny Doust and Matthew McInnes for helpful peer review comments.

2.8   References

Bossuyt PM, Lijmer JG, Mol BW. Randomised comparisons of medical tests: sometimes invalid, not always efficient. *Lancet* 2000; **356**: 1844–1847.

Chang SM, Matchar DB, Smetana GW, Umscheid CA. Methods guide for medical test reviews. Rockville, MD: Agency for Healthcare Research and Quality; 2012. Available at effectivehealthcare.ahrq.gov/sites/default/files/pdf/methods-guidance-tests_ overview-2012.pdf.

European Parliament and Council of the European Union. Regulation (EU) 2017/746 of the European Parliament and of the Council of 5 April 2017. Available at eur-lex.europa.eu/ legal-content/EN/TXT/PDF/?uri=CELEX:32017R0746&from=EN.

FDA-NIH Biomarker Working Group. BEST (Biomarkers, EndpointS, and other Tools) Resource. Silver Spring (MD): Food and Drug Administration (US). Co-published by National Institutes of Health (US), Bethesda (MD), 2016. Available at www.ncbi.nlm.nih. gov/books/NBK326791.

Ferrante di Ruffano L, Davenport C, Eisinga A, Hyde C, Deeks JJ. A capture-recapture analysis demonstrated that randomized controlled trials evaluating the impact of diagnostic tests on patient outcomes are rare. *Journal of Clinical Epidemiology* 2012a; **65**: 282–287.

Ferrante di Ruffano L, Hyde CJ, McCaffery KJ, Bossuyt PMM, Deeks JJ. Assessing the value of diagnostic tests: a framework for designing and evaluating trials. *BMJ* 2012b; **344**: e686.

Ferrante di Ruffano L, Dinnes J, Taylor-Phillips S, Davenport C, Hyde C, Deeks JJ. Research waste in diagnostic trials: a methods review evaluating the reporting of test-treatment interventions. *BMC Medical Research Methodology* 2017a; **17**: 32.

Ferrante di Ruffano L, Dinnes J, Sitch AJ, Hyde C, Deeks JJ. Test-treatment RCTs are susceptible to bias: a review of the methodological quality of randomized trials that evaluate diagnostic tests. *BMC Medical Research Methodology* 2017b; **17**: 35–35.

Gøtzsche PC, Jørgensen KJ. Screening for breast cancer with mammography. *Cochrane Database of Systematic Reviews* 2013; **6**: CD001877.

Hewitson P, Glasziou P, Irwig L, Towler B, Watson E. Screening for colorectal cancer using the faecal occult blood test, Hemoccult. *Cochrane Database of Systematic Reviews* 2007; **1**: CD001216.

Horvath AR, Lord SJ, StJohn A, Sandberg S, Cobbaert CM, Lorenz S, Monaghan PJ, Verhagen-Kamerbeek WD, Ebert C, Bossuyt PM. From biomarkers to medical tests: the changing landscape of test evaluation. *Clinica Chimica Acta* 2014; **427**: 49–57.

Ilic D, Neuberger MM, Djulbegovic M, Dahm P. Screening for prostate cancer. *Cochrane Database of Systematic Reviews* 2013; **1**: CD004720.

Lord SJ, Irwig L, Simes RJ. When is measuring sensitivity and specificity sufficient to evaluate a diagnostic test, and when do we need randomized trials? *Annals of Internal Medicine* 2006; **144**: 850–855.

Manser R, Lethaby A, Irving LB, Stone C, Byrnes G, Abramson MJ, Campbell D. Screening for lung cancer. *Cochrane Database of Systematic Reviews* 2013; **6**: CD001991.

National Institute for Health and Clinical Excellence. *Diagnostics assessment programme manual*. Manchester (UK): National Institute for Health and Clinical Excellence, 2011. Available at www.nice.org.uk/Media/Default/About/what-we-do/NICE-guidance/NICE-diagnostics-guidance/Diagnostics-assessment-programme-manual.pdf.

Odaga J, Sinclair D, Lokong JA, Donegan S, Hopkins H, Garner P. Rapid diagnostic tests versus clinical diagnosis for managing people with fever in malaria endemic settings. *Cochrane Database of Systematic Reviews* 2014; **4**: CD008998.

Schünemann HJ, Oxman AD, Brozek J, Glasziou P, Jaeschke R, Vist GE, Williams JW Jr, Kunz R, Craig J, Montori VM, Bossuyt P, Guyatt GH. Grading quality of evidence and strength of recommendations for diagnostic tests and strategies. *BMJ* 2008; **336**: 1106–1110.

3

Understanding the design of test accuracy studies

Patrick M. Bossuyt

KEY POINTS

- In the basic design for a test accuracy study, a single group of participants suspected of the target condition undergo the index test, the test under evaluation and the reference standard.
- The target condition can be a disease, a disease stage or any pathophysiological condition that has clinical consequences.
- The reference standard is usually the best available clinical method for finding out whether patients have the target condition.
- Instead of including a single group of participants, accuracy studies can also include two or more groups of participants, such as healthy controls or patients with a previously obtained diagnosis, without performing a reference standard in all participants.
- Test accuracy studies can rely on more than one reference standard. The reference standards can be a single test or procedure, a rule based on multiple procedures, a panel-based adjudication or can be based on latent class modelling.
- Comparative accuracy studies evaluate two or more index tests. The most valid designs are fully paired designs and randomized designs.

3.1 Introduction

Test accuracy studies evaluate the performance of a medical test: to what extent the test is able to distinguish patients with the target condition from those without. These studies do so by comparing the results of one or more index tests with the classification obtained with the reference standard, which typically is the best available clinical method for identifying patients with the target condition.

This chapter should be cited as: Bossuyt PM. Chapter 3: Understanding the design of test accuracy studies. In: Deeks JJ, Bossuyt PM, Leeflang MM, Takwoingi Y, editors. *Cochrane Handbook for Systematic Reviews of Diagnostic Test Accuracy*. 1st edition. Chichester (UK): John Wiley & Sons, 2023: 35–52.

Cochrane Handbook for Systematic Reviews of Diagnostic Test Accuracy, First Edition. Edited by Jonathan J. Deeks, Patrick M. Bossuyt, Mariska M. Leeflang and Yemisi Takwoingi.
© 2023 The Cochrane Collaboration. Published 2023 by John Wiley & Sons Ltd.

Estimates of test accuracy can be obtained from several types of studies. Before starting a review, review authors should understand what kind of primary study would ideally fit the review question. This helps in defining the search strategy and the eligibility criteria, and is essential for preparing evaluations of the risk of bias in included studies.

This chapter provides an overview of the most common designs used to assess test accuracy. It starts with a description of the basic study design for evaluating the accuracy of a single test, followed by a description of variations of this basic study design. It then identifies various types of reference standards. Another section describes designs for studies to evaluate and compare the accuracy of two or more tests.

3.2   The basic design for a test accuracy study

Systematic reviews of test accuracy studies are often performed to support clinical decisions and recommendations about the use of specific tests, in a well-defined context (Bossuyt 2020). To be informative, the studies included in such a review should match the intended use setting.

In the basic design for a test accuracy study, a single group of consecutive participants is included, all suspected of having the target condition. This study group should be representative for what we will refer to as the target population, or intended use population. This population consists of all patients in whom the test is currently used or will be used. For a new test, this will be the total group of patients in whom the test is considered in the future. For an existing test, the target population consists of all patients for whom the test is currently used. Ideally, the study eligibility criteria define the target population, while the study exclusion criteria specify those in the target population that cannot become a member of the study group.

In addition to sampling the study group from the target population, researchers should also recruit the study group in the intended use setting. The accuracy of many tests is known to vary across settings, and performance of the tests often differs in general practice compared to more specialized settings. For this reason, a test accuracy study should preferably be performed in the setting in which the test is used, or will be used.

Most medical tests intend to measure a specific quantity: the measurand. D-dimer assays, for example, intend to measure D-dimer, a fibrin degradation product: a small protein fragment present in the blood after a blood clot is degraded by fibrinolysis.

Very often, the purpose of testing is not so much the measurement itself, but a specific clinical purpose, such as making a diagnosis (see Chapter 2). Measuring D-dimer, for example, is used by clinicians to assist in the diagnosis of patients with suspected deep venous thrombosis or suspected pulmonary embolism.

More generally, we refer to the target condition: the condition to be detected with the test. Very often the target condition is a specific disease. Since many diseases vary in severity, it can also be a specific disease stage, as not all stages may be clinically consequential. In vascular medicine, for example, there have been discussions about the clinical relevance of subsegmental pulmonary embolism, and whether such emboli should be included in the definition of the target condition when evaluating tests for patients with suspected pulmonary embolism (Baumgartner 2020).

The target condition can also be a precursor of disease. An example is adenoma in the colon, which can develop into colon cancer. Tests to screen for colorectal cancer therefore aim to detect not only early cancer, but also other forms of neoplasia. The definition of what should be considered 'advanced neoplasia' has changed over time (Young 2016).

The target condition can also be a specific pathophysiological condition, such as hyperlipidaemia: abnormally elevated levels of any or all lipids or lipoproteins in the blood (Lord 2011).

In almost all cases, the target condition is a condition with clinical consequences. People with the target condition could benefit from treatment or from other actions, such as further testing. Detecting the target condition would therefore benefit those being tested, while missing the target condition could cause potential harm to those being tested.

All study group participants in a test accuracy study undergo the test that is being evaluated: the index test. This is the test for which estimates of accuracy will be reported. In a test accuracy study, this can be a single test, two or more tests or a test strategy, consisting of a specific sequence of medical tests.

Very shortly thereafter, or at the same time, all study group participants undergo a second procedure: the reference standard. The reference standard is usually the best available clinical method for finding out whether patients have the target condition. The reference standard can also be a single test or a combination of tests.

Like the target condition, what should be the reference standard is not always fixed; it can vary over time and may vary with changes in the definition of the target condition. See Section 3.5 for more information on the different types of reference standards.

In the analysis of a test accuracy study, the index test result of each study participant is then compared with the corresponding result, for the same participant, obtained with the reference standard. Once this cross-classification is done for every study group member, the comparisons are aggregated and expressed as an estimate of the accuracy of the index test, in that specific setting, for the target population. Accuracy expresses the clinical performance of medical tests: how well this test is able to identify those with the target condition in all who undergo testing. Chapter 4 discusses the various measures of test accuracy in more detail.

Figure 3.2.a shows a schema for the test accuracy study described in Box 3.2.a. The index test, a D-dimer test, is presented in light blue in Figure 3.2.a, the reference standard in orange. The same colours will be used in the other examples in this chapter. In this example, CT imaging is used as the reference standard. In another study for a different target condition, CT imaging may be the test under evaluation: one of the index tests, as shown in Figure 3.6.a and Figure 3.6.b.

In principle, questions about the accuracy of a medical test require a cross-sectional study design: we want to know how well the test performs in identifying patients *at the time of testing*, not whether the patients will develop the target condition in the near future (that would be a prognostic question), or whether the patients had a pulmonary embolism in the past (which may be relevant for answering questions about causality).

Since the question about test accuracy is essentially a cross-sectional one, it does not really matter whether the index test is performed first or the reference standard is performed first. Figure 3.2.b shows a different schema for the study summarized in Figure 3.2.a. In this case, the blood sample is taken shortly after CT imaging, instead

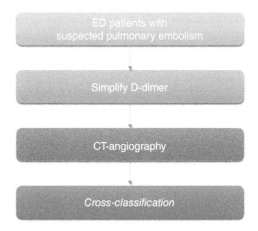

Figure 3.2.a An example of the basic design for a test accuracy study

of before CT imaging. CT imaging (in orange) is still the reference standard and D-dimer (in blue) the index test. The diagnostic accuracy estimates generated in this study will not be fundamentally different from those obtained with the study in Figure 3.2.a, provided the time interval between D-dimer testing and imaging is sufficiently short in both.

Because of the relatively recent interest in study designs for test accuracy studies, there is no agreed terminology to describe the different types of studies. Many terms borrowed from epidemiology are ill-fitted to describe this type of study. The study in Example 1 (see Box 3.2.a) is sometimes described as a cohort study, but we should keep in mind that, unlike cohort studies in epidemiology, the design of the study in Example 1

Box 3.2.a Example 1: Basic design of a test accuracy study

A research group wants to evaluate the diagnostic accuracy of the Simplify D-dimer in correctly identifying patients with pulmonary embolism presenting at the Emergency Department (ED) of a US hospital. The Simplify D-dimer is a point-of-care test that requires a drop of whole blood from the patient undergoing the test.

The researchers registered the study in a clinical trials registry before it started and obtained Institutional Review Board approval for the protocol. During the four years it took to complete the study, one of a group of emergency physicians identified ED patients with suspected pulmonary embolism based on presenting symptoms such as dyspnoea, chest pain or syncope, or physical signs such as a rapid pulse or low pulse oximetry reading that could not readily be explained by another disease process.

Eligible patients were invited to participate in the study and asked for informed consent. A data collection form was then completed, after which blood was drawn by a qualified respiratory therapist and the D-dimer test was performed. Immediately thereafter, patients underwent computed tomography (CT) angiography of the chest, the reference standard. The radiologist reading the CT images was unaware of the D-dimer results. After the study was completed, all D-dimer results were cross classified with the imaging results, to obtain estimates of the diagnostic accuracy of this Simplify D-dimer test.

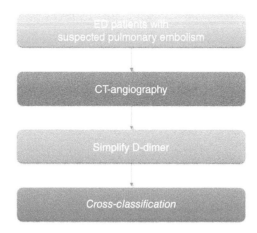

Figure 3.2.b A variation on the basic design for a test accuracy study

is not longitudinal but cross-sectional. The variation in Figure 3.2.b is sometimes called a case-control study (since the reference standard is performed shortly before the index test), but that term is misleading, and 'reverse flow' study design has been suggested as an alternative description (Rutjes 2005).

When the target condition is relatively rare, as in cancer screening, performing the index tests in all participants with the target condition and in all participants without the target condition may be inefficient: the second group may be much larger, generating a precision beyond what is needed for decision-making. In that case, performing the index test in all participants with the target condition and in a random subset of those without the target condition may be a more efficient alternative. This presents a variation on the study design in Figure 3.2.b.

An example is a study of DNA methylation-based detection, where a large group of patients had a CT scan for suspected lung cancer, with pathology in case lesions were detected (reference standard (Liu 2020)). The investigators recruited from this single group, after the CT results were known, 74 patients with pathological confirmation of non-small cell lung cancer and 27 patients with a non-cancer diagnosis. The investigators then reported the DNA methylation results in each group, but both these groups were selected from a single study group representing the target population: patients with suspected lung cancer. Even though only 101 participants were included in the analysis, there was a single set of study eligibility criteria, and every participant in this single study group had the same reference standard.

The basic design has a single group of participants, a single index test and a single reference standard. In the following sections we discuss variations on this basic design for each of these three components.

3.3 Multiple groups of participants

In the basic study design, there is a single set of eligibility criteria: one set of inclusion criteria that define the target population, the population from whom the study group is sampled and to whom the estimates of test accuracy are assumed to apply.

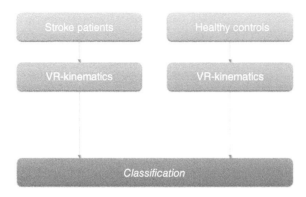

Figure 3.3.a A two-group (or two-gate) test accuracy study

In Example 1, these were patients presenting to the ED with suspected pulmonary embolism.

In having a single set of eligibility criteria, the basic test accuracy study design is similar to that of randomized trials, which also have a single set of inclusion and exclusion criteria. Anyone in the target population either has the target condition or not (pulmonary embolism in this case). In principle, the eligibility criteria are defined in such a way that anyone in the target population could have been included in the study group. The study group is therefore a truly random subset of the target population, and measures of test accuracy are assumed to apply to the target population.

A variation on the basic study design, which is commonly observed in test accuracy studies, is the study that uses two or more sets of eligibility criteria (Figure 3.3.a). In the study in Example 2 (see Box 3.3.a), the authors reported on the discriminative validity of VR-based kinematics by presenting estimates of sensitivity and specificity, which are common measures of test accuracy. They had two sets of eligibility criteria: one for stroke patients and a second set for the healthy controls. Each group was defined in a different way and participants in each group were recruited in a different way. Because of the two distinct groups, we refer to these studies as two-group studies or two-gate studies. Rutjes and colleagues have suggested the term "two-gate studies" for such

---

Box 3.3.a Example 2: Study with two groups of participants

A group of researchers wants to evaluate kinematic analysis using a virtual reality (VR) environment for evaluating motor function in stroke patients. They relied on two groups of participants:

- stroke patients with mild to moderate impairment; and
- healthy controls, recruited through a website.

The report estimates sensitivity and specificity. Sensitivity refers to the proportion of individuals with stroke diagnosis correctly identified as having stroke by the cut-off values for the kinematic variables. Specificity refers to the proportion of healthy controls who are correctly identified as controls by the cut-off values for the kinematic variables. This example is based on a study by Hussain and colleagues (Hussain 2018).

studies with two sets of eligibility criteria and "multiple-gate" as the more general term, for studies with two or more groups (Rutjes 2005). These labels have been somewhat slow to gain widespread acceptance, however, and there is as yet no agreed terminology for describing such studies.

Multiple-group accuracy studies may include three or more groups of study participants, for example additional groups of patients with a different diagnosis. The study in Example 2 could additionally have included patients with mild Parkinson's disease. A study of a test for detecting ovarian cancer may recruit a group of women with ovarian cancer, a second group of symptomatic patients with benign gynaecological conditions and a third group of healthy controls.

The distinguishing element between multiple-group studies and the standard accuracy design, as in Example 1, is that the two-group design does not have a single reference standard as part of the study protocol. While it may be tempting to think that a reference standard has been applied in order to designate included participants as stroke patients or healthy controls, this is not the case. The stroke patients in the study had objective tests to confirm their diagnosis before they were invited to participate in the study, but the healthy controls did not: they had a brief interview before joining the study, but no tests to exclude stroke. This means that the study in Example 2 is very different from the study in Example 1, where a single method (CT imaging) was used in all study participants to evaluate whether they truly had a pulmonary embolism.

Since most systematic reviews are performed to inform healthcare professionals and to support decisions about using the tests in practice, review authors should be careful when considering the inclusion of multiple-group studies in their review. The estimates usually do not correspond to a well-defined intended use population. In fact, neither of the two groups in Example 2 refers to a well-defined target population, the population in which this movement-based test may be used in the future. None of the healthy controls, obviously, was suspected of a recent stroke, and the stroke patients, who already had a stroke confirmed, may not represent the full spectrum of stroke patients in clinical practice.

Multiple-group studies are often used to test scientific hypotheses, not to evaluate the accuracy of the test in a clinical setting. Even when such studies present their results in terms of the accuracy of the test, their main objective is not to support decision-making about the test. The authors of the study on which Example 2 is based concluded that "individuals with mild and moderate stroke use longer time to perform the target task with their stroke-affected arm in a VR environment than healthy controls." This conclusion is not phrased in terms of the accuracy of VR kinematics as a test to detect stroke, even though the authors presented sensitivity and specificity in their report.

In the evaluation of tests, multiple-group studies can often be considered proof-of-principle or proof-of-concept studies, since they want to demonstrate the mere existence of a specific difference, in this case between stroke patients and healthy controls. This is typically done early in the development of a medical test, after the identification of a biomarker, and before embarking on larger accuracy studies that recruit patients from the target population, in the intended use setting (Sackett 2002).

We should distinguish two-group studies with two sets of study eligibility criteria, as in Figure 3.3.a, from studies in which two groups are defined within the study itself, based on a common reference standard, as in Figure 3.2.b.

The use of the term 'healthy controls' is a useful red flag in identifying multiple-group studies. Caution is needed, however, as the term is also used to refer to study participants who test negative on the reference standard in the standard basic accuracy design. In the report of the DNA methylation example, patients without a cancer diagnosis were labelled 'controls' (but not 'healthy controls').

In the past, many study and review authors have referred to two-group or two-gate designs as 'case-control' studies, and the QUADAS-2 instrument to evaluate risk of bias has as one of its signalling questions "Was a case-control design avoided?" (see Chapter 8). This question refers to the use of a multiple-group or multiple-gate design. The label 'case-control' study is increasingly used less often in test accuracy study reports and systematic reviews, because the term is somewhat ambiguous and its use may be misleading (Rutjes 2005). Test accuracy studies are cross-sectional in nature, unlike case-control studies in epidemiology, which are typically done for longitudinal questions about causality.

3.4 Multiple reference standards

The study in Example 1 – the basic study design – had a single reference standard: CT angiography to unequivocally identify the patients with pulmonary embolism. A test accuracy study can also have two or more reference standards, where patients undergo one of these, guided or not by a specific protocol.

The study on which Example 1 was based relied on a design that was slightly different from the flow presented in the example (Kline 2006). In the actual study, not all participants had CT pulmonary angiography. In principle, all study participants with a positive D-dimer result were expected to undergo CT imaging, but some participants had a contraindication for CT imaging. In the study, those who were allergic to iodinated contrast or had a serum creatinine measurement over 1.5 mg/dL underwent ventilation-perfusion scintillation lung scanning instead (V/Q scan), a different imaging procedure. A small group of 10 participants had conventional, non-CT pulmonary angiography, another imaging technique with high accuracy in detecting pulmonary embolism.

Only 350 of the 1612 participants with a negative D-dimer result underwent pulmonary vascular imaging. In all other participants, the findings from a 90-day follow-up were used, collected using a structured combination of telephone and medical record follow-up, described in the study protocol. If a pulmonary embolism diagnosis was made early during this follow-up period, the study participant was classified as having "definite pulmonary embolism" at the time of presentation. If no such pulmonary embolism diagnosis was made during follow-up, the participant was classified as having "no pulmonary embolism" at the time of presentation. In this way, events during follow-up were used as an alternative reference standard. So this study did not rely on one but on four reference standards: three imaging procedures (CT pulmonary angiography, ventilation-perfusion scintillation lung scanning, pulmonary angiography) and follow-up (Figure 3.4.a).

Although these four reference standards are related, they are not all exchangeable. Two reference standards for the same target condition can be called exchangeable only if they classify every participant in whom the target condition is suspected in the same

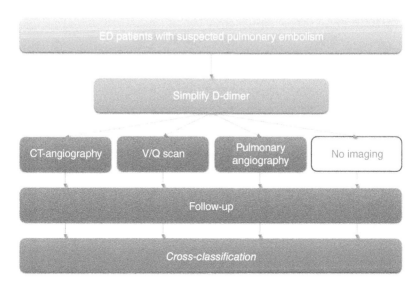

Figure 3.4.a   A test accuracy study with multiple reference standards

way. This may almost be the case for perfusion-ventilation scanning and CT pulmonary angiography, two imaging modalities, but is unlikely to be true for imaging and 90-day follow-up. Not every embolus identified on imaging would lead to a clinical event during follow-up. This implies that patients would not be classified in the same way as 'PE present' or 'PE absent' when evaluated with imaging or when evaluated based on follow-up.

Any interpretation of the presence or absence of the target condition will be more straightforward when only a single reference standard is used, or when reference standards are exchangeable. Caution should be applied whenever two or more reference standards are used, especially when these are not exchangeable. Depending on what measures are used to express test accuracy, the resulting estimates may be ambiguous and at risk of bias (see Chapter 8).

A special case of a study with multiple standards is a so-called management study, in which patients are managed on the basis of the index test results, with different management strategies for index test positive participants and for index test negative participants (Kruip 2006). A management study may present estimates of test accuracy, but the reference standard is different for test positive and for test negative participants. In a management study in patients with suspected pulmonary embolism, index test positive participants typically have imaging, and if the radiologist does not see signs of pulmonary embolism, the index test result is classified as a false positive (a true positive if the radiologist sees signs of pulmonary embolism). Index test negative participants are typically examined further to identify the origin of their complaints, and that may be without vascular imaging. If soon thereafter the work-up leads to a diagnosis of pulmonary embolism, the test result is classified as a false negative, and as a true negative in all other cases. Such management studies require careful consideration of the study design when presenting estimates of the test's accuracy (see Chapter 8).

3.5 More on reference standards

In the examples so far, the reference standard was performed at or around the time the index test was performed. More variations on the basic design are possible, however, and these will be encountered in systematic reviews of test accuracy studies.

3.5.1 Delayed verification

In the study in Figure 3.4.a, where multiple reference standards were available, the use of follow-up tied a cross-sectional study question (How good is this test in identifying patients with pulmonary embolism, here and now?) to a longitudinal study design: pulmonary embolism was presumed to be present at the time of testing if a clinical event, related to pulmonary embolism, occurred during the 90 days of follow-up after testing.

Relying on follow-up to confirm a diagnosis is known as 'delayed verification', and accuracy studies that rely on delayed verification have been called 'delayed cross-sectional' studies (Kline 2006). One other example is a study that evaluated a test for incipient Alzheimer's disease in patients with mild cognitive impairment. If a diagnosis of Alzheimer's disease was made during follow-up in a patient with a positive test result, this was considered a true positive finding (Hansson 2006).

3.5.2 Composite reference standard

In Example 1, the reference standard was a single procedure (CT pulmonary angiography) or one of a series of procedures: CT pulmonary angiography, perfusion-ventilation scanning or follow-up. It is also possible that the reference standard is based on a strategy in which multiple procedures are used, and a rule based on these procedures defines who has the target condition, or not. This is known as a composite reference standard.

An example is a study of the diagnostic performance of Xpert MTB/RIF, a cartridge-based nucleic acid amplification test, in the rapid identification of children with pulmonary tuberculosis (Nicol 2011). In this study, children aged 15 years or younger underwent sputum induction in a dedicated sputum induction room by a trained research nurse, after which automated liquid culture was done. In addition, all children were invited for a three-month follow-up visit. A child was defined as not having childhood pulmonary tuberculosis in case of negative tuberculosis cultures and documented resolution of symptoms and signs at three-month follow-up visit in children who did not receive treatment. Here there is a clear AND rule: only those with a negative culture AND resolution of symptoms were defined as not having tuberculosis.

3.5.3 Panel-based reference

A related type of reference standard, in which multiple procedures are used, is one in which a panel of experts decides on the final diagnosis. An example is the OPTIMA study, a diagnostic accuracy study of the accuracy of three imaging modalities to identify patients with urgent conditions in those presenting with acute abdominal pain at the ED (Laméris 2009) (Figure 3.6.a). Here, 1021 consenting patients with non-traumatic abdominal pain lasting two hours or more but less than five days who presented at one of six participating hospitals underwent three imaging modalities after clinical and laboratory examination: plain radiographs (upright chest and supine abdominal), abdominal ultrasonography and abdominal CT. Thereafter, patients were managed based on all findings from these examinations.

Study participants were followed up for at least six months, after which an expert panel consisting of two gastrointestinal surgeons and an experienced abdominal radiologist assigned a final diagnosis. These three panel members had not been involved in the imaging or management of the evaluated cases. The panel had a set of rules to assign a final diagnosis.

3.5.4 Latent class analysis

In some cases, no single test or procedure can act as the reference standard, as all are known to have imperfections. Schumacher and colleagues later analysed the study on Xpert MTB/RIF in a different way: not by evaluating the results against a composite reference standard, but by building a mathematical model. This is known as a latent class analysis (Schumacher 2016). More on latent class analysis and latent class meta-analysis can be found in Chapter 9 and Chapter 10.

3.5.5 Gold standard

In many reports of test accuracy studies, especially in older ones, the index test results are compared with a test that is labelled the 'gold standard'. The meaning of the gold standard is often identical or similar to what has been defined here as the reference standard: the best available method to identify the target condition.

Presenting a method as the 'gold standard' suggests that that method is error free. Since no testing procedure can be regarded as free of errors, several authors have argued that the term 'gold standard' should no longer be used, and its use in test evaluation has declined (Duggan 1992, Conti 1994). In evaluating tests for COVID-19, for example, some authors have referred to reverse transcription polymerase chain reaction (RT-PCR) as the gold standard for identifying a person with a SARS-CoV-2 infection, while others have criticised the use of this term (Dramé 2020, Hernández-Huerta 2021).

3.5.6 Clinical reference standard

Researchers sometimes refer to the reference standard as the clinical reference standard, to distinguish it from reference standards as they are known in metrology, the science of measurement, and from reference methods, as they are used in evaluations of the analytical performance of laboratory tests (Bossuyt 2015).

3.6   Comparative test accuracy studies

In the OPTIMA example (see Section 3.5.3), three imaging modalities were compared against the same reference standard (Laméris 2009). There are different study designs for comparing the accuracy of two or more index tests.

3.6.1 Paired comparative accuracy study

If all participants receive all the index tests in a comparative accuracy study, the study is sometimes referred to as a 'paired accuracy study': all combinations of testing can be evaluated in each study participant, against the reference standard. This means there is full exchangeability between the group that received the first test and the group that received the second test: they are one and the same, if all went well, and there is no risk of selection bias (see Chapter 8). All test results can be compared within the study participants. The OPTIMA study (Figure 3.6.a) presents an example of a paired comparative accuracy study with three imaging modalities.

3.6.2 Randomized comparative accuracy study

An alternative design for comparing index tests is one in which the study participants are randomly allocated to one of the groups. All participants in each of these groups receive the index test corresponding to that group, after which all participants undergo the same reference standard (taking into account the possible types of reference standard, as discussed in Section 3.5).

A randomized accuracy study can be considered if undergoing two or more index tests is considered too burdensome or too risky for study participants, for radiation reasons, for example, or if it is logistically not feasible.

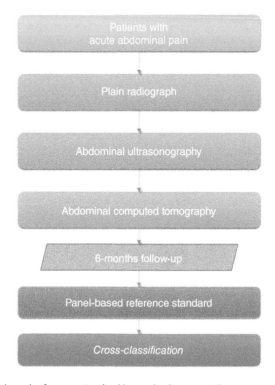

Figure 3.6.a A panel-based reference standard in a paired comparative accuracy study

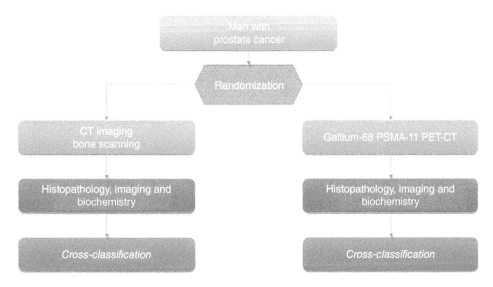

Figure 3.6.b An example of a randomized comparative accuracy study

In one multicentre study, men with biopsy-proven prostate cancer and high-risk features were recruited at 10 hospitals in Australia (Hofman 2020). Consenting participants, 302 men in total, were randomly assigned to one of two index tests to detect pelvic nodal or distant metastatic disease: conventional imaging with CT and bone scanning or gallium-68 prostate-specific membrane antigen (PSMA-11) positron emission tomography (PET)-CT. The reference standard was a composite one, based on histopathology, imaging and biochemistry at six-month follow-up (Figure 3.6.b).

3.6.3   Non-randomized comparative accuracy study

In some studies, the accuracy of two tests is evaluated in two separate groups: one group receives one index test and the reference standard, a second group receives the alternative index test and the same reference standard. The allocation of study partici-pants to the groups is done without randomization, such that the two groups may not be exchangeable: they could differ in baseline characteristics known to affect the detectability of the target condition. Such a non-randomized comparative accuracy study is therefore at risk of selection bias and may also suffer from a lack of representa-tiveness (see Chapter 8).

3.7   Additional aspects of study designs

So far, we have described the main study types based on how participants are recruited (single-group, two-group, multiple-group) and assigned to the various index tests (ran-domized or not, fully paired). A number of additional labels are used to describe test accuracy studies.

3.7.1   Prospective versus retrospective

In general, test accuracy studies in which the recruitment of study participants and all collection of data start after a protocol is finalized are preferred, since quality control measures can safeguard protocol adherence and the veracity and completeness of data. Such studies are prospective test accuracy studies. There are many other ways for a study to produce data of good quality and to generate results that are meaningful, without being fully prospective.

A test accuracy study can be performed on samples collected previously, for example in another study, from participants who had been recruited according to a well-defined protocol. Pepe and colleagues have suggested the term "prospective-specimen-collection, retrospective-blinded-evaluation" (PRoBE) for a design with prospective collection of specimens before any reference standard is applied, followed by applying the index test on specimens from randomly selected participants with the target condition and a second group of participants without the target condition (Pepe 2008). Both studies can generate valid and interpretable test accuracy results, but they have prospective and retrospective elements.

There is no uniform description in the clinical literature of what 'prospective' means, and there definitely is not one in test accuracy research. Similarly, 'retrospective' has no well-defined meaning in test accuracy research, and the use of 'prospective' or 'retrospective' in characterizing test accuracy studies provides limited information.

3.7.2   Pragmatic versus explanatory

Many studies of medical tests present results in terms of estimates of accuracy, such as sensitivity and specificity (see Chapter 4), yet not all these studies aim to inform clinical decisions and recommendations.

Schwartz and Lellouch introduced a distinction to structure debates about the design, analysis and interpretation of therapeutic trials, which can also be helpful in test accuracy studies (Schwartz 1967). Explanatory trials aim at verifying a biological hypothesis, whereas pragmatic trials intend to offer help in deciding between two treatment options.

In a similar way, explanatory accuracy studies are often designed to evaluate a scientific hypothesis that involves a medical test (Bossuyt 2020). They are typically selective in recruitment, may include 'healthy controls', and have a small sample size often recruited at a single centre. Explanatory studies may not consider representativeness, and the setting in which the study is conducted may differ greatly from the setting in which the test is usually conducted. Many of the two-group, or two-gate, studies discussed in Section 3.3 are explanatory studies.

In contrast, pragmatic accuracy studies are designed to guide decision-making. Ideally, they will recruit a single, large and representative group of participants, often at multiple sites, and will often present their results as estimates of sensitivity and specificity or predictive values at a pre-specified threshold for continuous test results. As such, pragmatic accuracy studies will try to mimic more closely how the index test is used in clinical practice. These studies aim to show how many patients with the target condition will be missed by the test, and how many patients without the target condition will be incorrectly classified as positive, the information most relevant for decision-making.

One cannot simply say that explanatory studies are 'wrong' and that pragmatic studies are 'right'. Each serves a different purpose and in performing systematic reviews one should keep the purpose of the review in mind. Distinguishing between explanatory and pragmatic test accuracy studies will typically require scrutiny of the study objectives and the conclusion drawn by the study authors. This is an emerging aspect of study design that has not reached sufficient maturity to guide inclusion and exclusion decisions in systematic reviews of test accuracy studies.

3.8 Concluding remarks

This chapter presented the main study designs for evaluating the accuracy of medical tests. Many more types of studies exist, but the ones described here are the ones that will most frequently be encountered in systematic reviews of test accuracy studies. Review authors – and all other readers – should be aware that the terminology for describing study designs is far from standardized.

It is worth recognizing that views about study design in test accuracy research are not static. In the twentieth century there was little recognition of the complexity of study designs to evaluate accuracy, and limited understanding of sources of bias. Many authors erroneously shared the idea that the accuracy of a test was a fixed, static characteristic, and it did not seem to matter much how one measured it. Similarly, authors of systematic reviews of test accuracy studies were keen to include every 2×2 classification table from any study that reported on the index test of interest, regardless of the actual design. We now know more about variations in study design, and how the design of a study can lead to results that are either not relevant or not valid for answering the review question.

Greater recognition of differences in the intended use of tests, with different target conditions and different reference standards, and increasing evidentiary demands from regulatory bodies and other decision makers will probably further stimulate the development of innovative and creative study designs in the clinical evaluation of medical tests.

3.9 Chapter information

Author: Patrick M. Bossuyt (*Department of Epidemiology and Data Science, University of Amsterdam, The Netherlands*).

Sources of support: The author declares no sources of support for writing this chapter.

Declarations of interest: The author declares no potential conflicts of interest relevant to the topic of this chapter.

Acknowledgements: The author would like to thank Christopher Hyde, Jenny Doust and Matthew McInnes for helpful peer review comments.

3.10   References

Baumgartner C, Tritschler T. Clinical significance of subsegmental pulmonary embolism: an ongoing controversy. *Research and Practice in Thrombosis and Haemostasis* 2020; **5**: 14–16.

Bossuyt PM, Reitsma JB, Bruns DE, Gatsonis CA, Glasziou PP, Irwig L, Lijmer JG, Moher D, Rennie D, de Vet HC, Kressel HY, Rifai N, Golub RM, Altman DG, Hooft L, Korevaar DA, Cohen JF. STARD 2015: an updated list of essential items for reporting diagnostic accuracy studies. *BMJ* 2015; **351**: h5527.

Bossuyt PM, Olsen M, Hyde C, Cohen JF. An analysis reveals differences between pragmatic and explanatory diagnostic accuracy studies. *Journal of Clinical Epidemiology* 2020; **117**: 29–35.

Conti CR. Confusing and sometimes meaningless terms used in cardiovascular medicine. *Clinical Cardiology* 1994; **17**: 53–54.

Dramé M, Tabue Teguo M, Proye E, Hequet F, Hentzien M, Kanagaratnam L, Godaert L. Should RT-PCR be considered a gold standard in the diagnosis of COVID-19? *Journal of Medical Virology* 2020; **92**: 2312–2313.

Duggan PF. Time to abolish 'gold standard'. *BMJ* 1992; **304**: 1568–1569.

Hansson O, Zetterberg H, Buchhave P, Londos E, Blennow K, Minthon L. Association between CSF biomarkers and incipient Alzheimer's disease in patients with mild cognitive impairment: a follow-up study. *Lancet Neurology* 2006; **5**: 228–234.

Hernández-Huerta MTP, Pérez-Campos Mayoral LP, Sánchez Navarro LM, Mayoral-Andrade GP, Pérez-Campos Mayoral EP, Zenteno EP, Pérez-Campos EP. Should RT-PCR be considered a gold standard in the diagnosis of COVID-19? *Journal of Medical Virology* 2021; **93**: 137–138.

Hofman MS, Lawrentschuk N, Francis RJ, Tang C, Vela I, Thomas P, Rutherford N, Martin JM, Frydenberg M, Shakher R, Wong LM, Taubman K, Ting Lee S, Hsiao E, Roach P, Nottage M, Kirkwood I, Hayne D, Link E, Marusic P, Matera A, Herschtal A, Iravani A, Hicks RJ, Williams S, Murphy DG. Prostate-specific membrane antigen PET-CT in patients with high-risk prostate cancer before curative-intent surgery or radiotherapy (proPSMA): a prospective, randomised, multicentre study. *Lancet* 2020; **395**: 1208–1216.

Hussain N, Alt Murphy M, Sunnerhagen KS. Upper limb kinematics in stroke and healthy controls using target-to-target task in virtual reality. *Frontiers in Neurology* 2018; **9**: 300.

Kline JA, Runyon MS, Webb WB, Jones AE, Mitchell AM. Prospective study of the diagnostic accuracy of the simplify D-dimer assay for pulmonary embolism in emergency department patients. *Chest* 2006; **129**: 1417–1423.

Kruip MJHA, Söhne M, Nijkeuter M, Kwakkel-Van Erp HM, Tick LW, Halkes SJM, Prins MH, Kramer MHH, Huisman MV, Büller HR, Leebeek FWG, Christopher Study Investigators. A simple diagnostic strategy in hospitalized patients with clinically suspected pulmonary embolism. *Journal of Internal Medicine* 2006; **260**: 459–466.

Laméris W, van Randen A, van Es HW, van Heesewijk JPM, van Ramshorst B, Bouma WH, ten Hove W, van Leeuwen MS, van Keulen EM, Dijkgraaf MGW, Bossuyt PMM, Boermeester MA, Stoker J. Imaging strategies for detection of urgent conditions in patients with acute abdominal pain: diagnostic accuracy study. *BMJ* 2009; **338**: b2431.

Liu B, Ricarte Filho J, Mallisetty A, Villani C, Kottorou A, Rodgers K, Chen C, Ito T, Holmes K, Gastala N, Valyi-Nagy K, David O, Gaba RC, Ascoli C, Pasquinelli M, Feldman LE, Massad

MG, Wang T-H, Jusue-Torres I, Benedetti E, Winn RA, Brock MV, Herman JG, Hulbert A. Detection of promoter DNA methylation in urine and plasma aids the detection of non–small cell lung cancer. *Clinical Cancer Research* 2020; **26**: 4339.

Lord S, Staub L, Bossuyt P, Irwig L. Target practice: choosing target conditions for test accuracy studies that are relevant to clinical practice. *BMJ* 2011; **343**: d4684.

Nicol MP, Workman L, Isaacs W, Munro J, Black F, Eley B, Boehme CC, Zemanay W, Zar HJ. Accuracy of the Xpert MTB/RIF test for the diagnosis of pulmonary tuberculosis in children admitted to hospital in Cape Town, South Africa: a descriptive study. *Lancet Infectious Diseases* 2011; **11**: 819–824.

Pepe MS, Feng Z, Janes H, Bossuyt PM, Potter JD. Pivotal evaluation of the accuracy of a biomarker used for classification or prediction: standards for study design. *Journal of the National Cancer Institute* 2008; **100**: 1432–1438.

Rutjes AW, Reitsma JB, Vandenbroucke JP, Glas AS, Bossuyt PM. Case-control and two-gate designs in diagnostic accuracy studies. *Clinical Chemistry* 2005; **51**: 1335–1341.

Sackett DL, Haynes RB. The architecture of diagnostic research. *BMJ* 2002; **324**: 539–541.

Schumacher SG, van Smeden M, Dendukuri N, Joseph L, Nicol MP, Pai M, Zar HJ. Diagnostic test accuracy in childhood pulmonary tuberculosis: a Bayesian latent class analysis. *American Journal of Epidemiology* 2016; **184**: 690–700.

Schwartz D, Lellouch J. Explanatory and pragmatic attitudes in therapeutical trials. *Journal of Chronic Diseases* 1967; **20**: 637–648.

Young GP, Senore C, Mandel JS, Allison JE, Atkin WS, Benamouzig R, Bossuyt PMM, Silva MD, Guittet L, Halloran SP, Haug U, Hoff G, Itzkowitz SH, Leja M, Levin B, Meijer GA, O'Morain CA, Parry S, Rabeneck L, Rozen P, Saito H, Schoen RE, Seaman HE, Steele RJC, Sung JJY, Winawer SJ. Recommendations for a step-wise comparative approach to the evaluation of new screening tests for colorectal cancer. *Cancer* 2016; **122**: 826–839.

4

Understanding test accuracy measures

Jonathan J. Deeks, Yemisi Takwoingi, Petra Macaskill and Patrick M. Bossuyt

---

KEY POINTS

- Tests may give binary results, ordered categories, counts or continuous measurements.
- To estimate test accuracy, test results should be dichotomized as positive and negative. For tests with non-binary results, this should be done by specifying a positivity threshold.
- Including and reporting test results that are inconclusive (often described as uninterpretable, intermediate or indeterminate) are essential to report test accuracy fully.
- Measures of test accuracy can be calculated from the frequencies of true positives, false positives, false negatives and true negatives in a 2×2 table, cross-classifying the results of the index test against the results of the reference standard.
- The most commonly reported measures of test accuracy are sensitivity and specificity, and positive and negative predictive values.
- Varying the positivity threshold induces a trade-off between sensitivity and specificity that can be visualized as a receiver operating characteristic (ROC) curve.
- The accuracy of two tests can be compared by computing absolute differences or ratios of their sensitivity and specificity.

4.1 Introduction

Before undertaking a test accuracy meta-analysis, it is necessary to understand the distinct types of data, as well as the presentation and meaning of statistical summaries of test accuracy reported in the primary studies. The accuracy of a test can be presented using several individual measures or pairs of measures. This chapter explains and illustrates the most commonly encountered measures. It can serve as a reminder for those already familiar with test accuracy research.

This chapter should be cited as: Deeks JJ, Takwoingi Y, Macaskill P, Bossuyt PM. Chapter 4: Understanding test accuracy measures. In: Deeks JJ, Bossuyt PM, Leeflang MM, Takwoingi Y, editors. *Cochrane Handbook for Systematic Reviews of Diagnostic Test Accuracy*. 1st edition. Chichester (UK): John Wiley & Sons, 2023: 53–72.

Cochrane Handbook for Systematic Reviews of Diagnostic Test Accuracy, First Edition. Edited by Jonathan J. Deeks, Patrick M. Bossuyt, Mariska M. Leeflang and Yemisi Takwoingi.

The most commonly reported test accuracy measures are computed from 2×2 tables where participants are cross-classified according to the result of the index test and the results of the reference standard (which classifies the participants into those who have the target condition and those who do not). The results of the cross-classification are most often presented as pairs of accuracy measures, which describe how well the test performs either in those with and without the target condition (sensitivity and specificity) or in those with positive and negative test results (positive and negative predictive values and likelihood ratios). Single measures provide overall expressions of accuracy.

The requirement of a 2×2 table for calculating test accuracy measures implies binary index test and reference standard results. This is not always the case, as an index test and/or reference standard may give results that cannot immediately be classified as positive or negative. The target condition being diagnosed may also have more than two categories or be a spectrum of severity measured on a continuum, as such test results may be ordinal or continuous. These issues create additional challenges that should be considered in primary studies and systematic reviews of test accuracy.

This chapter begins with an overview of types of test data (Section 4.2), followed by how to deal with inconclusive test results (Section 4.3) and a summary of issues in defining the target condition (Section 4.4). The remaining four sections focus on analysis, including the basic analysis of a primary test accuracy study (Section 4.5), thresholds for defining test positivity and their relationship with estimates of test accuracy (Section 4.6), generating and understanding receiver operating characteristic (ROC) curves (Section 4.7), and concluding with an analysis of comparative accuracy studies (Section 4.8).

4.2　Types of test data

Systematic reviews of the accuracy of diagnostic and screening tests can encounter test results that fall into the following data types.

Binary (dichotomous), in which the test result is reported as yes or no; positive or negative; normal or abnormal; and present or absent (for signs and symptoms). For example, immunochromatographic rapid tests for malaria provide a positive result when there is a colour change in the correct place on the test device.

Ordinal, in which the test result is reported on a set of ordered categories, often with verbal descriptors. For example, the main BI-RADS (Breast Imaging Reporting and Data System) assessment categories for mammography are 1 = negative, 2 = benign, 3 = probably benign, 4 = suspicious, 5 = highly suggestive of malignancy.

Counts, in which the test result is reported as a count, such as colony counts. For example, microbiologists report the number of colony-forming units per millilitre in urinalysis for suspected urinary tract infection.

Continuous, in which the test result is reported on a continuous scale, such as the concentration of a substance. For example, in prostate cancer diagnosis, PSA (prostate specific antigen) concentrations are reported on a continuous scale of nanograms of PSA per millilitre (ng/mL) of blood.

To compute the standard test accuracy measures, it is necessary to organize data of all types into binary categories related to whether a result is considered positive (indicating the likely presence of the target condition) or negative (indicating its absence).

Binary results should be relabelled as such, as either positive or negative. Ordinal, count and continuous test results are classified as positive or negative by applying a numerical threshold to dichotomize the results. Positivity thresholds and examination of accuracy at multiple thresholds are discussed in Section 4.6.

Many ordinal and binary categorizations arise – or can be conceptualized as arising – from underlying continuous phenomena categorized at one or more thresholds. For example, rapid diagnostic tests use lateral flow immunoassay technologies, which internally apply a threshold to change colour at a particular density of antibodies or antigens. Laboratory tests that report results as abnormal or normal typically involve a numerical measurement of a concentration that is categorized according to one or more pre-stated thresholds, while imaging tests may report an ordinal grade for the certainty of the presence of a feature or the stage of disease progression based on expert judgement.

4.3   Inconclusive index test results

To inform decision-making, researchers should report the results or outcome for all participants undergoing testing. For many tests, this means that researchers should also report the number of persons tested for whom a conclusive result – a clear positive or a clear negative – could not be obtained, and the reasons. Whenever possible, researchers should mention the proportion of participants with and without the target condition who received such inconclusive test results (Simel 1987, Shinkins 2013).

For some tests, it is possible that the procedure cannot be completed successfully. Spirometry, for example, is widely used in the assessment of lung function. Some patients are unable to expire long enough, even after repeated manoeuvres. Their results cannot be trusted and are sometimes called 'uninterpretable'. Acceptability criteria have been defined for spirometry and for many other tests (Graham 2019).

Depending on the intended use and the clinical setting, failed procedures should be excluded from the analysis, or classified as either positive or negative. Such classifications will often be guided by the consequences of the actions planned after positive and negative results, respectively.

When evaluating breath tests to rule out COVID-19, for example, only completed procedures that generate a 'negative' result are classified as negatives. All other outcomes, including failure to complete the manoeuvre and rejected results that do not meet the acceptability criteria, are classified as positives because in practice, the breath test would be used to refer likely infected people to a further diagnostic procedure.

Even when a test procedure was completed successfully, the result may be compromised. Haemolysis, the breakdown of red blood cells and other blood cells, is known to affect laboratory tests. It can cause clinically relevant bias in obtaining results through its interference with laboratory measurements. Most laboratories monitor haemolysis in their samples for clinical chemistry testing, but they differ in the extent to which they reject haemolyzed samples.

Primary studies that rely on not one but two thresholds will report some results as intermediate: in between the higher and the lower threshold. If higher values point to a greater likelihood of having the target condition, the lower threshold is typically used to rule out the target condition, and a higher one to rule in the target condition. Using both vvthresholds simultaneously, however, creates a third category, in addition to negatives (below the lower threshold) and positives (above the higher threshold): intermediate results. These studies deserve special attention.

In reviews of test accuracy studies, either threshold can be used to classify all test results as positive or negative, but only one threshold is typically used. Either the lower threshold is used, and intermediates are classified as positives, or the upper threshold is used, and intermediates are classified as negatives.

When analysing test accuracy, all study participants undergoing testing should in principle be included in the (re-)classification as positives or negatives. Depending on the application, inconclusive test results can be included in the analysis of a test accuracy study as either positives or negatives (see Chapter 7).

If such analyses were not done either as the main or sensitivity analyses in the primary studies, re-analysis by the review authors will be required depending on data availability. To generate a meaningful interpretation, representative of clinical management, a primary analysis should reflect the way in which inconclusive results are used in clinical practice, but the impact of their existence may be further assessed in a sensitivity analysis (see Chapter 7, Table 7.3.f).

4.4 Target condition

As discussed in Chapter 3, the accuracy of a test reflects the test's ability to detect the presence of a target condition.

In many cases, focusing on the presence or absence of a target condition is a simplification of the reality of diagnosis. The diagnosis may have more than two categories or constitute a spectrum of different severities of disease. For example, the severity of coronary artery disease (CAD) is defined according to the degree of stenosis seen in coronary arteries. As degree of stenosis is a continuous measure (often represented as a percentage), different thresholds for classifying the presence or absence of the target condition may have been used in different studies. A Cochrane Review found that some studies defined CAD as >50% stenosis and others as >70% stenosis (Wang 2011).

As explained in Chapter 5, the target condition should be defined in such a way that it can meaningfully inform clinical practice; it identifies the patients who will likely benefit from downstream actions, such as further testing, or starting effective treatment, while separating these from the ones who do not benefit, or do not benefit sufficiently.

It may not always be possible to have a reference standard result in all study participants, for the reasons discussed in Section 4.3. The reference standard may fail, for example. Participants may be unable to complete the procedure, or the result may not meet predefined acceptability criteria. Study authors should report the corresponding numbers in their study report.

4.5 Analysis of a primary test accuracy study

Having defined the target condition and chosen a particular threshold for test positivity, the data from a primary study can be presented in a 2×2 table showing the cross-classification of the reference standard result and the index test result, as in Table 4.5.a.

Table 4.5.a 2×2 cross-classification of index test results and reference standard

Index test result	Reference standard result		
	Target condition present (D)	**Target condition absent (D̄)**	**Total**
Index test positive (T+)	True positives (a)	False positives (b)	Test positives (a+b)
Index test negative (T−)	False negatives (c)	True negatives (d)	Test negatives (c+d)
Total	With target condition (a+c)	Without target condition (b+d)	N (a+b+c+d)

All study participants are classified in one of the four cells, depending on their index test result and the result of the reference standard. The true positives (upper left cell) had a positive index test result and were classified by the reference standard as having the target condition. The true negatives (lower right cell) had a negative index test result and were classified by the reference standard as not having the target condition. This means that both the true positives and the true negatives were correctly classified by the index test.

The false positives (upper right cell) had a positive index test result but were classified by the reference standard as not having the target condition. The false negatives (lower left cell) had a negative index test result but were classified by the reference standard as having the target condition. This means that the false positives and the false negatives were misclassified by the index test.

Measures of test accuracy are computed either as proportions of those with the target condition and those without the target condition (these are measures that are *conditional* on the target condition), or within those who tested positive and those who tested negative (these are measures that are *conditional* on the index test result), as described below.

4.5.1   Sensitivity and specificity

Sensitivity and specificity are measures that are conditional on the target condition status.

The sensitivity of a test is defined as the proportion of those with the target condition who test positive. In a test accuracy study, it is estimated using the numbers from Table 4.5.a as a/(a+c). It is expressed either as a proportion (with a range from 0 to 1) or a percentage. Sensitivity is sometimes referred to as the true-positive fraction.

The specificity of a test is defined as the proportion of those without the target condition who test negative. In a test accuracy study, it is estimated using the numbers from Table 4.5.a as d/(b+d). As with sensitivity, both proportions and percentages are used. Specificity is occasionally referred to as the true-negative fraction.

Some studies will summarize the results from the 2×2 table by referring to the proportion of those without the target condition with a false positive test result (b/(b+d)) and refer to this proportion (1−specificity) as the false positive fraction. This will be the case when we discuss ROC curves in Section 4.7.

Sensitivity is sometimes referred to as the true-positive rate and specificity is referred to as the true-negative rate. This is a misnomer, because a rate is a ratio of two quantities with different units of measure.

Sensitivity can also be interpreted as the conditional probability P(T+|D) of having a positive result (T+) for a randomly selected person with the target condition (D) in the intended-use population: the population for whom testing is considered. Similarly, specificity is interpreted as the conditional probability P(T−|$\overline{D}$) of having a negative result (T−) for a randomly selected person without the target condition ($\overline{D}$) in the population for whom testing is considered.

A test with high sensitivity will be positive in a high proportion of participants who have the target condition and may be used to rule out the presence of that target condition: false negatives are not likely, so any negative is probably a true negative.

A test with high specificity will be negative in most of those without the target condition and may be used for ruling in the target condition. As false positives are unlikely, most positive index test results will be true positives.

Nevertheless, the clinical utility of a test will always depend on both sensitivity and specificity, and will also be influenced by the proportion with the target condition among those tested. It is therefore crucially important always to report sensitivity and specificity in pairs: a high sensitivity may be achievable for many continuous tests, but if it comes at the cost of an extremely low specificity, the test may not be helpful – most of those with the target condition are classed as positives, but also many of those without the condition.

4.5.2   Predictive values

Predictive values are measures that are conditional on the index test results, as they are defined as proportions of the total with positive and the total with negative index test results.

The positive predictive value of a test is defined as the proportion of those with a positive index test who have the target condition. It is estimated using the numbers from Table 4.5.a as a/(a+b).

The negative predictive value of a test is defined as the proportion of those with a negative index test result who do not have the target condition. It is estimated using the numbers from Table 4.5.a as d/(c+d).

Like sensitivity and specificity, negative and positive predictive values are also reported either as proportions or percentages.

They can also be interpreted as probabilities. The positive predictive value P(D|T+) is the probability that a randomly selected person in the target population testing positive on the index test has the target condition. The negative predictive value P($\overline{D}$|T−) is the probability that a randomly selected person in the target population testing negative on the index test does not have the target condition. Studies may sometimes also report P(D|T−), the probability that a person with a negative test result has the target condition.

4.5.3   Proportion with the target condition

In test accuracy studies, reporting the proportion of persons tested who have the target condition, as detected by the reference standard, is an informative additional measure.

Studies can differ dramatically in the proportion of participants with the target condition. Such variability often indicates that studies were performed in a different population, or a different setting, or after pre-testing with other tests.

There is no specific term for referring to the proportion tested with the target condition. In many reports it has been referred to as the 'prevalence of the target condition', and this handbook occasionally uses this term in a similar way. Review authors should be aware, however, that prevalence has an accepted and different definition in epidemiology, where it is used to refer to the proportion of a population who have a disease, or a specific characteristic, at a given point in time or during a given period.

The proportion of participants undergoing testing who turn out to have the target condition may be substantially different from the prevalence of that target condition in the population. Testing for COVID-19, for example, is more often done in people with symptoms or recent exposure to others with a confirmed COVID-19 infection; in those being tested, the proportion with COVID-19 will be higher than the population prevalence of COVID-19 at the time the study was conducted.

4.5.4 Pre-test and post-test probabilities

Sensitivity and specificity, and positive and negative predictive value, are pairs of proportions that are computed within groups defined by (1) presence or absence of the target condition or (2) a positive or negative index test, respectively. We showed that these can also be interpreted as probabilities. Sensitivity, for example, can also be interpreted as the conditional probability of having a positive result for a randomly selected person with the target condition in the population for whom testing is considered.

The actual probability that a single person with the target condition will test positive may vary around the observed sensitivity. It is often influenced by other factors, such as that person's age, sex, comorbidities or duration of symptoms.

Something similar applies to the positive predictive value. While it can be interpreted as the probability that a randomly selected person in the target population testing positive on the index test has the target condition, the probability that a single person testing positive has the target condition is not necessarily equal to the positive predictive value.

That probability – often referred to as the post-test probability – will typically be different for a person with a high pre-test probability (a high suspicion of the target condition before being tested) than for someone with a low pre-test probability. In testing for COVID-19, for example, the post-test probability of being infected after a negative antigen test result will be higher for a person with fever and loss of sense of smell, in a household with many infected, than for another person testing negative who is free of symptoms.

Since random sampling rarely applies in clinical practice, sensitivity and specificity are preferably presented as group-based measures, expressed as proportions or percentages, rather than probabilities.

4.5.5 Interpretation of sensitivity, specificity and predictive values

The paired measures of sensitivity and specificity and positive and negative predictive values reflect proportions of patients undergoing testing who were correctly classified, but they do so in separate ways. Sensitivity and specificity focus on the presence of the target condition – if the target condition is an infectious disease, such as SARS-CoV-2 infection, the sensitivity of a rapid test for detecting SARS-CoV-2 infection informs us about the proportion of persons with the infection that the test correctly detects. Predictive values focus more on the consequences in specific groups after testing. For instance, the positive predictive value of the rapid test for patients with suspected SARS-CoV-2 infection refers to the proportion of those testing positive who turn out to have the infection.

Many of the older textbooks have taught that sensitivity and specificity are fixed test properties, in contrast to positive and negative predictive values. These authors expected sensitivity and specificity to be constant across different settings, while positive predictive values would be higher in situations where more persons being tested have the target condition.

It sounds plausible that, if many have the target condition, many of those will have a (true) positive result in a case of reasonable sensitivity. However, we now know that for many tests sensitivity and specificity also vary with the target population and with the role and context of testing (setting, earlier tests) and should not necessarily be considered fixed and stable test properties. When comparing individual studies in systematic reviews, researchers have seen that sensitivity and specificity sometimes vary as much as positive and negative predictive values, and sometimes even more (Leeflang 2012).

More primary accuracy studies seem to report and interpret results in terms of sensitivity and specificity, rather than in terms of positive and negative predictive values. Sensitivity and specificity are often preferred in the interpretation and communication of test results. In most testing applications, the reproducibility of results by the reference standard is also assumed to be better than that of the index test. For these reasons, the main emphasis in meta-analysis of test accuracy research is on meta-analysis of sensitivity and specificity. Predictive values are commonly computed from these meta-analytical estimates to explore how the test may perform across settings with different proportions of participants with the target condition, as observed in the primary studies, assuming that sensitivity and specificity are stable (see Chapter 11).

A notable exception is a situation where one reference standard is used for test positives (imaging, for example) and a different one for test negatives (follow-up, for example). In those cases, estimates of sensitivity and specificity are at risk of bias and reporting sensitivity and specificity may be misleading, while meta-analysis of predictive values may be more meaningful (see Chapter 8).

4.5.6 Confidence intervals

Sensitivity, specificity and positive and negative predictive values are estimates of proportions in a study population made in a sample from that population. Hence, there is uncertainty associated with them. Results from individual studies should be reported with confidence intervals for each measure to express this uncertainty (see Table 4.5.b).

A confidence interval is presented as a lower and an upper bound around the point estimate. This interval is likely to include the true value for the population with a certain degree of confidence (most often 95%), if the estimation process is repeated a large number of times, in similar samples of the same size, under similar circumstances.

As estimates of these proportions are often close to 1, methods that ensure appropriate asymmetrical confidence interval calculation when the proportion is equal to 1 or 0 should be used. This excludes commonly used methods based on normal approximations. An exact method called the Clopper–Pearson method is implemented in Review Manager 5 to provide estimates based on the binomial distribution (Clopper 1934), but is known to be conservative in some situations. Some software packages may use the alternative Wilson score interval (Wilson 1927, Brown 2001).

It is standard to present estimates with 95% confidence intervals, although intervals with greater or lesser coverage may be preferred in some circumstances. In Bayesian statistics, uncertainty is expressed using credible intervals. A 95% credible interval implies that the parameter value of interest has a 95% probability of falling within the range of values indicated by the interval.

4.5.7 Other test accuracy measures

Other measures that can be calculated using data from Table 4.5.a are briefly explained in this section. Several of these are presented for an example in Table 4.5.b.

Likelihood ratios are computed as the ratio of proportions of individuals with and without the target condition who receive a specific test result. The positive likelihood ratio describes how many times more likely positive index test results were in the group with the target condition compared to the group without the target condition. The positive likelihood ratio (LR+), which should be greater than 1 if the test is informative, is defined as

$$LR+ = P(T+|D)/P(T+|\bar{D}) = \text{sensitivity}/(1-\text{specificity}),$$

and is estimated as (a/(a+c)) / (b/(b+d)).

The negative likelihood ratio describes how many times less likely negative index test results were in the group with the target condition compared to the group without the target condition. The negative likelihood ratio (LR−), which should be less than 1 if the test is informative, is defined as

$$LR- = P(T-|D)/P(T-|\bar{D}) = (1-\text{sensitivity})/\text{specificity},$$

and is estimated as (c/(a+c)) / (d/(b+d)).

Likelihood ratios do not inform us directly about misclassifications. Instead, they reflect the information value of a specific test result. They are preferred by clinicians who like to use Bayes' theorem to calculate the post-test probability of having the target condition in a single patient, which they do so starting from a specific pre-test probability for that patient. If one assumes that the chances of having a positive or negative test result, conditional on the target condition, for that patient are identical to that of a randomly selected person in the target population, the post-test odds of having the target condition should equal the pre-test odds multiplied by the likelihood

Table 4.5.b Evaluation of the Innova lateral flow antigen test to detect SARS-CoV-2 infection in Liverpool, UK

		RT-qPCR reference standard			
		Positive	Negative	Void	Total
Innova LFT result	Positive	28 (TP: true positives)	3 (FP: false positives)	2	33
	Negative	42 (FN: false negatives)	5431 (TN: true negatives)	341	5814
	Void	4	18	0	22
	Total	74	5452	343	5869

Measure of test accuracy	Equation	Estimate	95% CI
Sensitivity	TP/(TP+FN)	0.400	(0.285 to 0.524)
Specificity	TN/(TN+FP)	0.999	(0.998 to 1.000)
Positive predictive value	TP/(TP+FP)	0.903	(0.742 to 0.980)
Negative predictive value	TN/(TN+FN)	0.992	(0.990 to 0.994)
Positive likelihood ratio	sensitivity/(1−specificity)	725	(226 to 2328)
Negative likelihood ratio	(1−sensitivity)/specificity	0.600	(0.496 to 0.727)
Diagnostic odds ratio	LR+/LR−	1207	(346 to 6311)

Data taken from García-Fiñana (2021).
If the control line of an LFT or RT-qPCR test fails to appear within 30 minutes, the result is recorded as void. All void results were excluded from the main analysis. In a secondary analysis, the study authors included void LFT results as test negatives. CI, confidence interval; LFT, lateral flow test; LR, likelihood ratio; RT-qPCR, quantitative reverse transcription polymerase chain reaction.

ratio of that test result. This is a simple result of the definition of conditional probabilities. For a test that is informative, the post-test probability should be higher than the pre-test probability if the test result is positive, while the post-test probability should be lower than the pre-test probability if the test result is negative. Considerations about the use of likelihood ratios in systematic reviews of test accuracy are explained in Chapter 11.

The values of sensitivity and specificity are sometimes combined in a single measure known as Youden's index, defined as *sensitivity + specificity − 1*. Youden's index is not a proportion and cannot be interpreted as a probability. Instead, it is a general index of test accuracy. Values close to 1 indicate high accuracy; a value of 0 means that the test cannot discriminate between those with and without the target condition. When the index is equal to 0 the proportion of true positives in those with the target condition is equal to the proportion of false positives in those without the target condition. This means that the test is not informative: a positive result is as likely in those with the target condition as in those without.

Youden's index combines sensitivity and specificity and, as a result, differences in the implications of misclassification between those with and without the target condition are lost. This makes it less informative for medical decision-making. However, it is not uncommon to encounter primary studies that claim to identify the 'optimal' threshold based on maximizing Youden's index. Such computations are only optimal under the unlikely assumption that the consequences of false negatives and false positives are the same, which often is not appreciated by those quoting these values.

Some test accuracy studies report the overall accuracy, computed as the total of true positives and true negatives divided by the total sample size. Again, this measure does not differentiate between the implications of false positive and false negative test errors and is therefore not recommended for any form of decision-making.

The diagnostic odds ratio (DOR) summarizes the diagnostic accuracy of the index test as a single number, which describes how many times higher the odds are of obtaining a positive test result in someone with the target condition, selected at random, than in someone without the target condition, also selected at random (Glas 2003). Alternatively, it can be defined as the odds of the target condition in test positives versus the odds of having the target condition in test negatives. The DOR is formally defined as

$$DOR = \frac{\frac{sensitivity}{1-sensitivity}}{\frac{1-specificity}{specificity}} = \frac{sensitivity \times specificity}{(1-sensitivity)\times(1-specificity)}$$

The DOR is also equal to LR+/LR−. It is estimated from Table 4.5.a as (ad)/(bc).

The same DOR may be achieved by different combinations of sensitivity and specificity, as shown in Figure 4.5.a, where the numbers circled in red indicate sensitivity–specificity combinations that have the same diagnostic odds ratio of 9. For example, a DOR of 9 could be achieved by a specificity of 90% and a sensitivity of 50%, or by a sensitivity of 90% and a specificity of 50%. The fact that it summarizes test accuracy

Specificity	Sensitivity						
	50%	60%	70%	80%	90%	95%	99%
50%	1	2	2	4	9	19	99
60%	2	2	4	6	14	29	149
70%	2	4	5	9	21	44	231
80%	4	6	9	16	36	76	396
90%	9	14	21	36	81	171	891
95%	19	29	44	76	171	361	1881
99%	99	149	231	396	891	1881	9801

Figure 4.5.a Diagnostic odds ratios achieved at different values of sensitivity and specificity

in a single number makes it popular with some authors. Like Youden's index and overall accuracy, it is uninformative about the nature of misclassifications. However, as will be explained in Chapter 9, the DOR has a particular role in meta-analysis models of test accuracy.

4.6   Positivity thresholds

In studies of the accuracy of tests with ordinal and continuous results, positive and negative test results are defined based on a threshold for test positivity and change if the threshold is altered. This dependence on threshold is a fundamental aspect of test accuracy evaluation. In the case of test sensitivity and specificity, the dependence induces a trade-off between the two quantities, one value increasing while the other decreases as the threshold for positivity is changed.

This is illustrated in the panels in Figure 4.6.a, which show the same hypothetical distributions of test results for those with and without the target condition on a continuous scale. The shaded areas show how the false negative fraction (red) and the false positive fraction (green) change as the positivity threshold varies. The panels vary in the numerical value of the threshold used to define test positive. At each threshold, the sensitivity of the test reflects the proportion of the area under the curve to the right of the threshold: those with the target condition. Similarly, the specificity reflects the proportion of the area under the curve to the left of the threshold.

As the threshold decreases from panel (a) to panel (e), the proportion of those with the target condition who are above the threshold – and hence have a positive test – increases from 69% to 99%. These values stand for the sensitivity of the test. At the same time, the corresponding proportion of those without the target condition who are below the threshold – and hence have a negative test result – decreases from 99% to 69%. These values stand for the specificity of the test.

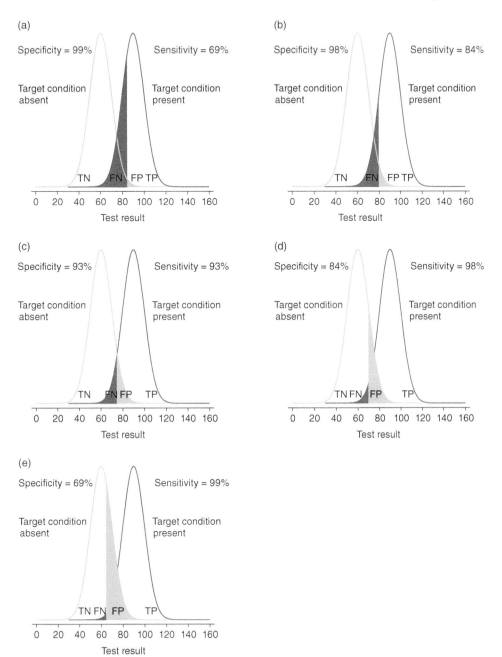

Figure 4.6.a Relationship between sensitivity, specificity and the positivity threshold

4.7   Receiver operating characteristic curves

Primary studies that evaluate a test at several thresholds sometimes present their findings as receiver operating characteristic (ROC) curves. The ROC curve of a test is the graph of the values of sensitivity and specificity that are obtained by varying the positivity threshold across all possible values. The graph plots sensitivity (true-positive fraction) against 1–specificity (false positive fraction).

The curve for any test moves from the point where sensitivity and 1–specificity are both 1 (the upper right corner), which occurs when the threshold classifies all partici-pants as test positive (there are no false negatives and all without the target condition are false positives), to a point where sensitivity and 1–specificity are both 0 (the lower left corner), which occurs when all participants are classified as test negative (giving no false positives and all with the target condition are false negatives). The shape and posi-tion of the curve between these two fixed points depend on the discriminatory ability of the test across all possible thresholds. The closer the curve lies to the top left-hand corner (where sensitivity and specificity are both 1), the more discriminatory the test.

In practice, the ROC curve is estimated from a finite sample of test results and hence will not necessarily be a smooth curve, as shown in Figure 4.7.a. Note that the horizon-tal axis for each ROC plot in Figure 4.7.a is labelled in terms of specificity decreasing from 1.0 to 0.0. This style of labelling is used in Cochrane Reviews and is equivalent to the usual labelling (1–specificity or the false positive fraction ranging from 0.0 to 1.0).

The position of the ROC curve depends on the degree of overlap of the distributions of the test results in those with and without the target condition. Where a test clearly discriminates between those with and without the target condition such that there is no or little overlap of distributions, the ROC curve will indicate that high sensitivity is achieved with a high specificity, i.e. the curve approaches the upper left-hand corner of the graph where sensitivity is 1 and specificity is 1 (Figure 4.7.a panel (a)). If the distribu-tions of test results in the two subgroups overlap completely, the test would be com-pletely uninformative, and its ROC curve would be the upward diagonal of the square (Figure 4.7.a panel (c)).

The ROC curves shown in Figure 4.7.a panel (a) to panel (c) are all symmetrical about the downward diagonal of the square, where sensitivity equals 1–specificity. It is also possible for ROC curves to be asymmetrical, as in Figure 4.7.a panel (d). Asymmetrical curves typically occur when the distribution of the test measurement in those with the target condition has more, or less, variability than the distribution in those without the target condition. Increased variability might occur, for example, if the target condition causes a biomarker both to rise and become more erratic; reduced variability might occur if the target condition lowers biomarker values to a bounding level, such as the lower level of detection.

The comparison of tests based on their ROC curves takes into consideration their accuracy across a range of thresholds and is aided by single summary measures. Several of these have been proposed in the literature. Most used among them is the area under the curve (AUC), which equals 1 for a perfect test and 0.5 for a completely uninformative test. The AUC is also sometimes referred to as the *c*-statistic.

The AUC can be interpreted as a probability: it reflects the chances that, in a pair of one with and one without the target condition, selected at random, the one with the target condition will have a test result that is more compatible with the target condition

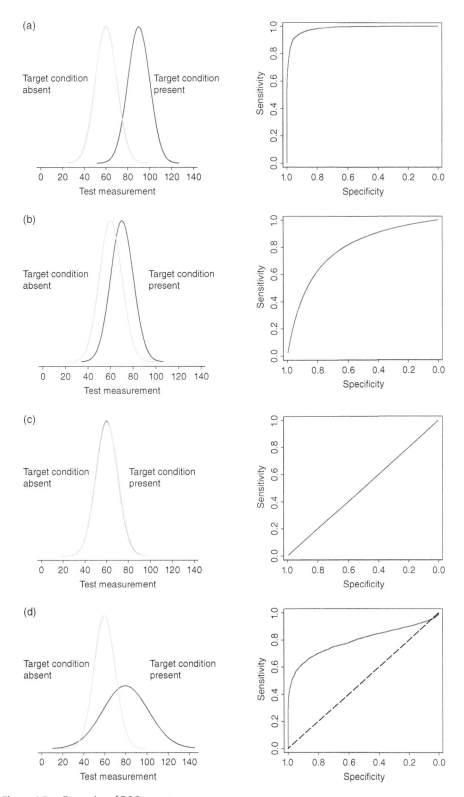

Figure 4.7.a Examples of ROC curves

than the other. If higher test results point to having the target condition, the AUC represents the probability that in that pair the one with the target condition will have a higher result than the one without the target condition.

The AUC can also be interpreted as an average sensitivity for the test, taken over all specificity values, or, equivalently, as the average specificity over all sensitivity values. Other summaries include partial areas under the curve, values of sensitivity corresponding to selected values of specificity (and the other way round) and operating points defined according to specified criteria (such as the Q* value, which is the point on the curve where sensitivity and specificity are equal).

4.8 Analysis of a comparative accuracy study

As explained in Chapter 3, robust comparative studies of diagnostic test accuracy use either a within-subject paired design, in which all patients undergo all tests together with a reference standard, or, more rarely, a between-subject randomized design, in which all patients undergo the reference standard test but are randomly assigned to have only one of the index tests (Takwoingi 2013). These designs have consequences for how the accuracy of two or more tests can be characterized.

For studies that use randomized comparisons, a separate 2×2 table will be created for the results in each arm of the study, and computation of test accuracy measures proceeds as before.

Point estimates will be the same if a paired design is analysed as a randomized design, but standard errors for comparisons will be inaccurate, leading to confidence intervals that are likely to be too large. Appropriate computations in studies using a paired design are more complex (Hayen 2010).

Table 4.8.a shows the joint classification of the results of two index tests from a study that used a paired design.

For two tests labelled A and B in Table 4.8.a, y_{11}^D is the number of patients with the target condition for whom both tests are positive; y_{00}^D is the number of patients with the target condition for whom both tests are negative; y_{10}^D is the number of patients with the target condition for whom test A is positive but test B is negative; and y_{01}^D is the number of patients with the target condition for whom test B is positive but test A is negative. For those without the target condition, the counts $y_{11}^{\bar{D}}$, $y_{00}^{\bar{D}}$, $y_{10}^{\bar{D}}$ and $y_{01}^{\bar{D}}$ can be interpreted in an equivalent manner.

For tests A and B, n_{A1}^D and n_{B1}^D are the numbers of true positives; $n_{A0}^{\bar{D}}$ and $n_{B0}^{\bar{D}}$ are the numbers of true negatives; n_{A0}^D and n_{B0}^D are the numbers of false negatives; and $n_{A1}^{\bar{D}}$ and $n_{B1}^{\bar{D}}$ are the numbers of false positives. If n_1 and n_0 represent the number of individuals with and without the target condition, respectively, then the sensitivity and specificity of the two tests can be estimated from the marginal frequencies as follows:

$$\text{Sensitivity}(A) = n_{A1}^D / n_1 : \text{Specificity}(A) = n_{A0}^{\bar{D}} / n_0$$
$$\text{Sensitivity}(B) = n_{B1}^D / n_1 ; \text{Specificity}(B) = n_{B0}^{\bar{D}} / n_0.$$

Table 4.8.b shows the results of two interferon gamma release assays (IGRAs) – T-SPOT. TB and a second-generation IGRA – for diagnosis of active tuberculosis cross-classified

Table 4.8.a Joint classification of paired index tests and reference standard results

		Target condition present			Target condition absent		
		Test A			Test A		
		Positive	Negative	Total	Positive	Negative	Total
Test B	Positive	y_{11}^D	y_{01}^D	n_{B1}^D	$y_{11}^{\bar{D}}$	$y_{01}^{\bar{D}}$	$n_{B1}^{\bar{D}}$
	Negative	y_{10}^D	y_{00}^D	n_{B0}^D	$y_{10}^{\bar{D}}$	$y_{00}^{\bar{D}}$	$n_{B0}^{\bar{D}}$
	Total	n_{A1}^D	n_{A0}^D	n_1	$n_{A1}^{\bar{D}}$	$n_{A0}^{\bar{D}}$	n_0

Adapted from Takwoingi (2016).

Table 4.8.b Comparison of T-SPOT.TB and second-generation IGRA for diagnosis of active tuberculosis

		Active TB present			Active TB absent		
		2nd-generation IGRA			2nd-generation IGRA		
		Positive	Negative	Total	Positive	Negative	Total
T-SPOT.TB	Positive	253	0	253	51	0	51
	Negative	16	33	49	19	296	315
	Total	269	33	302	70	296	366

Test accuracy measure	Estimate (95% CI)
Sensitivity of 2nd-generation IGRA	269/302 = 89.1% (85.0 to 92.43)
Sensitivity of T-SPOT.TB	253/302 = 83.8% (79.1 to 87.7)
Absolute difference in sensitivity (sensitivity of 2nd-generation IGRA– sensitivity of T-SPOT.TB)	5.30 (2.44 to 8.16) percentage points
Relative sensitivity (sensitivity of 2nd-generation IGRA/sensitivity of T-SPOT.TB)	1.06 (1.03 to 1.10)
Specificity of 2nd-generation IGRA	296/366 = 80.9% (76.5 to 84.8)
Specificity of T-SPOT.TB	315/366 = 86.1% (82.1 to 89.4)
Absolute difference in specificity (specificity of 2nd-generation IGRA– specificity of T-SPOT.TB)	−5.19 (−7.74 to −2.65) percentage points
Relative specificity (specificity of 2nd-generation IGRA/specificity of T-SPOT.TB)	0.93 (0.91 to 0.97)

Data taken from Whitworth (2019).
Borderline test results excluded. CI, confidence interval; IGRA, interferon gamma release assay; TB, tuberculosis.

among those with and those without the target condition. Although such a table of the joint classification of the results of two tests against those of the reference standard is potentially useful, many studies do not present results in this format, but rather give a separate 2×2 table of the results of each index test against the reference standard, as would be expected for a randomized design.

Absolute differences comparing the sensitivity and specificity of two tests can be estimated while relative comparisons can be estimated for most of the measures described in Section 5.5. (Full details of computations including confidence intervals are given in Hayen (2010)).

If the newer or experimental test is labelled as test A and the older test, or standard practice, as test B, then the absolute difference in sensitivity and specificity can be written as

$$\text{Absolute difference in sensitivity} = sensitivity(A) - sensitivity(B)$$
$$\text{Absolute difference in specificity} = specificity(A) - specificity(B).$$

These absolute differences describe the change in the proportion of those with the target condition who will be additionally detected using test A instead of test B (difference in sensitivity) and the absolute reduction in the numbers without the target condition given false positive results (difference in specificity).

The relative probabilities can be written as

$$\text{Relative sensitivity} = sensitivity(A) / sensitivity(B)$$
$$\text{Relative specificity} = specificity(A) / specificity(B).$$

It is more difficult to define a clear interpretation of the magnitude of relative sensitivity and specificity measures than of absolute differences. Ratios of 1-sensitivity and 1-specificity values describe multiplicative increases in the proportions misclassified (false negative and false positive fractions, respectively) and give a distinct perspective on the magnitude of differences. For example, if test A and test B have sensitivities of 99% to 90%, respectively, the ratio of sensitivities is 1.1 (a 10% increase), whereas the ratio of the equivalent false negative fractions of 1% with 10% is a 10-fold increase in false negatives.

Results may also be presented as odds ratios:

$$\text{Odds ratio}(\text{true positive}) = \frac{sensitivity(A)}{1 - sensitivity(A)} / \frac{sensitivity(B)}{1 - sensitivity(B)}$$

$$\text{Odds ratio}(\text{true negative}) = \frac{specificity(A)}{1 - specificity(A)} / \frac{specificity(B)}{1 - specificity(B)}.$$

These odds ratios are not equivalent to the DOR. Here the ratios compare the same measure (sensitivity or specificity) for one test to that of another test, while the DOR compares two groups (target condition present or absent) for one test

(Takwoingi 2016). The DORs of two tests can be compared and expressed as the relative DOR (RDOR).

If logistic regression models are used to compare the sensitivity and specificity of two or more tests, odds ratios are the natural output. However, odds ratios do not have an intuitive interpretation. Absolute differences and relative probabilities are more familiar to researchers and are straightforward to interpret; therefore, they are preferred measures of comparative accuracy.

The approximate relationship between odds ratios and relative risks that is exploited in epidemiology when events are rare (Altman 1998) is invalid in test research, because events (i.e. true positives or true negatives) are common.

Table 4.8.b shows the results of the comparison of the accuracy of the two IGRAs, in terms of absolute and relative differences in sensitivity and specificity. The relative sensitivity of 1.06 (95% confidence interval (CI) 1.03 to 1.10) indicates that the sensitivity of the second-generation IGRA is about 1.06 times or 6% higher than that of T-SPOT.TB. The 95% CI indicates that we are 95% confident that the sensitivity could be about 3% to 10% higher for the second-generation IGRA compared to T-SPOT.TB. The relative specificity of 0.94 (95% CI 0.91 to 0.97) indicates a 6% reduction in the specificity of the second-generation IGRA relative to that of T-SPOT.TB, and we are 95% confident that the decrease in sensitivity lies between 9% and 3%.

4.9   Chapter information

Authors: Jonathan J. Deeks (*Institute of Applied Health Research, University of Birmingham, UK*); Yemisi Takwoingi (*Institute of Applied Health Research, University of Birmingham, UK*); Petra Macaskill (*Sydney School of Public Health, University of Sydney, Australia*); Patrick M. Bossuyt *(Department of Epidemiology and Data Science, University of Amsterdam, The Netherlands)*.

Sources of support: Jonathan J. Deeks is a UK National Institute for Health Research (NIHR) Senior Investigator Emeritus. Yemisi Takwoingi is funded by a UK National Institute for Health Research (NIHR) Postdoctoral Fellowship. Jonathan J. Deeks and Yemisi Takwoingi are supported by the NIHR Birmingham Biomedical Research Centre at the University Hospitals Birmingham NHS Foundation Trust and the University of Birmingham. The views expressed are those of the authors and not necessarily those of the NHS, the NIHR or the Department of Health and Social Care. The authors declare no other sources of support for writing this chapter.

Declarations of interest: Jonathan J. Deeks, Yemisi Takwoingi and Petra Macaskill are members of Cochrane's Diagnostic Test Accuracy Editorial Team. Yemisi Takwoingi and Petra Macaskill are co-convenors of the Cochrane Screening and Diagnostic Tests Methods Group. The authors declare no other potential conflicts of interest relevant to the topic of this chapter.

Acknowledgements: The authors would like to thank Marta Roque and Gianni Virgili for helpful peer review comments.

4.10   References

Altman DG, Deeks JJ, Sackett DL. Odds ratios should be avoided when events are common. *BMJ* 1998; **317**: 1318.

Brown LD, Cai TT, DasGupta A. Interval estimation for a binomial proportion. *Statistical Science* 2001; **16**: 101–117.

Clopper C, Pearson ES. The use of confidence or fiducial limits illustrated in the case of the binomial. *Biometrika* 1934; **26**: 404–413.

García-Fiñana M, Hughes DM, Cheyne CP, Burnside G, Stockbridge M, Fowler TA, Fowler VL, Wilcox MH, Semple MG, Buchan I. Performance of the Innova SARS-CoV-2 antigen rapid lateral flow test in the Liverpool asymptomatic testing pilot: population based cohort study. *BMJ* 2021; **374**: n1637.

Glas AS, Lijmer JG, Prins MH, Bonsel GJ, Bossuyt PM. The diagnostic odds ratio: a single indicator of test performance. *Journal of Clinical Epidemiology* 2003; **56**: 1129–1135.

Graham BL, Steenbruggen I, Miller MR, Barjaktarevic IZ, Cooper BG, Hall GL, Hallstrand TS, Kaminsky DA, McCarthy K, McCormack MC, Oropez CE, Rosenfeld M, Stanojevic S, Swanney MP, Thompson BR. Standardization of Spirometry 2019 Update. An Official American Thoracic Society and European Respiratory Society Technical Statement. *American Journal of Respiratory and Critical Care Medicine* 2019; **200**: e70–e88.

Hayen A, Macaskill P, Irwig L, Bossuyt P. Appropriate statistical methods are required to assess diagnostic tests for replacement, add-on, and triage. *Journal of Clinical Epidemiology* 2010; **63**: 883–891.

Leeflang MM, Deeks JJ, Rutjes AW, Reitsma JB, Bossuyt PM. Bivariate meta-analysis of predictive values of diagnostic tests can be an alternative to bivariate meta-analysis of sensitivity and specificity. *Journal of Clinical Epidemiology* 2012; **65**: 1088–1097.

Shinkins B, Thompson M, Mallett S, Perera R. Diagnostic accuracy studies: how to report and analyse inconclusive test results. *BMJ* 2013; **346**: f2778.

Simel DL, Feussner JR, DeLong ER, Matchar DB. Intermediate, indeterminate, and uninterpretable diagnostic test results. *Medical Decision Making* 1987; **7**: 107–114.

Takwoingi Y, Leeflang MM, Deeks JJ. Empirical evidence of the importance of comparative studies of diagnostic test accuracy. *Annals of Internal Medicine* 2013; **158**: 544–554.

Takwoingi Y. Meta-analytic approaches for summarising and comparing the accuracy of medical tests [PhD]. Birmingham (UK): University of Birmingham, 2016.

Wang LW, Fahim MA, Hayen A, Mitchell RL, Baines L, Lord S, Craig JC, Webster AC. Cardiac testing for coronary artery disease in potential kidney transplant recipients. *Cochrane Database of Systematic Reviews* 2011; **12**: CD008691.

Whitworth HS, Badhan A, Boakye AA, Takwoingi Y, Rees-Roberts M, Partlett C, Lambie H, Innes J, Cooke G, Lipman M, Conlon C, Macallan D, Chua F, Post FA, Wiselka M, Woltmann G, Deeks JJ, Kon OM, Lalvani A, Abdoyeku D, Davidson R, Dedicoat M, Kunst H, Loebingher MR, Lynn W, Nathani N, O'Connell R, Pozniak A, Menzies S. Clinical utility of existing and second-generation interferon-gamma release assays for diagnostic evaluation of tuberculosis: an observational cohort study. *Lancet Infectious Diseases* 2019; **19**: 193–202.

Wilson EB. Probable inference, the law of succession, and statistical inference. *Journal of the American Statistical Association* 1927; **22**: 209–212.

Part Three

Methods and presentation of systematic reviews of test accuracy

5

Defining the review question

Mariska M. Leeflang, Clare Davenport and Patrick M. Bossuyt

KEY POINTS

- Systematic reviews of test accuracy should aim to address clinically relevant questions for which knowing a test's sensitivity and specificity, or other accuracy measures, is important.
- The objective of these systematic reviews is to collate evidence about the accuracy of a single test or to compare the accuracy of two or more tests for detecting the same target condition.
- Other objectives may be to study the differences in accuracy related to test characteristics, such as the type of assays, procedures or positivity thresholds, or to the setting where the tests can be used.
- The review question should contain information about the **P**opulation (including where and when they will be tested), **I**ndex tests (including competing tests) and **T**arget condition.
- Identifying the clinical pathway in which the index test(s) will be used helps to refine the review question.
- The eligibility criteria for studies should match the elements of the review question and include the acceptable reference standard(s) used to establish the presence or absence of the target condition.

5.1 Introduction

In Chapter 3 we discussed different study designs and terminology for designing a test accuracy study. In this chapter, we focus on how to formulate a review question for a systematic review of test accuracy, the objectives of the review and the eligibility criteria. These steps should consider the aim of the review: answering relevant questions for which knowing a test's sensitivity and specificity (or other accuracy measures) is important. That means that the objectives and the study eligibility criteria should address key issues such as the intended use of the test, the population to be tested, the role of the index test(s) in the clinical pathway, the relevant target condition and the acceptable reference standard(s).

Test accuracy is not a fixed property of a test: accuracy describes the performance of a test in specific circumstances. The accuracy of a test may therefore vary with the intended use (e.g. screening versus diagnosis), population (e.g. children versus adults), setting (rural health centre in a low-income country versus urban hospital), prior tests (e.g. only signs and symptoms, or also an X-ray before computed tomography (CT) scanning), level of training (novice versus expert readers) and many more elements. Since test accuracy is variable, review authors should be explicit in specifying the circumstances in the review question. The guiding principle is that the review question should flow from the clinical problem: the intended use of the index test, specified in sufficient detail.

In this chapter, we explain the aims of systematic reviews of test accuracy and their scope. We illustrate ways to derive the review question and we discuss setting the eligibility criteria.

5.2 Aims of systematic reviews of test accuracy

Systematic reviews of test accuracy studies can be used to guide policy and decision-making about the use of a test in current clinical practice. To serve this purpose, systematic reviews of test accuracy should aim to address clinically relevant questions, for which knowing a test's sensitivity and specificity, or other accuracy measures, is important. This includes comparisons of two or more tests, where decisions about selecting one or another test are guided by the differences in accuracy between the tests.

Some reviews will focus on whether a test is sufficiently sensitive and sufficiently specific to be used in a well-specified setting. This requires criteria that quantify the clinical performance that a new test must attain to achieve the desired health outcomes. These criteria will be guided by an exploration of the existing testing strategy, how the index test would fit in an alternative testing strategy, and the consequences of management actions based on the test results. This will require value judgements. Methods to define minimally acceptable criteria for accuracy have been suggested in the literature (Pepe 2016, Lord 2019).

Reviews could also explore the amount of variation in test accuracy that results from different test types (e.g. immunofluorescence versus enzyme-linked immunosorbent assays in autoimmune disease) or different samples (e.g. cervical swabs, vaginal swabs, or urine for chlamydia testing), which could help in selecting from the available test options.

In general, the aim of systematic reviews of test accuracy will be to inform decisions about the use of tests in defined populations based on the estimated test accuracy in that population. As discussed in Chapter 2, evaluating test accuracy is necessary but not sufficient to assess whether tests will benefit patients. Recommendations about testing will always require consideration of the downstream consequences of testing and test results on patient outcomes.

For these decision-making purposes, it is important that the review includes those studies that best answer the question and have a low risk of bias. Therefore, the eligibility criteria should ideally address both clinical relevance and methodological quality.

5.2.1 Investigations of heterogeneity

Heterogeneity is expected in systematic reviews of test accuracy and is typically higher than in intervention reviews. This may be partly due to calculation of point estimates of test accuracy, which are proportions akin to absolute risks in treatment or control groups in randomized controlled trials (RCTs). This could potentially make the estimates more heterogeneous than estimates of relative measures, in addition to differences in patient characteristics and other factors. Test accuracy studies may also be more diverse in design than RCTs, which may lead to heterogeneity.

Another explanation for heterogeneity is the diversity in target populations and disease severity in the study participants. Where intervention studies usually include participants with the same condition, test accuracy studies include participants who have the target condition and those who do not have the target condition. Furthermore, if a test is used in practice in a wide variety of situations and healthcare settings, then a systematic review about the accuracy of this test may also include studies done in different healthcare settings and thus studies that have included participants from different target populations. There is evidence that the accuracy of a test varies with the target population, and this leads to heterogeneity.

There may also be variation in the index test itself, for example because there may be variability in how the test is used and criteria for test positivity. Studies may also use different reference standards to verify the same target condition. These differences in the index test and reference standard may not always be clearly reported.

As heterogeneity is to be expected in systematic reviews of test accuracy, a relevant objective may therefore be to investigate potential sources of heterogeneity. In Chapter 9 and Chapter 10, we explain how these investigations can be done. Review authors need to realize that the value of these investigations depends on the number of studies included, how well the studies are reported and how consistently the variables are reported.

5.3 Identifying the clinical problem

The review question will guide the rest of the review process. It helps to define what studies to search for and what search terms to use, and guides the definition of the eligibility criteria. The review question also drives the tailoring of the signalling questions for assessing risk of bias and the applicability of the results from the studies included in the review.

5.3.1 Role of a new test

Test accuracy expresses the ability of a test to identify correctly persons with and without the target condition. For most target conditions, there will already be a testing strategy in place. The role of the index test should therefore be positioned relative to this existing strategy.

This also implies that clinical decisions about the use of a test require a comparison, explicit or implicit, between a testing strategy with and one without the index test. Few primary test accuracy studies will undertake a direct comparison between such strategies.

In general, three roles can be defined for a new test relative to an existing test: (1) to select patients for whom follow-up testing may be useful (triaging); (2) to increase the accuracy of a testing strategy, by adding an extra test to the existing strategy (add-on); and (3) to replace one or more tests in the existing strategy with the (new) index test (replacement) (Bossuyt 2006). These three roles will be discussed here.

In a situation where the current diagnostic testing strategy poses too high a burden for too many people, a triage test may select those persons who do not need to go through an existing, more extensive testing strategy (see Box 5.3.a). The accuracy of the testing strategy with the triage test should then be compared against the accuracy of the testing strategy without the triage test. For many triage tests, existing studies will only provide the accuracy of the triage test in isolation. In that case, the relevant question is: what accuracy is needed for this test to fulfil the role of triage test? If the aim of the triage test is to rule out disease, a sufficiently high sensitivity of the index test will be required, as the damage due to missed diagnoses may be high. A sufficient level of specificity is also needed, to justify using the triage test for reducing the number of people undergoing further testing. Box 5.3.a presents an example of a triage test. Alternatively the main aim of a triage test may be to rule in disease. In colorectal cancer screening, for example, a faecal occult blood test (FOBT) is often used as the first screening test, and FOBT positives are invited to undergo colonoscopy. The sensitivity of FOBT for cancer and its precursors is imperfect, but since colonoscopy is an invasive and costly procedure, for which there is limited capacity, using FOBT as a triage test is preferred.

Box 5.3.a Example of a triage question

Urine biomarkers to triage women who may need to undergo surgery for endometriosis

Endometriosis causes painful periods, chronic lower abdominal pain and difficulty conceiving. The most reliable way to diagnose it is to perform laparoscopic surgery and visualize the endometrial deposits inside the abdomen. Sending all women with complaints suggestive of endometriosis for surgical diagnosis immediately is undesirable. A non-invasive and easy-to-perform test that could identify women who do not need laparoscopy would minimize the diagnostic burden. Several urine tests are available to serve this purpose. This review investigated whether the proposed urine tests are sufficiently accurate for triaging these women. According to the authors of the review, a sensitivity of equal to or greater than 95% is required.

Source: Adapted from Lui 2015.

Another clinical need may arise in situations where the current testing strategy leads to a number of false positives that is considered too high. An extra test may then be added to the current testing strategy, to reduce the number of false positive test results. In such cases, an add-on test may be considered in those testing positive with the current strategy. In the example in Box 5.3.b, resectability was the target condition. Additional imaging was considered as an add-on staging test in patients (testing positive) qualifying for resection after conventional staging, to reduce the number of unnecessary surgical procedures in irresectable patients. Add-on tests do not necessarily have to reduce the number of false positives in an existing testing strategy. Alternatively, it is possible that too many patients may be missed by the existing testing strategy, leading to the wish to reduce the number of false negatives. In screening for breast cancer, for example, mammography is the standard procedure. For certain high-risk women, however, additional screening with magnetic resonance imaging is encouraged in some of the guidelines to reduce the number of cancers missed.

More straightforward review questions are those where the new test will replace an existing test, or where there is a choice between a number of tests for the same target condition, in the same setting. For example, many infectious diseases require microscopy, sophisticated molecular tests or culture to identify the relevant pathogen. In emergency settings and low-resource settings, rapid tests and point-of-care tests may be used to replace these more expensive tests, which also have longer turnaround times (Box 5.3.c).

Box 5.3.b Example of an add-on question

Different imaging modalities as add-on tests following CT scanning for assessing resectability in pancreatic and periampullary cancer

Periampullary cancer includes cancer of the head and neck of the pancreas, cancer of the distal end of the bile duct, cancer of the ampulla of Vater and cancer of the second part of the duodenum. If the tumour expands over an anatomical area that is too large, then it can no longer be surgically removed. Before starting such a surgical operation, the surgeons need to know if a resection of the tumour is possible. CT scanning is the preferred method to assess resectability, but it underestimates the extent to which periampullary cancer has expanded, leading to the decision to operate while the tumour is no longer resectable (false positive test result). Here, the review question is whether other imaging methods such as magnetic resonance imaging (MRI), positron emission tomography (PET), PET-CT and endoscopic ultrasound (EUS) can be used as an add-on test after CT scanning. The expectation is that when these other methods are used in patients who were thought to have a resectable tumour (CT positive), they may indicate further which patients' tumours are indeed resectable (true positives) and which tumours turn out to be not resectable (false positives) based on the add-on imaging test.

Source: Adapted from Tamburrino 2016.

Box 5.3.c Example of a replacement question

Rapid tests to replace blood culture for diagnosing enteric fever

Enteric fever may be caused by the bacteria *Salmonella typhi* (typhus) or *Salmonella paratyphi A* (paratyphus). The currently preferred tests are time consuming and either invasive (bone marrow culture) or relatively insensitive (blood culture or the Widal test, a serological measurement). The review authors wanted to assess which rapid tests would be sufficiently accurate to replace blood culture in the daily clinical setting as the World Health Organization (WHO)–recommended main diagnostic test for enteric fever.

Source: Adapted from Wijedoru 2017.

Sometimes it is not clear whether a test will replace an existing test or be placed before (triage) or after (add-on) an existing test strategy. Or the new test opens up a completely new test–treatment pathway. In these situations, the systematic review may be used in a more exploratory way and the clinical pathway may not (yet) be clear. Possible new pathways may be used as a starting point for defining the review questions.

5.3.2   Defining the clinical pathway

In specifying the clinical question, it may be helpful to draw the existing and alternative testing strategies. Cochrane Reviews of test accuracy studies contain a section called 'Clinical pathway' within the Background, in which the review author is invited to explain how and where the test under evaluation is to be used, relative to other tests for the same target condition in the same population.

Drawing a clinical pathway will provide the review team with the information needed to formulate the review question and the study eligibility criteria. It will also help to specify the actions following testing, as well as the respective consequences of these actions for patients, and may therefore help with the interpretation of the review results (Gopalakrishna 2013). This way, describing the clinical pathway facilitates thinking about the effects of the test on patient-important outcomes, providing a useful description of context that is relevant for the methods and results of the review.

Review authors are asked to provide a description, either graphical or narrative, of the current pathway that patients follow just before and after testing (Gopalakrishna 2016). A description of the clinical pathway should contain the following elements: (1) the setting and patient groups to be tested, including relevant prior testing; (2) the index test and any comparator index tests; and (3) subsequent steps after testing, driven by the test result, such as further testing or treatment.

Setting and population
Here, we will start with defining the clinical setting, the purpose of testing and the people who will be tested with the index test. For a systematic review on triage tools for severe neck injuries in children after an accident (Slaar 2017), the review authors took the emergency department as the starting point (Figure 5.3.a). They distinguished

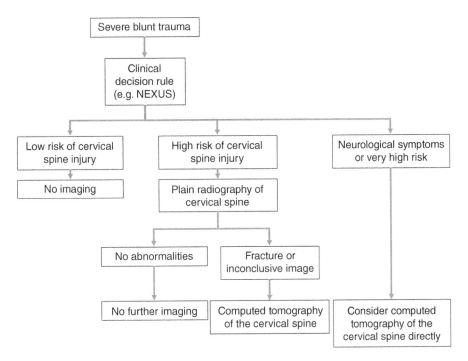

Figure 5.3.a **Clinical pathway for neck injuries in children (<18 years).** The setting (emergency department) is not shown in the figure but is stated in the text. Source: Adapted from Slaar 2017.

between children under 8 years old versus children between 8 and 18, as each age group has different injury patterns.

The purpose of the testing may differ. For example, a molecular rapid test for tuberculosis may be intended as a screening test in persons without any symptoms or proposed as a diagnostic test for evaluating symptomatic patients. The purpose of testing should be specified explicitly, as well as the intended use population (asymptomatic people versus symptomatic people). The performance of rapid tests for tuberculosis may differ in people with HIV versus people without HIV, in adults versus children, or in patients pre-selected after imaging versus all-comers. Figure 5.3.b shows the clinical pathway for a molecular test for tuberculosis in a screening situation.

The reference standard in evaluations of test accuracy may or may not be part of current clinical practice. The clinical pathway may therefore not be the same as the research study design for the included studies. For example, in current clinical practice only some patients may receive the reference standard (often only index test positives), whereas the study design to estimate sensitivity and specificity requires that all participants (index test positive and index test negative) receive a reference standard. In Figure 5.3.a, children with severe neck trauma will first be assessed using a clinical rule (e.g. the National Emergency X-Radiography Utilization Study (NEXUS) rule) and if that indicates cervical spine injury, the child will be referred for radiography first and, if necessary, CT scans afterwards. The clinical rules are the index tests. Radiographs and CT (either separately or combined) could be the reference standard, but have a different role in the pathway.

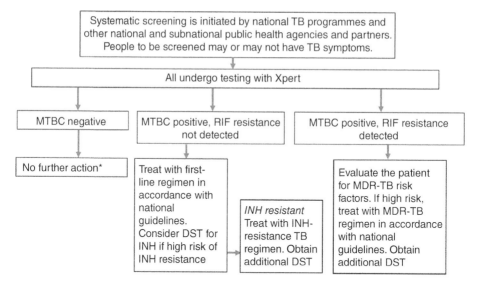

Figure 5.3.b **Clinical pathway for a molecular WHO-recommended rapid diagnostic test to screen for pulmonary tuberculosis, irrespective of signs and symptoms.** *If an individual has symptoms, evaluate clinically for TB in accordance with national guidelines. DST, drug susceptibility testing; INH, isoniazid; MDR-TB, multidrug-resistant TB; MTBC, *Mycobacterium tuberculosis* complex; RIF, rifampicin; TB, tuberculosis; Xpert, Xpert MTB/RIF or Xpert MTB/RIF Ultra. Source: Adapted from Shapiro 2021.

Index test(s)

The next element in specifying the clinical pathway is identifying the tests of interest: one or more index tests. For the molecular WHO-recommended rapid diagnostic test for screening for tuberculosis example, the review authors were interested in Xpert MTB/RIF and Xpert MTB/RIF Ultra, the next generation of the test. For the review about triage tests for neck injuries in children, the authors focused on tests that may be used to decide whether children should be referred for further imaging. These index tests are usually combinations of findings at physical examination or history taking. Two such tests were already in use in clinical practice (NEXUS and DTM) and so the focus was on these two tools.

Subsequent steps for test positives and test negatives

After defining the tests of interest, the steps after the index test results need to be speci-fied. What will happen if the index test result is positive? What will happen if the index test is negative? Is there a third option, such as a middle 'unclear' or 'intermediate' test result? What if the test fails? These steps may sometimes be difficult to define, as there may be variability in practice patterns.

In the example of a blood test for fungal disease in immunocompromised patients, the next step after a positive test is usually referral for high-resolution CT scanning. Some hospitals, however, may decide upon treatment based on the blood test, or patients may be referred for radiographs before undergoing CT scanning. Where rele-vant, the clinical pathway should contain information on all alternative next steps following index test results.

Management decisions to be made after testing will help to decide what the minimally acceptable performance of a test should be. For example, if the disease is lethal, but has a good prognosis when treated in time, then minimizing the number of false negatives may be far more important than minimizing the number of false positives. Alternatively, when the treatment may cause severe adverse events or when the follow-up test is invasive, then minimizing the number of false positives may be at least equally important.

5.3.3   Unclear and multiple clinical pathways

If the intended use (for example diagnosis or screening) or role (add, replace, triage) of one or more of the index tests is unclear, it may be helpful to draw multiple versions of the clinical pathway to clarify changes in the pathway related to different contexts of use.

A single test may be used for different purposes, in different populations, in distinct roles relative to existing tests, and at various positions in the clinical pathway. As accuracy is not fixed, the participants and setting of an informative accuracy study should correspond to those in the clinical problem. Depending on the clinical question, different accuracy studies may be relevant.

Each intended use, and each role, will require inspection of the pathway following the steps in Section 5.3.2. Review authors may then need to consider whether these multiple clinical problems can be dealt with in a single systematic review, or whether multiple reviews should be performed, each focusing on a specific use, role, setting and/or index test.

If multiple reviews address clinical questions that are linked, because they consider the same test or the same target condition, then their development may be supported by a generic protocol, which will aim to address all relevant questions in a single protocol. Such a protocol will specify the questions that will be addressed in each review, report the generic methodology for all planned reviews, and may explain potential differences in methods between the reviews. The resulting reviews may refer to one another, to emphasize similarities and common ground. Ideally, review authors would summarize the reviews in an overview of reviews, addressing all relevant questions in one document.

To ensure that review questions address relevant healthcare problems, to understand the clinical pathways and to define appropriate review questions, it is desirable to involve healthcare professionals with expert knowledge. These may include clinicians who order and interpret the test, as well as those who provide the results, such as laboratory professionals, radiologists or pathologists. It is also desirable to include patient and public representatives, inviting them to clarify the importance of the question and their experience with testing and its consequences. Priority-setting exercises may be used to make the review more relevant for stakeholders (Chalmers 2014). With most triage and screening tests in low-prevalence settings, for example, the majority of those tested will not have the target condition. In some applications, such as population screening, the general public will be a relevant stakeholder.

Sometimes, the context of use for a new test is not (yet) well defined. This may happen when the role of a new test in a clinical pathway is not clear, or when a test is proposed to detect a novel target condition. In these situations, a systematic review of test accuracy may be used to inform policy makers and healthcare professionals about the potential use of the test, considering its accuracy. For example, a systematic review may be used to make an inventory of early-stage biomarkers, or biomarker combinations, to identify those that should be considered for further evaluation.

5.4 Defining the review question

Having identified the clinical problem as a choice between well-specified testing strategies in well-defined circumstances, review authors will then define the informative review question.

Those familiar with intervention reviews may know the **PICO** format for formulating review questions. The PICO format has four components: **p**atients, **i**ntervention, **c**omparator, **o**utcome. PICO is also useful for questions on the impact or effectiveness of testing on patient-relevant outcomes, for example when summarizing test–treatment randomized controlled trials or randomized screening trials.

Using the PICO format for *accuracy* questions is not straightforward, however. Unlike questions about interventions that aim to influence health outcomes – reducing the risk of avoidable outcomes, for example, or improving favourable outcomes – the target condition in a test accuracy question is the condition we want the index test to detect, not a health outcome resulting from testing.

In addition, there is not necessarily a comparator (C in PICO) in a test accuracy question: a review question could very well address the accuracy of a single index test. It should be noted that the reference standard is not the comparator, in the PICO sense, in a test accuracy question. Although sometimes the index test may be considered as a replacement for the reference standard, this is not the general rule. The reference standard in test accuracy research is primarily used for evaluating test accuracy, i.e. it establishes how well the index test performs in detecting the target condition in those undergoing testing.

We prefer the alternative acronym **PIT** for test accuracy questions, where the three letters refer to population, index test(s) and target condition. **P** describes the persons for whom the test is considered, and may include the healthcare setting and tests done prior to using the index test. We prefer 'population' rather than 'patients', because tests may also be used in asymptomatic persons, as in population screening programmes. **I** describes the index test(s). **T** describes the target condition. These three elements are further explained below.

5.4.1 Population

A test may perform differently in distinct groups of people. This depends on the spectrum of disease in those with the target condition, as well as on the range of alternative conditions in those without the target condition.

Faecal immunochemical tests (FIT), for example, are used as tests to detect colorectal cancer, both in screening and in clinical settings. Like many other tests, their sensitivity varies depending on stage of disease, with better sensitivity for more advanced stages of disease severity (Niedermaier 2020). As a consequence, FIT sensitivity in detecting colorectal cancer will vary depending on whether it is used in screening or in a diagnostic or surveillance setting. Population screening programmes invite asymptomatic members of the public and aim to detect cancer or its precursors. If cancer is detected, it is more likely to be early-stage disease. In contrast, an oncology clinic will typically manage symptomatic patients, who more often will have advanced-stage cancers. FIT sensitivity in detecting colorectal cancer will therefore be lower in asymptomatic people invited to participate in a population screening programme than in symptomatic patients evaluated in a diagnostic or surveillance setting.

D-dimer, a test used in patients with suspected pulmonary embolism, typically has a lower specificity in inpatients compared to outpatients, even when the same assay is used, with the same cut point to define positive test results (Schrecengost 2003). Hospitalized patients can have a range of conditions, other than pulmonary embolism, that lead to elevated levels of D-dimer, including prolonged immobilization itself. Results may be positive even if these patients do not have pulmonary embolism. Because of the higher proportion of false positive results in those without pulmonary embolism, specificity will be markedly lower in inpatients compared to outpatients.

The description of the population should therefore take into consideration the context of use, the setting, any prior testing and how those tested present (asymptomatic or with signs and symptoms). In addition, age and sex may also be important: will the test be used in children, in adults or in all? Women, for example, have a longer list of differential diagnoses when they present with abdominal pain than do men.

The authors of the review on Xpert MTB/RIF and Xpert MTB/RIF Ultra for screening for pulmonary tuberculosis and rifampicin resistance considered several populations. The review referred to people living with HIV, high-risk groups such as people residing in prisons and household contacts of people with tuberculosis, and the general population without specific risk factors. In these populations, the review authors analysed and presented test accuracy results separately.

5.4.2   Index test(s)

The 'I' in PIT stands for index test(s). A single test could be considered, or two or more tests, either used separately or in combination, to form a testing strategy.

As explained in Section 5.3.1, a substantial part of systematic reviews of test accuracy will focus on a comparison between two or more index tests or testing strategies. An example can be found in Box 5.3.c, where a number of rapid tests (index tests) were compared to find the best replacement for blood culture (the test in current practice) to diagnose enteric fever.

5.4.3   Target condition

A question for a systematic review of test accuracy studies should specify the target condition (see Chapter 3, Section 3.2), while the study eligibility criteria should specify which methods to define the target condition (and reference standard) are acceptable and therefore eligible.

The target condition may not necessarily be the disease for which the patient will ultimately be treated; it could also relate to a characteristic of patients that determines the need to be referred for further testing. For example, for initial diagnosis the exact stage of cancer is less relevant than the detection of cancer at any stage. The reference standard for this initial diagnosis question therefore does not need to indicate the exact stage of cancer: it must detect in a reliable way whether there is a malignant tumour present or not.

5.4.4   The review question: PIT

With the components of population, index test(s) and target condition one can define the review question. For example, the systematic review on triage tools for detecting severe injuries in the neck of children after an accident (Figure 5.3.a) asked: "What is the accuracy of clinical decision rules, based on findings at physical examination and history, in detecting serious neck injuries in children presenting at the emergency department after trauma?" (Slaar 2017).

The systematic review about urinary markers as a triage tool to surgery for endometriosis (Box 5.3.a) aimed "To provide summary estimates of the diagnostic accuracy of urinary biomarkers for the diagnosis of pelvic endometriosis against surgical diagnosis as a reference standard" (Liu 2015).

Note that both questions include the term 'accuracy'. Alternative question formulations could have been 'Do clinical decision rules accurately detect serious neck injuries in children presenting at the emergency department after trauma?' or 'Are urinary biomarkers sufficiently sensitive in detecting endometriosis in women of reproductive age with complaints that may indicate endometriosis?'

5.4.5   From review question to objectives

The starting point for the author teams of systematic reviews of test accuracy is the healthcare problem at hand. This clinical problem can be illustrated using a clinical pathway, which informs review authors and readers about the population, index test(s) and target condition that are relevant to the review question.

The review question then leads to the objectives of the review. These describe the necessary information for addressing the review question, to help solve the clinical problem. The objectives define measurable outcomes and may include a definition of minimally required sensitivity or specificity of the index tests to fulfil their role (Korevaar 2019).

The primary objective will typically refer to the accuracy of the index test(s) for the diagnosis of the target condition in the relevant population. It may or may not refer to a comparative test accuracy question.

Secondary objectives can provide more detail to the review question, for example by referring to differences in accuracy between subgroups, or variations on the index test, such as manufacturer or operator skill, or different test positivity thresholds. However, such secondary objectives should be addressed with caution, as the included studies may be a selective group of studies or because few of the studies have low risk of bias and low applicability concerns. Table 5.4.a provides examples of aims and objectives from three reviews.

Table 5.4.a Examples of aims and objectives of systematic reviews of test accuracy

	Galactomannan detection for invasive aspergillosis in immunocompromised patients (Leeflang 2015)	Triage tools for detecting cervical spine injury in paediatric trauma patients (Slaar 2017)	Diagnostic tests for autism spectrum disorder in preschool children (Randall 2018)
Review question	Is measuring galactomannan in blood (I) sufficiently sensitive to serve as a triage test for fungal disease (T) in immunocompromised patients (P)?	Do clinical decision rules (I) accurately detect serious neck injuries (T) in children presenting at the emergency department after trauma (P)?	Which diagnostic tool (I) is most accurate in detecting autism spectrum disorders (T) in preschool children (P)?
Primary objectives	To assess the diagnostic accuracy of galactomannan detection in serum for the diagnosis of invasive aspergillosis in immunocompromised patients, at different cut-off values for test positivity.	To evaluate the diagnostic accuracy of the NEXUS criteria and the Canadian C-spine rule in a paediatric population evaluated for cervical spine injury following trauma.	To identify which diagnostic tools most accurately diagnose ASD in preschool children when compared with multidisciplinary team clinical judgement.*
Secondary objectives	To study several possible sources of heterogeneity: subgroups of patients, different interpretations of the EORTC/MSG criteria as the reference standard and study design features.	To explore heterogeneity due to: 1. differences in healthcare settings and designs; 2. age-related differences.	To evaluate whether any diagnostic test has greater accuracy for age-specific subgroups within the preschool age range.

* Slightly modified because in the original review a number of primary objectives were stated. ASD, autistic spectrum disorders; I, index test; P, population; T, target condition.

5.4.6 Broad versus narrow questions

Every component of the review question (population, index test(s), target condition) can be broad or narrow. In all cases, the review authors will need to decide the scope of the review. If the components of the question are defined too narrowly, the review may not be clinically useful, as the narrowly defined population or index tests may not be representative of clinical practice, or there may be too few studies available to answer the review question. If the question is defined too broadly, applicability may be jeopardized, since accuracy inevitably varies across populations and types of index tests, and for different definitions of the target condition. In addition, interpretation will be compromised by the wide heterogeneity.

   In practice, a somewhat broad, clinically informative question is a good place to start. It is easier to split or refine a broad review if this becomes unfeasible, compared to broadening an initially narrow review. For example, a broad review, covering multiple tests, may be more useful than a series of narrow reviews of separate tests. The latter would force readers to cross-reference multiple reviews, possibly with slightly different methodological approaches, before they can decide which test may be best for a target condition. It is also impractical and less valid to evaluate a range of index tests in separate reviews when the overarching question is a comparative one. One way to manage this is the development of a generic protocol for a suite of reviews and questions (see Section 5.3.3) and the production of an overview of reviews afterwards, summarizing the complete suite of reviews in a single report.

Reviews developed with generic protocols can be found in the *Cochrane Database of Systematic Reviews,* which includes, for example, a suite of systematic reviews on the accuracy of tests for diagnosis and screening for different types of skin cancer, in different clinical settings (for example Chuchu 2018, Dinnes 2018, Ferrante di Ruffano 2018). The *Cochrane Database of Systematic Reviews* also contains a suite of accuracy reviews of tests for diagnosing COVID-19 (Dinnes 2021, Islam 2021).

5.5 Defining eligibility criteria

Once the review question has been formulated, one can define the eligibility criteria for the review. Defining inclusion and exclusion criteria at the protocol stage ensures that all review authors in the team are aware of the focus of the review, increases the efficiency of searches and evaluations of eligibility, and acts as a safeguard against bias.

After the initial inclusion of studies, some studies may be excluded on further inspection, because they do not address the review question. Reasons for exclusion at later stages in the review process may be, for example, not reporting the necessary data for inclusion in a meta-analysis, or not fulfilling certain methodological quality criteria.

Balancing between stricter eligibility criteria and broader criteria will likely require expert knowledge of the available literature. Reviews should aim to collect the best available evidence, meaning that they should aim to restrict their eligibility criteria to applicable studies with low risk of bias. If one expects that a sufficiently high number of high-quality studies will be available, then more biased study designs can be safely excluded.

5.5.1 Types of studies

In a typical test accuracy study, a single group of patients receives one or more index tests and undergoes the reference standard. Chapter 3 presented several variations on this basic study design. There may be reasons not to include some of these study design variations in the review. The main reason may be that specific study designs are more likely to generate biased results. The example in Box 5.5.a included cross-sectional studies irrespective of how eligible participants were identified.

Some studies do not include a single group of patients in whom the target condition is suspected, but recruit separate groups instead. In the example of the blood test for invasive fungal disease (Table 5.4.a), researchers may decide to include one group of immunocompromised patients with previously confirmed invasive fungal disease to estimate sensitivity and a second group of healthy study participants, who may not even be immunocompromised, to estimate specificity. As discussed in Chapter 3 and in Chapter 8, such studies are known to generate biased estimates of test accuracy: there may be too few false negatives and far fewer false positives, compared to a study in which only a single group of participants, all immunocompromised and all suspected of having invasive fungal disease, would be included. For this reason, such multiple-group

---

Box 5.5.a Example of specification of eligible study designs

Fluorine-18-fluorodeoxyglucose (FDG) positron emission tomography (PET) computed tomography (CT) for the detection of bone, lung and lymph node metastases in rhabdomyosarcoma

"All cross-sectional studies that report the diagnostic accuracy of 18F-FDG-PET/CT in diagnosing lymph node involvement or bone or lung metastases or a combination of these metastases in patients with confirmed rhabdomyosarcoma were eligible for inclusion."

Source: Adapted from Vaarwerk 2021.

---

studies – especially the ones with healthy 'controls' – may not be considered eligible for the review.

If the review addresses a question that concerns multiple index tests, the review authors need to decide whether to include only primary studies with a direct comparison between the tests or also any evaluations of only one of the tests. If they opt for studies with comparisons, inclusion will be limited to fully paired or randomized designs and studies that evaluate only one of the index tests would not be eligible.

5.5.2 Participants

The inclusion criteria for eligible studies should preferably correspond to the population in the review question. This includes the relevant clinical characteristics or presentations of those patients in whom testing may be considered. We use the plural 'presentations' to allow for reviews covering a range of presentations of interest.

For example, a systematic review on first-rank symptoms for schizophrenia in participants with psychotic symptoms specified how psychosis may have been defined in the included studies, for example by hallucinations, delusions and grossly disorganized behaviour (Soares-Weiser 2015). By contrast, the review on galactomannan testing for aspergillosis (Table 5.4.a) purposefully included distinct groups of participants, as one of the objectives was to investigate whether these distinct groups might result in different accuracy estimates (Leeflang 2015).

The setting in which the test will be used in practice should be specified and there should be explicit consideration of whether the review will be limited to one setting or include studies regardless of setting (see the example in Box 5.5.b). As discussed in Section 5.4.1, the accuracy of many tests is known to vary between clinical settings, and between screening and diagnosis. Even if all settings are relevant, it is useful to make this explicit, for example by including an investigation of the difference in accuracy between settings as a secondary objective.

If applicable, review authors should describe what prior tests, if any, participants will have had and how that redefines the range of presentations of interest. This is particularly important if the index test is to be used after other tests. For example, a new test may only be of interest in people in whom a prior test has been negative. The accuracy of the test in studies where patients have been filtered by previous test results may be

---

Box 5.5.b Example of the definition of patient populations to be included or excluded

Triage tools for detecting cervical spine injury in paediatric trauma patients

"We included children between the age of 0 and 18 who underwent blunt trauma evaluation in the emergency department. We excluded patients with a history of previous surgery of the cervical spine or congenital cervical spine anomalies, or both. In case of studies with mixed populations, e.g. that included some participants in the groups and that could not be separated from the eligible participants, we tried to contact the study author to provide the data for the group of interest."

Source: Slaar 2017

---

different from the accuracy of the test in studies where included participants have not been filtered by such tests.

Review authors should be aware of the poor reporting in many test accuracy studies. Many studies fail to specify the actual inclusion criteria for their test accuracy study, which means that decisions about eligibility must sometimes be based on reported patient characteristics.

5.5.3   Index test(s)

Many index tests come in different forms, and review authors need to consider carefully whether they can all be included in the review, or whether the review will be restricted to a well-defined subclass (see the example in Box 5.5.c).

For many markers, multiple assays are available for measurement. For example, the biomarker D-dimer can be measured using commercially available, qualitative point-of-care assays, but also with one of the several available quantitative laboratory assays. The analytical performance and diagnostic accuracy of these assays vary. Authors considering a systematic review of evaluations of D-dimer have to decide whether they want to study all available D-dimer assays or, for example, only the point-of-care assays.

Similar concerns apply to imaging tests. CT scanners build images based on 64 up to 640 slices. MRI scanners differ in their magnetic field. Review authors should decide if

---

Box 5.5.c Example of variation in the use of an index test

Galactomannan detection for invasive aspergillosis in immunocompromised patients

"A commercially available galactomannan sandwich ELISA (Platelia©) was the test under evaluation. We only included studies concerning galactomannan detection in serum. We excluded studies addressing detection in BAL fluid, a number of other body fluids, such as CSF or peritoneal fluid, and tissue. We also excluded studies evaluating in-house serum galactomannan tests."

Source: Leeflang 2015

---

they want to include all variations in CT scanners or MRI scanners, or whether they want to focus on a subset or compare variations in test versions.

The collection of samples and the preferred matrix also should be considered. Antigen tests for SARS-CoV-2 infection, for example, can be performed using different samples: from a nose swab, a throat swab or in saliva. Samples can be taken by trained professionals or by the persons taking the test themselves. Here also, review authors should consider not just the assay but also the pre-analytical elements.

The continuous results from some index tests may be dichotomized to present positive and negative test results. For this dichotomization, a threshold is applied (see Chapter 4, Section 4.6). Different researchers may have used different thresholds, and different thresholds may be used in practice. Review authors need to be aware of the use of thresholds in practice and of the implications this may have for their review question. Sometimes, focusing on one or a few thresholds reflects clinical practice best. In other cases, results are reported on a continuous scale or with multiple thresholds. The application of thresholds in clinical practice will have consequences for which thresholds to include in the review: review authors may wish to include all available studies or only studies that report results using the clinically relevant thresholds.

General principles here are that the clinical problem guides the review question and that review authors should not narrow the index test eligibility criteria too much. One reason is that the *Cochrane Database of Systematic Reviews* is used worldwide, in different healthcare environments. It is possible to evaluate, in the analysis phase, differences between index test technologies, training, timing, samples or other potential sources of heterogeneity in test accuracy, in a subgroup analysis or stratified analysis. The use of different thresholds may also be accommodated at the analysis phase (see Chapter 9, Section 9.4.5).

5.5.4 Target condition

In defining the study eligibility criteria, review authors will also need to define the target condition of interest with sufficient precision (see the example in Box 5.5.d).

A single disease may encompass a wider range of target conditions. For example, if review authors are interested in testing for tuberculosis, the review could cover tuberculosis disease or tuberculosis infection. The aim for detection of tuberculosis

---

Box 5.5.d Example of a target condition that covers multiple subconditions

Diagnostic tests for autism spectrum disorder (ASD) in preschool children

"The target condition was autism spectrum disorder in preschool children. Autism spectrum disorder can be diagnosed according to DSM-5. Diagnostic subgroups of autism (childhood autism (ICD-10) or autistic disorder (DSM-IV)); pervasive developmental disorder (atypical autism (ICD-10), pervasive developmental disorder, unspecified (ICD-10), or pervasive developmental disorder – not otherwise specified (PDD-NOS) (DSM-IV)); and Asperger syndrome or Asperger disorder were grouped together as ASD."

Source: Randall 2018.

infection is to identify people for preventive treatment, or to stop or limit progression to tuberculosis disease, whereas the aim for detection of tuberculosis disease is to provide benefits for individual patients (e.g. earlier diagnosis and the opportunity to begin earlier, appropriate treatment, decrease morbidity and mortality) and opportunities for public health (e.g. interrupt tuberculosis transmission).

Similarly, review authors should specify what the target condition will be when evaluating tests in screening for colorectal cancer. These tests aim to detect colorectal cancer as well as precursor stages, and readers need to know if these stages will be included in the review. If one disease covers a range of target conditions or stages, review authors should also specify what defines the presence of the target condition (e.g. stages IV and V) versus absence of the target condition (e.g. stages I, II or III).

5.5.5   Reference standard

Review authors not only need to define the target condition, they also should specify the preferred or acceptable reference standard(s) to identify patients with that target condition (see the example in Box 5.5.e).

For many conditions, multiple procedures can be used to establish the presence or absence of the target condition. They may or may not be interchangeable: some reference standards may be better at identifying the target condition of interest. Reference standards may also differ in the way they verify the presence or absence of the target condition.

In the evaluation of tests for children with suspected cervical spine injury, both imaging and follow-up were used as reference standards (Slaar 2017). Similarly, biopsy followed by histopathology as well as follow-up and clinical findings were the reference standards considered to verify suspected distant metastases and lymph node involvement in patients with rhabdomyosarcoma. This was necessary, as metastases that are not seen in initial images cannot be biopsied.

Box 5.5.e Example of different reference standards

Fluorine-18-fluorodeoxyglucose (FDG) positron emission tomography (PET) computed tomography (CT) for the detection of bone, lung, and lymph node metastases in rhabdomyosarcoma

"The optimal reference standard for suspected distant metastases and lymph node involvement in rhabdomyosarcoma patients would be confirmation by histopathology obtained by biopsy. For both ethical and practical reasons, this cannot be done for every suspected lesion. When biopsy results were not available, the results of the 18F-FDG-PET/CT should have been compared with the judgement of a multidisciplinary tumour board, where experts had the knowledge of a patient's clinical findings, results from conventional imaging, and histological data. Clinical follow-up and imaging follow-up could also be used to support the final diagnosis of nodal involvement and bone and lung metastases. In general, after nine weeks of chemotherapy, tumour response was evaluated with imaging including an X-ray of the thorax."

Source: Adapted from Vaarwerk 2021.

Review authors should define up front the reference standard(s) to be included in the review. They should also explain whether variations or combinations of reference standards will be considered acceptable for inclusion.

5.6   Chapter information

Authors: Mariska M. Leeflang (*Department of Epidemiology and Data Science, University of Amsterdam, The Netherlands*), Clare Davenport (*Institute of Applied Health Research, University of Birmingham, UK*), Patrick M. Bossuyt (*Department of Epidemiology and Data Science, University of Amsterdam, The Netherlands*).

Sources of support: The authors declare no sources of support for writing this chapter.

Declarations of interest: Mariska M. Leeflang and Clare Davenport are members of Cochrane's Diagnostic Test Accuracy Editorial Team. Mariska M. Leeflang is co-convenor of the Cochrane Screening and Diagnostic Tests Methods Group. The authors declare no other potential conflicts of interest relevant to the topic of this chapter.

Acknowledgements: The authors thank Rob J. Scholten and Chris Hyde for contributions to a previous version of this chapter. The authors would like to thank Karen R. Steingart and Ingrid Arevalo-Rodriguez for helpful peer review comments.

5.7   References

Bossuyt PM, Irwig L, Craig J, Glasziou P. Comparative accuracy: assessing new tests against existing diagnostic pathways. *BMJ* 2006; **332**: 1089–1092.

Chalmers I, Bracken MB, Djulbegovic B, Garattini S, Grant J, Gülmezoglu AM, Howells DW, Ioannidis JP, Oliver S. How to increase value and reduce waste when research priorities are set. *Lancet* 2014; **383**: 156–165.

Chuchu N, Takwoingi Y, Dinnes J, Matin RN, Bassett O, Moreau JF, Bayliss SE, Davenport C, Godfrey K, O'Connell S, Jain A, Walter FM, Deeks JJ, Williams HC. Smartphone applications for triaging adults with skin lesions that are suspicious for melanoma. *Cochrane Database of Systematic Reviews* 2018; **12**: CD013192.

Dinnes J, Deeks JJ, Grainge MJ, Chuchu N, Ferrante di Ruffano L, Matin RN, Thomson DR, Wong KY, Aldridge RB, Abbott R, Fawzy M, Bayliss SE, Takwoingi Y, Davenport C, Godfrey K, Walter FM, Williams HC, Cochrane Skin Cancer Diagnostic Test Accuracy G. Visual inspection for diagnosing cutaneous melanoma in adults. *Cochrane Database of Systematic Reviews* 2018; **12**: CD013194.

Dinnes J, Deeks JJ, Berhane S, Taylor M, Adriano A, Davenport C, Dittrich S, Emperador D, Takwoingi Y, Cunningham J, Beese S, Dretzke J, Ferrante di Ruffano L, Harris IM, Price MJ, Taylor-Phillips S, Hooft L, Leeflang MM, Spijker R, Van den Bruel A, Cochrane COVID-19 Diagnostic Test Accuracy Group. Rapid, point-of-care antigen and molecular-based tests for diagnosis of SARS-CoV-2 infection. *Cochrane Database of Systematic Reviews* 2021; **3**: CD013705.

Ferrante di Ruffano L, Takwoingi Y, Dinnes J, Chuchu N, Bayliss SE, Davenport C, Matin RN, Godfrey K, O'Sullivan C, Gulati A, Chan SA, Durack A, O'Connell S, Gardiner MD, Bamber J, Deeks JJ, Williams HC, Cochrane Skin Cancer Diagnostic Test Accuracy G. Computer-assisted diagnosis techniques (dermoscopy and spectroscopy-based) for diagnosing skin cancer in adults. *Cochrane Database of Systematic Reviews* 2018; **12**: CD013186.

Gopalakrishna G, Langendam MW, Scholten RJPM, Bossuyt PMM, Leeflang MMG. Guidelines for guideline developers: a systematic review of grading systems for medical tests. *Implementation Science* 2013; **8**: 78.

Gopalakrishna G, Langendam MW, Scholten RJPM, Bossuyt PMM, Leeflang MMG. Defining the clinical pathway in Cochrane diagnostic test accuracy reviews. *BMC Medical Research Methodology* 2016; **16**: 153.

Islam N, Ebrahimzadeh S, Salameh JP, Kazi S, Fabiano N, Treanor L, Absi M, Hallgrimson Z, Leeflang MM, Hooft L, van der Pol CB, Prager R, Hare SS, Dennie C, Spijker R, Deeks JJ, Dinnes J, Jenniskens K, Korevaar DA, Cohen JF, Van den Bruel A, Takwoingi Y, van de Wijgert J, Damen JA, Wang J, McInnes MD. Thoracic imaging tests for the diagnosis of COVID-19. *Cochrane Database of Systematic Reviews* 2021; **3**: CD013639.

Korevaar DA, Gopalakrishna G, Cohen JF, Bossuyt PM. Targeted test evaluation: a framework for designing diagnostic accuracy studies with clear study hypotheses. *Diagnostic and Prognostic Research* 2019; **3**: 22.

Leeflang MM, Debets-Ossenkopp YJ, Wang J, Visser CE, Scholten RJ, Hooft L, Bijlmer HA, Reitsma JB, Zhang M, Bossuyt PM, Vandenbroucke-Grauls CM. Galactomannan detection for invasive aspergillosis in immunocompromised patients. *Cochrane Database of Systematic Reviews* 2015; **12**: CD007394.

Liu E, Nisenblat V, Farquhar C, Fraser I, Bossuyt PM, Johnson N, Hull ML. Urinary biomarkers for the non-invasive diagnosis of endometriosis. *Cochrane Database of Systematic Reviews* 2015; **12**: CD012019.

Lord SJ, St John A, Bossuyt PM, Sandberg S, Monaghan PJ, O'Kane M, Cobbaert CM, Röddiger R, Lennartz L, Gelfi C, Horvath AR. Setting clinical performance specifications to develop and evaluate biomarkers for clinical use. *Annals of Clinical Biochemistry* 2019; **56**: 527–535.

Niedermaier T, Balavarca Y, Brenner H. Stage-specific sensitivity of fecal immunochemical tests for detecting colorectal cancer: systematic review and meta-analysis. *American Journal of Gastroenterology* 2020; **115**: 56–69.

Pepe MS, Janes H, Li CI, Bossuyt PM, Feng Z, Hilden J. Early-phase studies of biomarkers: what target sensitivity and specificity values might confer clinical utility? *Clinical Chemistry* 2016; **62**: 737–742.

Randall M, Egberts KJ, Samtani A, Scholten R, Hooft L, Livingstone N, Sterling-Levis K, Woolfenden S, Williams K. Diagnostic tests for autism spectrum disorder (ASD) in preschool children. *Cochrane Database of Systematic Reviews* 2018; **7**: CD009044.

Schrecengost JE, LeGallo RD, Boyd JC, Moons KG, Gonias SL, Rose CE, Jr., Bruns DE. Comparison of diagnostic accuracies in outpatients and hospitalized patients of D-dimer testing for the evaluation of suspected pulmonary embolism. *Clinical Chemistry* 2003; **49**: 1483–1490.

Shapiro AE, Ross JM, Yao M, Schiller I, Kohli M, Dendukuri N, Steingart KR, Horne DJ. Xpert MTB/RIF and Xpert Ultra assays for screening for pulmonary tuberculosis and rifampicin resistance in adults, irrespective of signs or symptoms. *Cochrane Database of Systematic Reviews* 2021; **3**: CD013694.

Slaar A, Fockens MM, Wang J, Maas M, Wilson DJ, Goslings JC, Schep NW, van Rijn RR. Triage tools for detecting cervical spine injury in pediatric trauma patients. *Cochrane Database of Systematic Reviews* 2017; **12**: CD011686.

Soares-Weiser K, Maayan N, Bergman H, Davenport C, Kirkham AJ, Grabowski S, Adams CE. First rank symptoms for schizophrenia. *Cochrane Database of Systematic Reviews* 2015; **1**: CD010653.

Tamburrino D, Riviere D, Yaghoobi M, Davidson BR, Gurusamy KS. Diagnostic accuracy of different imaging modalities following computed tomography (CT) scanning for assessing the resectability with curative intent in pancreatic and periampullary cancer. *Cochrane Database of Systematic Reviews* 2016; **9**: CD011515.

Vaarwerk B, Breunis WB, Haveman LM, de Keizer B, Jehanno N, Borgwardt L, van Rijn RR, van den Berg H, Cohen JF, van Dalen EC, Merks JH. Fluorine-18-fluorodeoxyglucose (FDG) positron emission tomography (PET) computed tomography (CT) for the detection of bone, lung, and lymph node metastases in rhabdomyosarcoma. *Cochrane Database of Systematic Reviews* 2021; **11**: CD012325.

Wijedoru L, Mallett S, Parry CM. Rapid diagnostic tests for typhoid and paratyphoid (enteric) fever. *Cochrane Database of Systematic Reviews* 2017; **5**: CD008892.

6

Searching for and selecting studies

René Spijker, Jacqueline Dinnes, Julie Glanville and Anne Eisinga

---

KEY POINTS

- Review teams should include an information specialist or at least one co-author with expertise in searching.
- Search strategies should be developed by the information specialist in close collaboration with review authors with clinical and technical knowledge of, and expertise in, the index test(s) and target condition(s) under investigation.
- Test accuracy questions can be complex and the optimal search strategy may use several combinations of key concepts combined into one overall database query (multi-stranded) to capture the different ways in which relevant studies may be described.
- Methodological search filters should not be added to the final set of search results, as they may result in studies being missed. They could, however, be used within the search as part of a multi-stranded approach.
- In addition to MEDLINE and Embase, a range of bibliographic databases including subject-specific (e.g. DiTA (physiotherapy), CINAHL) and regional databases (e.g. LILACS) should be searched. The references of retrieved studies, forward citation searches, the 'similar articles' feature in electronic databases, grey literature and internet searches should also be considered.
- The proposed search strategy for at least one database should be included in the protocol of the review to enable peer review at an early stage in review production.
- Full details of the search process should be reported in the final review, including the full details of each search as conducted. Complex searches should be explained in a narrative way so that the logic of their construction is clear.

This chapter should be cited as: Spijker R, Dinnes J, Glanville J, Eisinga A. Chapter 6: Searching for and selecting studies. In: Deeks JJ, Bossuyt PM, Leeflang MM, Takwoingi Y, editors. *Cochrane Handbook for Systematic Reviews of Diagnostic Test Accuracy*. 1st edition. Chichester (UK): John Wiley & Sons, 2023: 97–130.

Cochrane Handbook for Systematic Reviews of Diagnostic Test Accuracy, First Edition. Edited by Jonathan J. Deeks, Patrick M. Bossuyt, Mariska M. Leeflang and Yemisi Takwoingi.
© 2023 The Cochrane Collaboration. Published 2023 by John Wiley & Sons Ltd.

6.1   Introduction

Conducting an effective search for studies to determine the diagnostic accuracy of tests is a crucial and challenging task in preparing a systematic review of test accuracy. Search strategies for test accuracy studies can be particularly complex and knowledge of a range of resources may be needed. This chapter is designed to help review authors gain a better understanding of the search process as a whole and of the key role played by the information specialist on the review team. An online technical supplement to Chapter 4 of the *Cochrane Handbook for Systematic Reviews of Interventions*, aimed at those actually carrying out the search process, provides more detail on searching methods (Lefebvre 2021). It is accompanied by an appendix listing a wide range of potential resources to search and search tools to aid in the review process. This is regularly updated. To support decisions on how best to optimize searching, there is further evidence-based information, including appraisals of published research, on the SuRe Info portal (www.sites.google.com/york.ac.uk/sureinfo/home), which is updated twice a year. There is a specific section dedicated to diagnostic test accuracy.

This chapter provides an overview of approaches for searching for test accuracy studies. It starts with the general principles for searching for studies and sources to search, followed by considerations for designing search strategies and documenting and reporting the search process. The process of selecting relevant studies and a summary of future developments completes the chapter.

6.2   Searching for studies

The aim of the literature search is to generate as extensive a list as possible of studies that may be suitable for answering the review question, within available resource constraints. Key decisions include the type of literature that may be relevant, the identification of relevant sources of literature and the design of a search strategy that will identify as many relevant reports as possible in the most efficient way, without creating an unmanageable volume of records for title and abstract screening.

The literature typically encompasses published and unpublished study reports, including journal articles, dissertations, conference proceedings and reports (see Chapter 7), the importance of which will vary depending on the review question. Sources include a range of electronic bibliographic databases, web-based topic-specific resources (such as the Cochrane COVID-19 Study Register (www.covid-19.cochrane.org)) and other search approaches such as handsearching journals, citation tracking and contacting experts, other research groups and test manufacturers (Section 6.4). The selection of sources to search, particularly when resources are scarce, should be guided by evidence whenever possible from information retrieval research and systematic reviews of similar topics. Although publication bias is a more complex issue in systematic reviews of test accuracy than in intervention reviews (see Section 6.4.7 and Chapter 12, Section 12.3.1.5), a well-planned search strategy, for example including searching conference abstracts, trials registries and checking for test accuracy study protocols, may provide information about unpublished evidence and mitigate potential publication or reporting bias (Zarei 2018, Glanville 2021).

Box 6.2.a Performance measures for search strategies

Search recall (search sensitivity) is defined as the number of relevant records identified by a search strategy divided by the total number of relevant records on a given topic. It is a measure of the comprehensiveness of the search method. Strategies with high recall tend to have low levels of precision and the other way round. The challenge in estimating the effectiveness of search recall is that we rarely know how many relevant records are available to be identified.

Precision is defined as the number of relevant records identified by a search strategy divided by the total number of records identified. It is a measure of the ability of a search to exclude irrelevant reports. Its inverse (1/precision) represents the number of records we need to read to find one relevant report (number needed to read, NNR).

Source: Adapted from Bachmann 2002.

Search strategies need as an aim to identify all relevant records, but without retrieving too many irrelevant records. Therefore we need to balance optimum recall with manageable precision; see Box 6.2.a. Another term for recall is (search) sensitivity. However, as this handbook is about systematic reviews of test accuracy, and sensitivity is also a performance measure of tests, we use the term recall instead of (search) sensitivity in this chapter.

Depending on the research question (see Chapter 5) and the possible ways in which relevant studies have been designed and described (see Chapter 3), strategies for identifying test accuracy studies may use a number of different combinations of concepts from the research question. The starting point for most reviews will be to structure the search using terms related to two key concepts: the test(s) of interest (index test) and the condition to be detected (target condition). Other concepts, including the population to be tested, the reference standard or accuracy measures, may also be used in combination with either one or both of these key concepts. Depending on how exactly they will be combined, these additions may increase search recall (to minimize the risk of missing relevant studies) or may be used to improve precision (to minimize the retrieval of irrelevant records) if a simple two-concept search is producing unmanageable numbers of records.

For some topics, a combination of several search queries may be needed, each representing different combinations of key concepts (Whiting 2006). To determine the optimal approach, review authors need to explore how relevant test accuracy studies have been reported in the literature and indexed in databases (see Section 6.3 and Section 6.4). Reporting guidelines for studies of diagnostic test accuracy (STARD) have been developed (Bossuyt 2015, Cohen 2017), including standards designed for specific subject areas, such as diagnostic accuracy studies in dementia (Noel-Storr 2014) and those evaluating tests that make use of artificial intelligence (STARD-AI) (Sounderajah 2021). These standards, if adhered to, should help to make studies more discoverable by systematic searches. There is some evidence that adoption of the STARD reporting guideline for diagnostic accuracy studies (Bossuyt 2015) has begun to improve reporting standards (Korevaar 2014b, Korevaar 2015), but abstracts can still be poorly reported, leading to inadequate indexing (Cohen 2019, Gurung 2020). Search strategies therefore should not only rely on subject headings assigned by database indexers, but include text word searches of the record title, abstract and authors' keywords. These search options can differ across databases, so a good working knowledge of the features of the major databases as well as search query design is essential (Section 6.4.7).

6.2.1 Working in partnership

There are many advantages for systematic review teams that include review authors with a range of expertise. Ideally, review author teams should include an information specialist or at least one author with equivalent experience of systematic review searching. This expertise includes more than just an extensive knowledge of possible search terms. Knowledge of the types of documents that may contain the required evidence and knowledge of the databases and other places where these documents may be found are needed to design and execute good search strategies. Planning, designing and conducting the complete search process constitute a team effort. Although the electronic searching will typically be carried out by one individual with experience in designing electronic search strategies, other search types, such as manually checking reference lists or identifying grey literature, may be done by other review authors. Box 6.2.b provides examples of the type of information that might be provided by review authors with clinical and technical knowledge and the contributions that can be provided by an information specialist. Above all, the involvement of an information specialist in the review should improve the quality of various aspects of the search process (Rethlefsen 2015, Meert 2016, Metzendorf 2016).

Box 6.2.b Range of review author roles for systematic review searching

Review authors with clinical and technical knowledge about the index test(s) and target condition(s) can:

- explain and clearly describe each of the key concepts of the review;
- advise on terminology, for example where tests may have different names or can be referred to using different abbreviations, or if the names for diseases have changed over time;
- provide known relevant studies to help develop search strategies and validate search results;
- suggest specialized sources (such as journals, databases, registries, etc.) to search;
- provide advice on the relevance of records retrieved during search iterations or when responding to peer reviewer comments to clarify whether proposed search terms are appropriate;
- identify related systematic reviews for information on helpful sources to search, terminology used and potentially relevant citations;
- provide information about potentially eligible commercial tests or test manufacturers; and
- provide any other information relevant to searching the literature, such as advice on different uses of clinical terms, how far back to search, which study authors or research groups are known experts in the topic area, etc.

Information specialists can:

- provide feedback on the clarity or scope of the review question in relation to the reports expected to be found;
- provide feedback and advice on the types of reports to be included;
- support the team by providing insight on types of report likely to be found and how this relates to the question and the types of report the team may wish to identify;
- select sources to search;
- design, develop, test, adapt and run search strategies in each selected database;
- provide a draft search narrative to include search sources and master strategy and any key outputs/deliverables (e.g. search narrative and EndNote file of search results) for sign-off before beginning the definitive searches;
- save search results;
- remove duplicates;
- send results to the team in a format compatible with the team's chosen reference management software where possible;
- provide a detailed search log to assist with fully documenting and reporting the search process;
- assist in locating the full text of documents; and
- contribute to writing the review, with specific emphasis on writing up the search methods and search results.

6.2.2 Advice for review teams that do not include an information specialist

If for any reason it is not possible to include an information specialist on the review team, author teams can contact an information specialist or medical/healthcare librarian at their own institution. Many university (medical) libraries and specialized research institutes employ qualified staff who will have experience in systematic review search approaches. Alternatively, the team can contact resources such as Cochrane task exchange (taskexchange.cochrane.org) or independent search specialist services.

6.3 Sources to search

6.3.1 Bibliographic databases

Thousands of electronic bibliographic databases exist. Some, such as MEDLINE and Embase, cover a wide range of areas of health care and index journals from around the world, while others index journals from specific regions, focus on specific areas of health care or on specific document types.

Choosing the most appropriate databases to search is an essential component of designing a search. Review authors with topic expertise should share with the information specialist any knowledge they have regarding specialized sources of research that may be useful, as these may yield relevant studies not held in mainstream databases. Topic experts should also provide a list of relevant journals in the field, as these can be used to make an informed decision about the bibliographic databases to be searched. Sources such as Ulrichsweb (www.ulrichsweb.serialssolutions.com) list all the bibliographic databases that index a specific journal. The online technical supplement to the *Cochrane Handbook for Systematic Reviews of Interventions* provides a selective list of possible resources that can be searched, together with a regularly updated appendix of additional resources (Lefebvre 2021).

There is overlap between different databases with regard to the journals indexed and the records retrieved. For example, Embase now includes all MEDLINE records. Differences in the way in which the two databases index records, using different indexing systems and rules, mean that some articles that are difficult to identify from one database may be retrieved more easily from the other. In addition, database providers of MEDLINE and Embase present different search interfaces with differing functionality, which may also explain why some records may be retrieved from one interface to the database and not another. Because of the overlap between databases, one of the first steps of the selection process is deduplication of the retrieved articles. This can often be automated, but needs to be checked by a human (see online technical supplement, Section 4.3 in Lefebvre 2021).

6.3.1.1 MEDLINE, PubMed and Embase

MEDLINE, the US National Library of Medicine's database of citations and abstracts, currently indexes over 5200 journals in about 40 languages. Its subject scope is biomedicine and health. MEDLINE is available free via PubMed, on subscription from a number of online database providers, such as Ovid, or can be accessed through Embase (see later). The Ovid search interface and others offer advanced search facilities that can help increase search precision.

MEDLINE is the primary component of **PubMed** (www.pubmed.ncbi.nlm.nih.gov), a search engine supporting the retrieval of literature from MEDLINE. PubMed also includes records from journals that are not indexed for MEDLINE and records considered 'out of scope' from journals that are only partially indexed for MEDLINE. Using PubMed is free of charge and does not require registration, which is why many review authors use PubMed as their primary way to search MEDLINE. However, PubMed does not currently have advanced search techniques such as proximity operators, genuine phrase searching, wildcards and the ability to limit truncation, which are useful tools to optimize the balance between search recall and precision in information retrieval.

Embase, a biomedical and pharmacological bibliographic database published by Elsevier, indexes over 8200 journals in over 30 languages. Embase also includes conference abstracts from 2010 onwards. Embase includes records from MEDLINE from 1966 to date, thus allowing both databases to be searched simultaneously. Embase is only available by subscription and can be accessed through a number of interfaces, including Ovid and Embase.com.

Both Embase and MEDLINE have an indexing system (also known as a 'controlled vocabulary'): EMTREE for Embase and Medical Subject Headings (MeSH) for MEDLINE. These indexing systems are topic based and use a preferred term to describe a concept that might be described by authors in many different ways using many different terms. This can help to increase recall, for example if a record does not mention a specific term. The preferred term is assigned by the indexer to all the records covering that concept, irrespective of how the authors have described the concept in the article. Every article is labelled with multiple indexing terms to describe concepts such as the population, disease or condition, outcomes and tests. Other indexing terms are used to retrieve particular publication types such as letters and comments, and still others are designed to retrieve particular types of study design, for example test accuracy studies (see Section 6.5.2).

The PubMed and Ovid interfaces also have 'similar articles' or 'find similar' features, where an algorithm is used to find articles that may be similar in subject to the studies already retrieved. This can be a useful tool when building a set of relevant articles to help design and test a search strategy (see Section 6.4.7).

6.3.1.2 National and regional databases

Country- or region-specific databases, such as the Latin American and Caribbean Health Sciences Literature (LILACS) database or China National Knowledge Infrastructure (CNKI), record the literature produced in these geographical areas and often include publications not indexed elsewhere. Record abstracts may be in English or other languages, in which case searches need to be performed in the region-specific language(s). Many such databases are available free of charge on the internet, while others are available by subscription or on a 'pay-as-you-go' basis. The complexity and consistency of database indexing vary by database, as does the sophistication of the search interface. Examples are included in the online technical supplement of the Cochrane Handbook for Systematic Reviews of Interventions and an extensive list is given in the supplementary appendix of resources (Lefebvre 2021).

Region-specific databases can be an important source of additional studies, particularly as tests are not always used in the same way across countries and regions, and test accuracy can vary according to the population tested or role of the test in the clinical pathway. A case study by Cohen and colleagues compared two systematic reviews of anti-cyclic citrullinated peptide for diagnosing rheumatoid arthritis (Cohen 2015). One review, which included Chinese databases in its search strategy, resulted in the identification of 100 additional studies compared to the other review. Supplementing a search of MEDLINE and Embase with databases from other regions may therefore be particularly important for systematic reviews of test accuracy.

6.3.1.3 Subject-specific databases

Subject-specific databases index literature according to fields of research, for example CINAHL indexes nursing and allied health literature, PsycINFO covers psychology and psychiatry, and BIOSIS Previews covers biological sciences and related areas. Searching subject-specific databases may add unique records from journals not indexed in MEDLINE or Embase (Whiting 2008, Rice 2016). For example, PsycINFO may include additional studies on the measurement of instrument performance.

Evidence of the impact of searching extensively, for example including subject-specific databases compared to restricting the search to one or two main biomedical sources, on the estimates of sensitivity and specificity in syntheses of test accuracy is sparse (van Enst 2014, Glanville 2021) or has not been conducted as part of exploratory studies to improve search efficiency (Preston 2015). Searching for test accuracy studies in subject-specific databases should be considered as part of a careful search strategy plan to minimize the risk of missing potentially relevant studies for Cochrane Reviews of diagnostic test accuracy. Further evidence is needed on the impact on accuracy estimates of extensive compared to restrictive searching for studies of test accuracy.

Most of the main subject-specific databases are only available on a subscription or 'pay-as-you-go' basis. Access may therefore be limited to those databases that are available through review authors' institutions or medical libraries. Some of the main subject-specific databases are listed in the online technical supplement of the Cochrane Handbook for Systematic Reviews of Interventions and an extensive list is given in the supplementary appendix of resources (Lefebvre 2021). Some subject-specific databases with relevant studies for syntheses of test accuracy are accessible to search for free.For physiotherapists, there is a subject-specific database of primary studies and systematic reviews of test accuracy related to physiotherapy practice (DiTA; www.dita.org.au) (Kaizik 2019, Kaizik 2020).

During the COVID-19 pandemic other sources such as online COVID-19 data sets or research repositories emerged as potentially useful sources of studies relevant to syntheses of test accuracy being conducted in response to COVID-19. Examples include the Cochrane COVID-19 Study Register (www.covid-19.cochrane.org), the WHO database of global literature on COVID-19 (search.bvsalud.org/global-literature-on-novel-coronavirus-2019-ncov/), the Epistemonikos Foundation COVID-19 Living Overview of Evidence (L-OVE; www.app.iloveevidence.com/topics) and the COVID-19 Living Evidence database (www.ispmbern.github.io/covid-19/living-review) from the University of Bern.

6.3.1.4 Dissertations and theses databases

Some studies have found that dissertations and theses are more likely to be published in a journal article if the results are positive (Smart 1964, Vogel 2000, Zimpel 2000) and that, on average, dissertations that remain unpublished have lower effect sizes than the published literature (Smith 1980). It is not yet known whether dissertations about test accuracy research follow a similar publication pattern, but to minimize possible effects of publication bias, review authors should consider searching for dissertations and theses. Specific databases for theses and dissertations include Open Access Theses and Dissertations (OATD; www.oatd.org), ProQuest Dissertations and Theses Global (PQDT; www.about.proquest.com/en/products-services/pqdtglobal) and DART-Europe (www.dart-europe.eu/basic-search.php). Some subject-specific databases, including CINAHL and PsycINFO, also index dissertations relevant to their respective fields (Lefebvre 2021). A list of selected dissertations and theses can be found in Section 1.1.5 of the online technical supplement of the Cochrane Handbook for Systematic Reviews of Interventions (Lefebvre 2021).

6.3.2 Additional sources to search

Even a very sensitive search strategy may miss a proportion of relevant studies indexed in general biomedical databases. Studies may not have been indexed correctly, may not have an informative title and abstract (Cohen 2019) or may not (yet) be formally published at all. Additional methods to identify studies, such as checking references (see Section 6.3.2.1), handsearching (see Section 6.3.2.2), forward citation searching and co-citation searches (see Section 6.3.2.3), web search engines (see Section 6.3.2.4), grey literature databases and preprint servers (see Section 6.3.2.5), trial registries (see Section 6.3.2.6) and more informal sources (see Section 6.3.2.7) may therefore need to be considered.

6.3.2.1 Related reviews, guidelines and reference lists as sources of studies

Checking the reference lists of primary studies (particularly those identified for inclusion in the review) and of existing reviews and meta-analyses can be an effective method of identifying additional studies (Greenhalgh 2005, Bayliss 2007, Horsley 2011). Whiting (2008) found that the majority of relevant test accuracy studies not found from database searches were identified by checking reference lists. Preston (2015) found that in a convenience sample of nine Health Technology Assessment systematic reviews of test accuracy, of the 46 (15%) included studies not retrieved by the published searches of MEDLINE and Embase, 24 (8%) could be found by checking the reference lists of the included studies. Reference lists also point to reviews and discussion articles on the subject or closely related topics (Devillé 2002a, Devillé 2002b). It may also be helpful to update and rerun the electronic search if additional search terms are identified from studies discovered from these other sources.

Guidelines or other guidance assessing diagnostic tests, such as Health Technology Assessments, may also prove useful as sources of studies, for example the Diagnostics Guidance produced by the UK National Institute for Health and Care Excellence (www. nice.org.uk/guidance/published?ngt=Diagnostics%20guidance&ndt=Guidance).

Sources of reviews, guidelines and other guidance are listed in the online technical supplement of the Cochrane Handbook for Systematic Reviews of Interventions and added to in the supplementary appendix of resources (Lefebvre 2021).

6.3.2.2 Handsearching

Handsearching is the systematic screening of the contents of every issue of a relevant journal published within a defined time period. Evidence from one study suggests that handsearching for systematic reviews of test accuracy with well-constructed search strategies may not identify additional studies if the index test is well defined and study records are consistently assigned a database indexing term (Glanville 2012). The expected benefits from handsearching must be offset against the time and resources required to do it well. Handsearching may be best justified in cases where a key journal likely to be of interest is not indexed in the major bibliographic databases.

6.3.2.3 Forward citation searching and co-citation searching

Forward citation searching or 'forward snowballing' looks for studies that have cited one or more key articles of interest to a review question. Forward citation searching can provide a means of identifying additional relevant studies or, like the "See All Similar Articles" option in PubMed and the "Find Similar" option in Ovid, can be a useful tool when building a set of relevant articles to help design and test a search strategy. A number of online resources allow forward citation searching, including Web of Science and Scopus (both of which require a paid subscription) and Google Scholar (which is available free of charge). Evidence on the added value of these search strategies in systematic reviews of test accuracy is currently lacking.

Co-citation is a method designed to find articles that might be of interest because they are frequently cited together in reference lists of other articles. It is different from forward citation searching. For example, an eligible study A is cited by studies C, D and E. Another study B is also cited by studies C, D and E. Study A and B have a co-citation relationship. Some studies are co-cited more frequently than others and can be ranked accordingly. For example, CoCites (www.cocites.com) is a novel interface for searching within PubMed that not only retrieves the 100 most recent citations of an article of interest, but also extracts all other titles in their respective reference lists, counting how often each title appears and ranking results by frequency (Janssens 2020). It has been noted that some types of studies, particularly grey literature such as conference proceedings and studies in progress, cannot reliably be identified using citation analysis methods. This may be because authors rarely cite them or the citation databases do not index them, making these methods susceptible to publication bias (Belter 2016). Citation analysis methods should not be used to replace database searching for test accuracy studies. It is not known whether citation analysis methods, when used as an adjunct to database searching, may identify additional test accuracy studies for Cochrane systematic reviews.

6.3.2.4 Web searching

Searching the web in a systematic way for test accuracy studies is challenging. It is likely to involve using general search engines, such as Google Search, and accessing selected websites likely to cover relevant topics, such as those belonging to charitable organizations, research funders, diagnostic test manufacturers or regulatory agencies, health technology assessment agencies, test accuracy research groups and other professional societies. These resources are usually not designed to enable advanced search techniques for retrieving potentially relevant studies from within their wide range of content and so are problematic to search efficiently. There is, however, some evidence that eligible and even 'unique' studies, not identified by other search methods, can be found by web searching (Eysenbach 2001, Ogilvie 2005, Stansfield 2014, Godin 2015, Bramer 2017). When using search engines, review authors need to be aware that search results can be personalized, for example when logged in to Google, and efforts should be made to ensure that searches are as reproducible as possible by 'logging out' prior to carrying out searches.

Google Scholar, a specialized version of Google Search, offers a way of searching the scholarly literature on the web, including published and grey literature. It can be a useful tool to use alongside bibliographic database searching, not just for citation searching but also for the option to search the full text of studies, an advantage in tracking down studies not indexed in, or not retrieved by searches of, bibliographic databases. Some evidence indicates that using Google Scholar can identify unique studies using similar or the same search terms as used in bibliographic databases (Bramer 2017). At the same time, empirical work has particularly highlighted Google Scholar for the lack of reproducibility of searches that could not be explained by 'natural' database growth (Gusenbauer 2020). Although web searching has its challenges, as already outlined, it has potential usefulness as a supplement to the other types of searching, but should not be used as the single source for a systematic review of test accuracy. More detail on web searching methods and a list of search engines can be found in Section 1.3.5 of the online technical supplement of the Cochrane Handbook for Systematic Reviews of Interventions (Lefebvre 2021).

Although internet searches are increasingly used as a resource for systematic reviews, reporting standards are generally poor and a number of authors have provided guidance to improve the transparency and reproducibility of internet searches (e.g. Briscoe 2015). Options include saving a local electronic copy with details about any possibly relevant study found. Notetaking software such as Evernote or OneNote, or website logging software such as Zotero, should be used in preference to 'bookmarking' the site in case the record of the study is removed or altered at a later stage. Briscoe (2015) suggests that in addition to this type of record-keeping, a minimum set of information should be recorded both for websites (name, URL, dates searched, search terms, including any specific sections searched and results) and for specific search engines (name, dates searched, search terms, and how the results were selected).

6.3.2.5 Grey literature databases

Grey literature generally refers to documents that are not formally published in accessible sources such as books or journals. Examples may be conference abstracts, reports by non-governmental organizations, policy briefs, national registries, etc. Grey literature has been shown to contribute about 10% of the studies referenced in Cochrane systematic reviews of intervention (Mallett 2002). Grey literature is more likely to concern studies reporting non-significant results than are healthcare journal articles (McAuley 2000, Hopewell 2005, Hopewell 2007). Thus, failure to include studies from the grey literature may threaten the validity of a systematic review. More research is needed across a range of diagnostic accuracy topic areas to determine whether studies of diagnostic accuracy exhibit similar publication biases (Brazzelli 2009, Wilson 2015, Korevaar 2016); there are some indications that this may be the case for imaging studies (Brazzelli 2009).

Forms of grey literature that have become more accessible in recent years are preprints and open access archives. These reports are accessible through the websites and preprint databases of commercial publishers (e.g. medRxiv, bioRxiv or SSRN), but also through open access platforms, such as Zenodo and OpenScience framework (www.osf.io). The status of these reports may vary, from first drafts with typos and mistakes to peer-reviewed manuscripts almost ready to be formally published. Review authors need to be aware of the level of rigour of the preprints that are retrieved and should keep track of version numbers, as information is subject to change. It is advisable to check the latest version and contact authors of any selected preprints deemed eligible for inclusion in the review before submitting the review for publication.

6.3.2.6 Trial registries

Awareness of the existence of a possibly relevant ongoing study can affect decisions about when to conduct or update a review. Information on research projects in progress, as well as completed project records that may contain study results or references to publications, can be found in online registers maintained by professional associations or national governments. No single, central register of ongoing test accuracy evaluations currently exists, but such studies are increasingly being included in existing trials registers (Hooft 2011) and regulatory agency data sets. A website listing some key registers and how to search them is available at sites.google.com/a/york.ac.uk/yhectrialsregisters/home.

For Cochrane Reviews, information about possible relevant ongoing studies should be included in the 'Characteristics of ongoing studies' table.

6.3.2.7 Contacting colleagues, study authors and manufacturers

Colleagues can be an important source of information about unpublished studies and informal channels of communication may be the only means of identifying unpublished data. Authors of relevant studies or other experts in the field may know about completed but unpublished studies (Reveiz 2006). Conference reports on topics of interest may be a source of potential authors and experts. One approach is to send a request for information to the contact author of reports of included studies, together with a list of relevant articles already identified and the eligibility criteria for the review, and ask whether they know of additional studies (published, unpublished or ongoing) that might be relevant. A similar request could be sent to test manufacturers.

6.4   Designing search strategies

Searches for test accuracy studies are often more challenging to design compared to searches for randomized controlled trials of interventions. Not all databases have subject headings for measures of accuracy or publication-type indexing for test accuracy studies. Where those are available, they may not always be applied consistently or have been available for a long period of time (Gurung 2020). For example, the methodological MeSH terms 'Sensitivity and Specificity', introduced to MEDLINE in 1991, may refer to test accuracy measures, but may also refer to the lowest concentration that can be measured of a certain compound (Wilczynski 1995). Authors also do not consistently report measures of accuracy in article titles and abstracts, and older studies are less likely to contain abstracts, which reduces the efficiency of indexing and text word searching and can lead to missed studies (Doust 2005, Leeflang 2006, Ritchie 2007).

Cases of incomplete reporting of test accuracy studies, a lack of relevant indexing terms in some databases and variation in applying existing indexing terms may all contribute to low search recall (see Section 6.4.7). Multi-stranded approaches to searching may be needed, which in turn may lower precision. Search strategies may also pass through many iterations as the information specialist tests out different approaches to achieve the best balance between search recall and precision.

The initial set of search terms used to develop a draft search strategy will be informed by discussions between the information specialist and other review authors with clinical or topic expertise, and by the information specialist's knowledge and expertise. A number of other techniques can be used to build up a set of candidate search terms (Lefebvre 2013, Lefebvre 2021). Putting together a set of known relevant studies is a good starting point. Searching each database for this set of known studies can identify relevant subject indexing and may be particularly useful when the test name is not standardized or to capture all components of a composite test. Relevant studies 'missed' by the preliminary searches should be searched for using the author names, terms from the title or other bibliographic data. If a 'missed' study is found, its subject headings and text words can be noted and any that are deemed potentially useful can be incorporated into the search strategy.

Usually, a series of preliminary searches using a range of subject headings and text words is conducted and records for retrieved studies are examined to identify relevant text words and their variants (synonyms, abbreviations, spelling variants, common mis-spellings) as well as subject headings assigned by the database indexers. Some database search interfaces have a facility for mapping keyword searches to subject headings (see Section 6.3.1.1), and tools such as PubMed PubReMiner (www.hgserver2.amc.nl/cgi-bin/miner/miner2.cgi) and the Yale MeSH Analyzer (www.mesh.med.yale.edu) can also help to identify MeSH from known relevant records.

After adding terms, it may be necessary to test the search strategy to ensure it is achieving an appropriate balance of recall and precision. The set of known relevant studies that would be expected to be retrieved can be used to test the recall of the search and to check how these studies have been indexed in different databases. During these preliminary searches, it is important to note which topic concepts are being described by the authors and captured by the database indexers so that the structure of the search strategy can be designed to maximize retrieval of relevant studies.

This iterative process can be followed to identify a wide range of search terms and the key concepts of the research topic.

6.4.1 Structuring the search strategy

Chapter 5 outlines the essential components or 'concepts' of a review question. Information specialists need to have a good understanding of these key concepts to allow them to identify the most useful concepts to include in a search strategy. It is not usually necessary to search on every aspect of the review question, as some concepts may not appear in article titles or abstracts or may not be well indexed with subject headings (van der Weijden 1997, Fielding 2002, Vincent 2003, Korevaar 2015). Depending on the complexity of the topic(s) and/or the complexity of the ways in which the topic(s) are described in records, one or more search strategies may be developed.

- *A single-stranded approach based on a single key concept* – only suitable for index tests that are well defined and consistently described. An example can be found in a Cochrane Review of diagnostic test accuracy about the Informant Questionnaire on Cognitive Decline in the Elderly (IQCODE) for the detection of dementia within community dwelling populations (Quinn 2021).
- *A single-stranded approach combining two key concepts*, most commonly but not limited to (1) index test(s) AND (2) target condition(s) (e.g. a review of the use of ultrasound for confirmation of gastric tube placement combined terms related to 'ultrasound' with key terms related to 'stomach tube' (Tsujimoto 2017)).
- *A single-stranded approach involving three key concepts* (e.g. (1) index test(s) AND (2) target condition(s) AND (3) population) – only suitable if this can focus the search without unduly compromising search recall. For example, clinical assessment for diagnosing congenital heart disease in newborn infants with Down syndrome (see Figure 6.4.a).

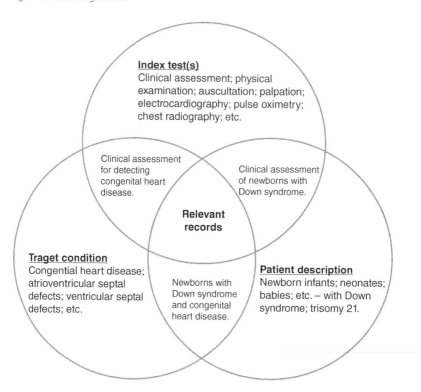

Figure 6.4.a **Combining concepts as search sets in a simple structure.** Example: Clinical assessment for diagnosing congenital heart disease in newborn infants with Down syndrome

- *A multi-stranded approach* whereby a number of different single-stranded approaches are applied to optimize search recall. This approach might be taken where a diagnostic question can be conceptualized in a number of different ways, or where the search terms from relevant concepts are not always present in all records (so a permutation of concepts is required). Multiple single-stranded approaches are developed, each capturing a different way in which the relevant literature might be described by combining key concepts in different ways. The individual single-stranded approaches are then combined to create the final search strategy. For example, a review of physical examination for low back pain ultimately combined four single-stranded searches, each of which combined two or more sets of search terms related to either physical examination, specific tests that could be included in a physical examination, low back pain, the relevant causes of low back pain and diagnostic accuracy terms (van der Windt 2010). A simplified example of this type of complex search structure is provided in Table 6.4.a.

6.4.2   Controlled vocabulary and text words

Several database producers index records using standard keywords or subject headings. Well-known examples of subject headings include MeSH for MEDLINE and EMTREE for Embase. The indexing terms are a controlled vocabulary and are database specific,

Table 6.4.a Multi-stranded search to find brief psychometric instruments to identify depression in prison or offender populations

Search strand	Concept 1	Concept 2	Concept 3
1	General screening instruments	AND Depression	AND People who committed a crime
	Index tests (general)	*AND Target condition*	*AND Population*
2	Specific terms for depression screening instruments		AND People who committed a crime
	Index test/Target condition concept merged		*AND Population*
3	Specific depression screening instruments for offender populations		
	Index test/Target condition/Population concept merged		
4	General diagnostic terms	AND Depression	AND People who committed a crime
	Diagnostic filter	*AND Target condition*	*AND Population*
5	1 OR 2 OR 3 OR 4		

Within each of these search queries a range of search terms and search techniques will be used to maximize retrieval of relevant studies and minimize retrieval of irrelevant studies.

Source: Adapted from Hewitt 2011.

i.e. the subject headings used are not identical across databases and the approach to indexing may also differ. Embase records are often indexed in greater depth than MEDLINE records and in recent years Elsevier has increased the number of subject headings assigned to each Embase record. Searches of Embase may therefore retrieve additional articles that were not retrieved by a MEDLINE search, even if the records were present in both databases. Retrieving more records does not necessarily mean retrieval of more relevant records, and it is important that search strategies are custom-ized for each database searched (Falck-Ytter 2004).

Text word searches will automatically 'map' to relevant database subject headings when using PubMed as an interface. The mapping should be checked to make sure the mapping terms presented are appropriate for the search topic (they may be broader or narrower than required). If mapping is not providing correct results, mapping in PubMed can be prevented by careful use of field tags. Other interfaces, such as Embase. com and Ovid, offer options to look up the subject heading based on entering an exam-ple, which provides the user with more control over the search strategy and the results retrieved. Again, careful inspection of the headings available and the broader and nar-rower headings around a specific heading is important to ensure efficient searches and to achieve a good balance of search recall and precision. Subject headings can also be identified using other search tools provided with the database, such as the Permuted Index under Search Tools in Ovid or the MeSH database (www.ncbi.nlm.nih.gov/mesh) for PubMed. Database thesauri may offer the facility to 'explode' subject headings that have more specific terms associated with them. For example, the MeSH term 'Prenatal Diagnosis' has several lower-level terms covering more specific types of prenatal diagnosis such as 'Amniocentesis' or 'Chorionic Villi Sampling'. 'Explosion' of a higher-level subject heading such as 'Prenatal diagnosis' captures all of these more specific terms and so searches for several terms at once. If the review is about amniocentesis, then articles on amniocentesis should only be indexed with the specific term 'Amniocentesis', and the search should include the heading 'Amniocentesis'. However, in practice some records may receive the more general term 'Prenatal Diagnosis' rather than 'Amniocentesis', so if that is found to be the case, it would also be necessary to search for 'Prenatal Diagnosis' unexploded. If the review is about all prenatal diagnosis tests, then it would be best to search using the exploded heading 'Prenatal Diagnosis'. It is always important to check the impact of an explosion to ensure that precision does not suffer. The information specialist should seek clarification from clinical and technical specialists about whether to include all of the terms grouped under the highest-level term or only some of them.

Older publications are harder to identify than recent ones. For example, MEDLINE does not generally include abstracts for articles published before 1976, so only text word searches can be used on titles for this period. In addition, MEDLINE subject headings relating to study design and methodology were not available before the 1990s, so text word searches are necessary to retrieve older records (Wilczynski 1995, Vincent 2003).

6.4.3 Text word or keyword searching

A sensitive search strategy includes a range of text words for each concept to be searched and it is important to consider alternative ways of specifying the same concept, for example via synonyms (e.g. 'newborn' or 'neonate'), using related terms (e.g. 'Down Syndrome' or 'Downs syndrome' or 'trisomy 21') and variant spellings (e.g. 'paediatric' or 'pediatric'). Depending on the service provider and the search concept, some types of variations can also be captured using truncation (e.g. electrocardiogra* for electrocardiogram, electrocardiograph, electrocardiography, etc.) or wildcards (e.g. wom?n for woman or women). These features differ across database interfaces and can also change over time, so database interface help files should be checked. It is crucial to describe fully each concept deemed important to be searched to ensure that when all these concepts are combined in a multi-stranded approach, the risk of missing studies is kept to a minimum (see Figure 6.4.a).

Once defined, search terms (including both subject headings and text words) are combined using Boolean operators or 'connecting words', the basic ones being 'AND' and 'OR' (see Figure 6.4.a). Terms within the same search concept (e.g. all the search terms for the index test(s)) are usually combined using 'OR', while 'AND' is used to combine sets of search terms for two or more concepts (e.g. index test AND target condition).

Some search interfaces allow the use of additional operators (known as proximity operators) to specify how close to each other words must be (e.g. occurring within a certain number of words of each other). Proximity operators, where available and in suitable cases, can be very useful for improving the precision of searches.

The third Boolean operator, the 'NOT' operator, can be used to exclude records indexed with certain terms (for example, to carefully exclude records related exclusively to research on animals). Extreme care should be taken when using the NOT operator to avoid inadvertently removing relevant records from the search result. Further details about use of Boolean operators can be found in the online technical supplement of the Cochrane Handbook for Systematic Reviews of Interventions (Lefebvre 2021).

6.4.4 Search filters

The accuracy of a diagnostic test can be expressed in a number of ways: sensitivity and specificity, positive and negative predictive values, positive and negative likelihood ratios, diagnostic odds ratio, receiver operating characteristic (ROC) curve and area under the curve (AUC). These terms can be included in a search string as words in the title and abstract, and as standard index terms, such as the MeSH terms, for example 'Sensitivity and Specificity'. A combination of these terms can be used as a methodological search filter to focus searches on the studies that are most likely to report test accuracy data.

A number of filters have been developed and published, but none has sufficiently high levels of reliability that would justify its use as a sound method to optimize precision without compromising search recall for Cochrane Reviews of diagnostic test accuracy. The filters have not attained the proven level of efficiency that the randomized controlled trial filters have, for example.

A routine reliance on methodological search filters for systematic reviews of test accuracy is therefore not recommended. Evaluations have shown that even the most sensitive filters miss relevant studies, do not perform consistently across subject areas and study designs (Doust 2005, Mitchell 2005, Leeflang 2006, Ritchie 2007, Beynon 2013) and do not significantly reduce the number of studies that have to be screened (Leeflang 2006, Ritchie 2007). A methodological filter should only be used as part of a multi-stranded approach to searching (see Section 6.4.1). Search filters can be identified from the InterTASC Information Specialists' Sub-Group (ISSG) Search Filter Resource (www.sites.google.com/a/york.ac.uk/issg-search-filters-resource/home). Further evidence-based information on the performance of test accuracy search filters can be found within the diagnostic accuracy section of the SuRe info portal (www.sites.google.com/york.ac.uk/sureinfo/home/diagnostic-accuracy).

6.4.5 Language, date and type of document restrictions

Further research is needed to determine whether studies of test accuracy are at risk of language and other reporting biases (see Section 6.4.7). Although language restrictions are not recommended, restricting the search to particular dates might be worthwhile if the diagnostic test of interest was introduced from a particular date or has been substantially improved over time and the review focuses only on the most recent versions.

Excluding records based on document type is not recommended. Letters may report test accuracy data from the correspondents' own institution, and some journals publish short reports of studies as a research letter. Letters and errata may also report clues to additional studies or new information about a study that is not reported elsewhere. Further research is needed to determine the importance of letters or other types of document, such as case reports, as a source of test accuracy data.

6.4.6   Identifying fraudulent studies, other retracted publications, errata and comments

It is important to check at the initial search stage – before data extraction – whether eligible studies have been corrected or retracted, and also at the review update stage for any retractions or corrections since initial publication. Reports of retracted studies in MEDLINE are assigned the Publication Type 'Retracted Publication'. However, journal editors do not always retract studies that warrant this sanction (Elia 2014) or do not do so promptly, so corrections, errata, comments and expressions of concern should also be examined. Another source to identify retractions is Retraction Watch (www.retractionwatch.com) and the related Retraction Watch Database (www.retractiondatabase.org). Some reference management software links with the Retraction Watch database and sends an automatic notification when the reference to a study matches a retraction in the database. Information on how to search for retracted publications, errata and expressions of concern can be found in the online technical supplement of the Cochrane Handbook for Systematic Reviews of Interventions, Section 3.9 (Lefebvre 2021).

Identifying fraudulent studies is challenging (Boughton 2021). For guidance, consult the Cochrane Policy for Managing Potentially Problematic Studies (www.cochranelibrary.com/cdsr/editorial-policies#problematic-studies) and the accompanying implementation guidance (documentation.cochrane.org/display/EPPR/Policy+for+managing+potentially+problematic+studies%3A+implementation+guidance).

6.4.7   Minimizing the risk of bias through search methods

Systematic reviews are distinct from traditional narrative reviews. Systematic reviews set out to identify as many relevant studies as possible and document searches in a transparent way and with sufficient detail to be reproduced. These features help to minimize bias and increase the reliability of review findings (Easterbrook 1991, Egger 1998, Song 2000, Dickersin 2005).

Bias resulting from the search process could arise when studies with certain results (often the more positive results) are easier to find than others and the search strategy has not sufficiently accounted for this phenomenon. However, most of the evidence for possible bias comes from work on systematic reviews of the effectiveness of interventions, and it is not yet clear whether publication and reporting biases exist in the same way for test accuracy studies. There is evidence of test accuracy studies failing to achieve full publication (Brazzelli 2009, van Enst 2015, Korevaar 2016) or being subject to selective reporting (Rifai 2008). Higher accuracy has been shown to be associated with faster publication of diagnostic imaging studies (van Enst 2015, Cherpak 2019, Treanor 2021). However, whether there is a general relationship between study results, study size and time to publication is uncertain. Language bias and bias in the reporting of certain subgroups or results within test accuracy publications require further research.

The risk of introducing bias from the search can be minimized by searching several electronic databases and using additional methods to retrieve published and unpublished studies (Whiting 2008). A search of MEDLINE alone is generally not considered adequate for systematic reviews and may lead to bias (van Enst 2014). Even if relevant records are in MEDLINE, it can be difficult to retrieve them efficiently; by extending the search to other sources, some of these records may be retrieved elsewhere (Golder

2006, Whiting 2008). For intervention reviews, searching Embase in addition to MEDLINE has been shown to affect the estimate of effectiveness (Sampson 2003), probably partly due to its broader coverage of languages other than English. Evidence about the impact of restricting a search to MEDLINE alone on sensitivity and specificity estimates in syntheses of test accuracy is sparse (van Enst 2014). Some analyses have suggested that searching MEDLINE alone (van Enst 2014, Rice 2016) or MEDLINE and Embase, together with reference checking (Preston 2015), may be sufficient for systematic reviews of test accuracy. These findings, however, may not be representative, as they are based on small, selected or exploratory convenience samples; have had to rely on known sets of test accuracy studies, where the search strategies of the original meta-analyses were not able to be replicated and their original performance is unknown; or had included test accuracy search filters, which may have reduced their sensitivity.

Some studies may be recorded in specialist databases instead of in MEDLINE, for example according to topic (such as the Cumulative Index to Nursing and Allied Health Literature, CINAHL) or geographical area (such as the Latin American and Caribbean Health Sciences Literature, LILACS) (Pereira 2019). There is some evidence to suggest that other databases that might yield additional studies for systematic reviews of test accuracy include the Science Citation Index, BIOSIS and LILACS (Whiting 2008), Scopus, PsycINFO and Embase (Rice 2016). Relying exclusively on a MEDLINE search may retrieve a set of reports unrepresentative of those that would have been identified through a more extensive search of additional sources (Rice 2016).

Supplementary search methods, beyond database searches, include checking reference lists (Greenhalgh 2005, Horsley 2011), forward citation searches, co-citation analysis (Janssens 2015, Belter 2016, Belter 2017, Janssens 2020), handsearching and contacting experts, other research groups and test manufacturers. Additional approaches are needed to detect unpublished test accuracy studies. Although they are not generally required to be recorded in trial registries such as ClinicalTrials.gov and are less often registered than other study types (Korevaar 2014a), prospective registration of test accuracy studies in existing public registries has been encouraged and a minimal data set has been suggested of the key information needed to describe test accuracy studies within registries, including study type, index test(s) and target condition (Korevaar 2017). Consistently populating these specific data fields for test accuracy studies would also help make the records more discoverable. Searching trial registries for test accuracy studies may therefore prove helpful (Glanville 2021), as may checking for test accuracy study protocols (Zarei 2018). Conference abstracts may also point review authors to ongoing or completed but (as yet) unpublished studies (Cherpak 2019, Korevaar 2020).

6.5   Documenting and reporting the search process

It is crucial to document and report the search process clearly, with enough detail to indicate how extensive the search strategy is, which in turn can be a marker of how methodologically sound the review's evidence base is likely to be. Thorough documentation and transparent reporting can also aid in the reproducibility of the search strategy and facilitate future updates of the review, as well as provide a resource of potentially useful search terms and their combinations for other researchers of similar reviews to consider.

Consensus has been reached on a minimum set of items to report when documenting the search process in systematic reviews (PRISMA-S), including specific guidance for reviews of diagnostic test accuracy (PRISMA-DTA and PRISMA-DTA for Abstracts). PRISMA for Searching (PRISMA-S) (Rethlefsen 2021) is an extension to the PRISMA (Preferred Reporting Items for Systematic Reviews and Meta-Analyses) Statement, and specifically addresses the reporting of search strategies in systematic reviews. PRISMA-S can be used in conjunction with the PRISMA Statement for Diagnostic Test Accuracy, PRISMA-DTA (McInnes 2018), and its accompanying explanation and elaboration article (Salameh 2020), as well as the corresponding checklist, explanation and elaboration PRISMA article for journal and conference abstracts, PRISMA-DTA for Abstracts (Cohen 2021).

Incomplete reporting of the search process in systematic reviews has been noted (Sampson 2008, Roundtree 2009, Niederstadt 2010), including in reviews of test accuracy (Salameh 2019), and can undermine confidence in the research itself. A study measuring the completeness of reporting of 100 systematic reviews of test accuracy against the PRISMA-DTA reporting checklist found there was a need for improvement. The sources searched were reported by 87 of the 100 reviews analysed, the last date the search was run by 33 of 100 and the complete search strategies by 42 of 100 (Salameh 2019). In the same study, measuring against the PRISMA-DTA for Abstracts checklist, improvements were also found to be needed, for example in reporting the databases searched (63 of 100) and the last date the search was run (42 of 100).

6.5.1 Documenting the search process

Documenting the search process involves keeping a careful record of each step taken by the searcher and will help make the final reporting of the search in the review much easier and less likely to be incomplete. This internal record-keeping of the search process includes documenting all sources searched, on which date, search terms used, the full strategies as they were run, the yield for each source, details about contacting experts or test manufacturers, searching reference lists, scanning websites and search iterations. Careful documentation is especially important for systematic reviews of test accuracy as methods are still being refined. Searches that are carefully documented can be more easily reported, while good reporting will provide future insight into the best sources of studies and the effects of search strategies on likely sources of bias.

6.5.2 Reporting the search process

6.5.2.1 Reporting the search process in the protocol

Any protocol of a systematic review of test accuracy submitted for publication should report the intended search strategy, ideally for each electronic database but at least for one major bibliographic database. Protocols for Cochrane Reviews of diagnostic test accuracy are formally peer reviewed before they are published and before the actual review process starts. Peer reviewing the search strategy at this early stage by information specialists with expertise in searching for reviews of test accuracy is very important, as it is the starting point for retrieving the evidence included in the review. Authors of Cochrane Reviews of diagnostic test accuracy are therefore advised to report the complete search strategy in the protocol of at least one database, including the verbatim search strings so that these can be peer reviewed. Any later changes to the search strategy, and additional search strategies for additional databases, should be described in the final review.

6.5.2.2   Reporting the search process in the review
In the final review report, the searches for systematic reviews should be reported in the review abstract, methods and results sections, with relevant detail provided as supplementary appendices. Again, this enables peer review of the search strategy, which is an important quality check for the review as a whole.

The PRISMA for Diagnostic Test Accuracy Statement (PRISMA-DTA) should be followed (McInnes 2018). PRISMA-DTA provides a 27-point checklist including recommendations for reporting of four items relating to searching, covering (1) what should be reported in the abstract by referring to PRISMA-DTA for Abstracts (Cohen 2021); (2) all information sources used (their coverage and dates last searched); (3) full search strategies for each source searched (any limits); and (4) study selection, ideally presented as a flow diagram through the search process. The PRISMA-DTA for Abstracts recommends that key databases and the dates when each was last searched be included in the search methods section of an abstract (Cohen 2021). Review authors may also wish to refer to the PRISMA extension for searching that covers reporting of literature searches in systematic reviews of all types (PRISMA-S) (Rethlefsen 2021).

Full search strategies (preferably copied and pasted from the original saved search strategies rather than retyped) should be included as an appendix to the review. All other resources used should also be reported, including grey literature resources, handsearching, online searches, citation tracking (forward and backward citation searching and co-citation searches) and any contact with study authors, experts or commercial organizations, such as test manufacturers. Complex searches, such as the use of multistranded approaches in searching for test accuracy studies, should be explained in a narrative way so that the logic of their construction is clear and so that they can be understood and replicated (Cooper 2018).

The dates on which the searches were done may be different from the dates until which the searches were done. For example, review authors may restrict searches to complete years (e.g. until 1 January 2021) instead of to the actual date of the search (e.g. conducted on 3 March 2021). Both dates should be reported in the review. The starting year for the search should also be reported, especially if the database was not searched from its inception date onwards (e.g. the starting date is dictated by the availability of the index test). Reporting the relevant dates of the search strategy and the search conduct enables readers and peer reviewers to assess how relevant the current review may be. Although guidelines for search dates may differ between tests and target conditions (a test that evolves rapidly may need a more up-to-date search than a test that remains stable for decades), a rule of thumb is for searches to have been conducted within the 12 months before publication of the review.

The results section of the review should include a comprehensive summary of the result of the search, including the total number of citations identified and the number of records remaining after deduplication; the number of records included after title and abstract screening; and the number of reports that were finally included in the review after full text assessment. The PRISMA Statement recommends reporting the flow of citations through the systematic review process in a flow diagram (see Figure 6.5.a). PRISMA 2020 flow diagram templates for both new reviews and

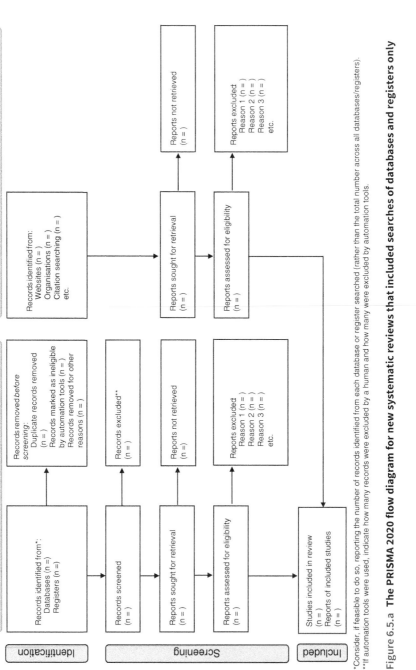

Figure 6.5.a **The PRISMA 2020 flow diagram for new systematic reviews that included searches of databases and registers only**

*Consider, if feasible to do so, reporting the number of records identified from each database or register searched (rather than the total number across all databases/registers).
**If automation tools were used, indicate how many records were excluded by a human and how many were excluded by automation tools.

review updates can be downloaded from the PRISMA Statement website (www.prisma-statement.org) and edited to suit. Flow diagrams can also be generated using a Shiny App (www.eshackathon.org/software/PRISMA2020.html).

6.6   Selecting relevant studies

Once initial searches of bibliographic databases have been completed, the next stage of the selection process, manual judgement for relevancy, can begin. In parallel, searching of additional resources (e.g. handsearching, web searching or finding grey literature) can continue, as this may take longer. Ongoing studies identified by the searches may be completed during the course of the review, so can be judged later on during the review process. Checking reference lists of included studies can only start after these studies have been identified.

Starting with the bibliographic database searches, all search results should be merged using reference management software and duplicate records of the same study report removed, so that one set of initially retrieved unique records can be defined. Reference management software, such as EndNote (www.endnote.com), Mendeley (www.mendeley.com), RefWorks (www.proquest.com/products-services/refworks.html) and Zotero (www.zotero.org), use different algorithms for automated detection of duplicate records, and open-source software programs have been developed for this purpose (Jiang 2014, Rathbone 2015). No consensus has been reached on the optimal process for deduplication and a combination of automated methods and visual inspection is common. For a list of selected reference management software, see Section 4.1 of the online technical supplement of the Cochrane Handbook for Systematic Reviews of Interventions (Lefebvre 2021). For more detail on methods for removing duplicates using reference management software or the use of open-source software programs, see Section 4.3 of the online technical supplement (Lefebvre 2021).

The initial screening phase is based on an examination of titles and abstracts. In this phase, obviously irrelevant records should be removed, for example reports about completely different target conditions or studies obviously answering a different question than an accuracy question. Reviews, overviews and editorials should also be removed but, where relevant to the review question, may be flagged for checking the reference lists. It is important to be aware that titles and abstracts are not always good reflections of the study described in the full report. It is therefore not advisable at this stage in the process to exclude records because eligible index test(s) are not mentioned in the title or abstract. Some studies may have compared multiple index tests, but reported only one in the abstract.

Screening of titles and abstracts can be done in reference management software, in online software applications specifically designed for literature reviews or in spreadsheet software such as Excel. The benefit of online software applications is that deduplicated search results can be uploaded and screened online and reports that pass the first stage (title and abstract screening) are automatically forwarded to the next stage (full-text screening). Some applications allow lists of relevant or irrelevant keywords to be added and their appearance highlighted on each record to aid screening decisions, while others sort the order of screening based on the potential relevance of the record using machine learning algorithms. More information about these techniques and about further automation of the selection process through machine learning and text mining can be found in Section 4.6.6 of the *Cochrane Handbook for Systematic Reviews of Interventions*.

Although title and abstract screening can be carried out by one review author alone – especially when this author is over-inclusive – it is recommended that at least two review authors examine every title and abstract independently from each other. This way errors can be minimized and bias from subjective exclusions reduced.

Review authors who are used to screening for intervention reviews may be surprised, first by the initial number of records to be screened for a review of test accuracy, and subsequently by the number of reports remaining for full-text assessment. The frequent complexity of searches for test accuracy studies (see Section 6.4) can lead to retrieval of large numbers of records. The variety of study designs that may be used to evaluate the accuracy of tests (see Chapter 3) makes it difficult to define preferred designs to help narrow study selection. Authors of diagnostic accuracy reviews should expect a relatively high workload in the screening and selection process (Petersen 2014).

6.6.1   Examine full-text reports for compliance of studies with eligibility criteria

After the first round of selection based on title and abstract, the next phase is to examine full-text reports to identify studies that meet the review eligibility criteria. In this phase the decision will be made to either include or exclude records, therefore every record should be assessed by two review authors independently from each other. A pre-specified list of reasons for exclusion should be used and at least one explicit reason for exclusion should be documented for every excluded study. Disagreements may be solved by discussion, or by a third person or 'arbiter'.

The information that is needed to assess study eligibility is often not available in the abstract and may sometimes be 'hidden', or not explicitly stated, even in the full text of the study report. For example, studies do not always report what reference standard was used to define the presence of the target condition or provide key details about how it was applied in the study. In these situations, review authors have to make judgement calls about study inclusion, e.g. if the reference standard (or other key aspect of the study) is not clear, will studies be included or not? Ideally, potentially difficult decisions like this should be addressed a priori in the review eligibility criteria; however, it is not possible to anticipate every nuance in advance and independent screening of every full-text report helps ensure consistency in decision-making.

Although time consuming, correspondence with investigators of potentially relevant studies, for example to ask whether the correct reference standard was used or to clarify other aspects of study eligibility, can be very fruitful and help ensure all relevant studies are included (see Chapter 7, Section 7.2.2).

During this phase, review authors may also encounter multiple reports of the same study, or multiple studies in one study report (see also Chapter 7, Section 7.2.1). As the studies, and not the reports, are the unit of analysis in a systematic review, it is important to find out whether multiple reports from the same studies have been published and to link together multiple reports of the same study. It is possible, for example, that a study was designed as a comparative study, but that the data for each test were reported in a separate publication.

Studies are often excluded because complete 2×2 tables could not be derived. However, if the study meets all the other eligibility criteria for a review, then it may be important to flag how many studies could have been summarized but did not provide the required data.

6.7   Future developments in literature searching and selection

One problem in searching for and selecting test accuracy studies is the lack of relevant index terms to capture the study design in some bibliographic databases. Another problem is that relevant information may be reported in various study designs (see Chapter 3). In the long term it is hoped that there will be a mechanism for re-tagging test accuracy studies in MEDLINE with a specific suitable Publication Type (similar to the way in which randomized controlled trials are now labelled) to facilitate searching. Such a term, 'diagnostic test accuracy study', was introduced in Embase in 2011 (Cochrane Community 2011) as a check tag, a designated term for indexers to use to denote study types. However, 'diagnostic test accuracy study' retrieves only about half of the test accuracy studies in Embase (Gurung 2020) published since 2011, and obviously none before that date.

More promising developments include crowdsourcing and solutions involving the use of artificial intelligence, such as machine learning. Searching for thousands of test accuracy studies using a very broad and sensitive search is one thing, but these records need to be screened for relevance as well. Cochrane is exploring innovative methods including crowdsourcing techniques (where many volunteers contribute their time to screen records) to assist in the screening of otherwise unmanageable numbers of records and to minimize the risk of missing relevant studies. So far, crowd screening has been mainly used to identify randomized controlled trials (Noel-Storr 2021), but it is hoped that this screening approach could be developed to identify studies for systematic reviews of diagnostic test accuracy and generate a sufficiently large data set from which to develop a test accuracy study classifier, similar to the Cochrane RCT Classifier (Thomas 2021) and the recently validated Cochrane COVID-19 Study Classifier, using machine learning techniques (Shemilt 2022). New techniques, including text mining or deep learning methods, have applications for search strategy design, for screening the results for systematic reviews and for data extraction and quality assessment. Research has shown that these approaches may improve the efficiency and accuracy of these tasks (Marshall 2019, Norman 2019). These approaches may be especially helpful for review updates, although the final performance of the technique chosen strongly depends on careful data preparation (data pre-processing) (Lange 2021). These are fast-moving areas of research and development, and review authors are advised to keep an eye on such techniques and approaches, to be able to take advantage of developments as they become available.

6.8   Chapter information

Authors: René Spijker (*Cochrane Netherlands, Utrecht University; Medical Library, University of Amsterdam, The Netherlands*), Jacqueline Dinnes (*Institute of Applied Health Research, University of Birmingham, UK*), Julie Glanville (glanville.info, York, UK), Anne Eisinga (Cochrane UK, Oxford, UK).

Sources of support: Jacqueline Dinnes is supported by the NIHR Birmingham Biomedical Research Centre at the University Hospitals Birmingham NHS Foundation Trust and the University of Birmingham. The views expressed are those of the authors and not necessarily those of the NHS, the NIHR or the Department of Health and Social Care. No other authors declare sources of support for writing this chapter.

Declarations of interest: René Spijker is an Information Specialist with Cochrane Netherlands. Jacqueline Dinnes is a member of Cochrane's Diagnostic Test Accuracy Editorial Team. Julie Glanville was a co-convenor of the Cochrane Information Retrieval Methods Group at the time of writing the chapter, and is co-producer of several websites and resources mentioned in the chapter: ISSG Search Filters Resource, SuRe Info and a Clinical Trials Registers resource. Anne Eisinga is an Information Specialist with Cochrane UK. The authors declare no other potential conflicts of interest relevant to the topic of their chapter.

Acknowledgements: This chapter re-uses and builds on material included in the following chapters of the *Cochrane Handbook for Systematic Reviews of Interventions* to ensure consistency in guidance for authors of Cochrane Reviews: (1) Lefebvre C, Glanville J, Briscoe S, Littlewood A, Marshall C, Metzendorf M-I, Noel-Storr A, Rader T, Shokraneh F, Thomas J, Wieland LS. Chapter 4: Searching for and selecting studies. In: Higgins JPT, Thomas J, Chandler J, Cumpston M, Li T, Page MJ, Welch VA (editors). *Cochrane Handbook for Systematic Reviews of Interventions* version 6.2 (updated February 2021). Cochrane, 2021. (2) Lefebvre C, Glanville J, Briscoe S, Littlewood A, Marshall C, Metzendorf M-I, Noel-Storr A, Rader T, Shokraneh F, Thomas J, Wieland LS. Technical supplement to Chapter 4: Searching for and selecting studies. In: Higgins JPT, Thomas J, Chandler J, Cumpston M, Li T, Page MJ, Welch VA (editors). *Cochrane Handbook for Systematic Reviews of Interventions* version 6.2 (updated February 2021). Cochrane, 2021. We are grateful to the authors for kindly sharing pre-publication drafts with us.

The authors thank Lotty Hooft, Madhukar Pai, Yngve Falck-Ytter, Lucas Bachmann, Fritz Grossenbacher, Mark Bruyneel, Ruth Mitchell, Henrica CW de Vet, Ingrid I Riphagen, Bert Aertgeerts, Daniel Pewsner and the many information specialists for contributions to a previous version of this chapter.

The authors would like to thank April Coombe, Anna Noel-Storr and the Cochrane Information Specialist Executive for helpful peer review comments.

6.9   References

Bachmann LM, Coray R, Estermann P, Ter Riet G. Identifying diagnostic studies in MEDLINE: reducing the number needed to read. *Journal of the American Medical Informatics Association* 2002; **9**: 653–658.

Bayliss S, Davenport C. Locating systematic reviews of diagnostic studies: how five specialist review databases measure up [abstract]. Fourth Annual Meeting of Health Technology Assessment International (HTAi); 2007 Jun 17-20; Barcelona, Catalonia, Spain.

Belter CW. Citation analysis as a literature search method for systematic reviews. *Journal of the Association for Information Science and Technology* 2016; **67**: 2766–2777.

Belter CW. A relevance ranking method for citation-based search results. *Scientometrics* 2017; **112**: 731–746.

Beynon R, Leeflang MM, McDonald S, Eisinga A, Mitchell RL, Whiting P, Glanville JM. Search strategies to identify diagnostic accuracy studies in MEDLINE and EMBASE. *Cochrane Database of Systematic Reviews* 2013; **9**: MR000022.

Bossuyt PM, Reitsma JB, Bruns DE, Gatsonis CA, Glasziou PP, Irwig L, Lijmer JG, Moher D, Rennie D, de Vet HC, Kressel HY, Rifai N, Golub RM, Altman DG, Hooft L, Korevaar DA, Cohen JF. STARD 2015: an updated list of essential items for reporting diagnostic accuracy studies. *BMJ* 2015; **351**: h5527.

Boughton SL, Wilkinson J, Bero L. When beauty is but skin deep: dealing with problematic studies in systematic reviews. *Cochrane Database of Systematic Reviews* 2021; **6**: ED000152.

Bramer WM, Rethlefsen ML, Kleijnen J, Franco OH. Optimal database combinations for literature searches in systematic reviews: a prospective exploratory study. *Systematic Reviews* 2017; **6**: 245.

Brazzelli M, Lewis SC, Deeks JJ, Sandercock PA. No evidence of bias in the process of publication of diagnostic accuracy studies in stroke submitted as abstracts. *Journal of Clinical Epidemiology* 2009; **62**: 425–430.

Briscoe S. Web searching for systematic reviews: a case study of reporting standards in the UK Health Technology Assessment programme. *BMC Research Notes* 2015; **8**: 153.

Cherpak LA, Korevaar DA, McGrath TA, Dang W, Walker D, Salameh J-P, Dehmoobad Sharifabadi A, McInnes MDF. Publication bias: association of diagnostic accuracy in radiology conference abstracts with full-text publication. *Radiology* 2019; **292**: 120–126.

Cochrane Community. EMBASE introduces diagnostic test accuracy study as an indexing term 2011. community.cochrane.org/news/embase-introduces-diagnostic-test-accuracy-study-indexing-term.

Cohen JF, Korevaar DA, Wang J, Spijker R, Bossuyt PM. Should we search Chinese biomedical databases when performing systematic reviews? *Systematic Reviews* 2015; **4**: 23.

Cohen JF, Korevaar DA, Gatsonis CA, Glasziou PP, Hooft L, Moher D, Reitsma JB, de Vet HC, Bossuyt PM. STARD for Abstracts: essential items for reporting diagnostic accuracy studies in journal or conference abstracts. *BMJ* 2017; **358**: j3751.

Cohen JF, Korevaar DA, Bossuyt PM. Diagnostic accuracy studies need more informative abstracts. *European Journal of Clinical Microbiology and Infectious Diseases* 2019; **38**: 1383–1385.

Cohen JF, Deeks JJ, Hooft L, Salameh J-P, Korevaar DA, Gatsonis C, Hopewell S, Hunt HA, Hyde CJ, Leeflang MM, Macaskill P, McGrath TA, Moher D, Reitsma JB, Rutjes AWS, Takwoingi Y, Tonelli M, Whiting P, Willis BH, Thombs B, Bossuyt PM, McInnes MDF. Preferred reporting items for journal and conference abstracts of systematic reviews and meta-analyses of diagnostic test accuracy studies (PRISMA-DTA for Abstracts): checklist, explanation, and elaboration. *BMJ* 2021; **372**: n265.

Cooper C, Dawson S, Peters J, Varley-Campbell J, Cockcroft E, Hendon J, Churchill R. Revisiting the need for a literature search narrative: a brief methodological note. *Research Synthesis Methods* 2018; **9**: 361–365.

Devillé W, Buntinx F. Guidelines for conducting systematic reviews of studies evaluating the accuracy of diagnostic tests. In: JA Knottnerus, editor. *The evidence base of clinical diagnosis*. London: BMJ Books; 2002a.

Devillé WL, Buntinx F, Bouter LM, Montori VM, de Vet HC, van der Windt DA, Bezemer PD. Conducting systematic reviews of diagnostic studies: didactic guidelines. *BMC Medical Research Methodology* 2002b; **2**: 9.

Dickersin K. Publication bias: recognizing the problem, understanding its origins and scope, and preventing harm. In: Rothstei H, Sutton A, Borenstein M, editors. *Publication bias in meta-analysis: prevention, assessment and adjustments*. Chichester (UK): John Wiley & Sons; 2005.

Doust JA, Pietrzak E, Sanders S, Glasziou PP. Identifying studies for systematic reviews of diagnostic tests was difficult due to the poor sensitivity and precision of methodologic filters and the lack of information in the abstract. *Journal of Clinical Epidemiology* 2005; **58**: 444–449.

Easterbrook PJ, Berlin JA, Gopalan R, Matthews DR. Publication bias in clinical research. *Lancet* 1991; **337**: 867–872.

Egger M, Smith GD. Bias in location and selection of studies. *BMJ* 1998; **316**: 61–66.

Elia N, Wager E, Tramèr MR. Fate of articles that warranted retraction due to ethical concerns: a descriptive cross-sectional study. *PloS One* 2014; **9**: e85846.

Eysenbach G, Tuische J, Diepgen TL. Evaluation of the usefulness of Internet searches to identify unpublished clinical trials for systematic reviews. *Medical Informatics and the Internet in Medicine* 2001; **26**: 203–218.

Falck-Ytter Y, Motschall E. New search filter for diagnostic studies: Ovid and PubMed versions not the same (rapid response) 2004. www.bmj.com/rapid-response/2011/10/30/new-search-filter-diagnostic-studies-ovid-and-pubmed-versions-not-same.

Fielding AM, Powell A. Using Medline to achieve an evidence-based approach to diagnostic clinical biochemistry. *Annals of Clinical Biochemistry* 2002; **39**: 345–350.

Glanville J, Cikalo M, Crawford F, Dozier M, McIntosh H. Handsearching did not yield additional unique FDG-PET diagnostic test accuracy studies compared with electronic searches: a preliminary investigation. *Research Synthesis Methods* 2012; **3**: 202–213.

Glanville J, Higgins C, Holubowich C, Spijker R, Fitzgerald A. Diagnostic accuracy. In: SuRe Info: Summarized Research in Information Retrieval for HTA. Last updated 24 October 2021. www.sure-info.org//diagnostic-accuracy.

Godin K, Stapleton J, Kirkpatrick SI, Hanning RM, Leatherdale ST. Applying systematic review search methods to the grey literature: a case study examining guidelines for school-based breakfast programs in Canada. *Systematic Reviews* 2015; **4**: 138.

Golder S, McIntosh HM, Duffy S, Glanville J, Centre for Reviews and Dissemination and Cochrane Centre Search Filters Design Group. Developing efficient search strategies to identify reports of adverse effects in MEDLINE and EMBASE. *Health Information and Libraries Journal* 2006; **23**: 3–12.

Greenhalgh T, Peacock R. Effectiveness and efficiency of search methods in systematic reviews of complex evidence: audit of primary sources. *BMJ* 2005; **331**: 1064–1065.

Gurung P, Makineli S, Spijker R, Leeflang MMG. The Emtree term 'diagnostic test accuracy study' retrieved less than half of the diagnostic accuracy studies in Embase. *Journal of Clinical Epidemiology* 2020; **126**: 116–121.

Gusenbauer M, Haddaway NR. Which academic search systems are suitable for systematic reviews or meta-analyses? Evaluating retrieval qualities of Google Scholar, PubMed, and 26 other resources. *Research Synthesis Methods* 2020; **11**: 181–217.

Hewitt CE, Perry AE, Adams B, Gilbody SM. Screening and case finding for depression in offender populations: a systematic review of diagnostic properties. *Journal of Affective Disorders* 2011; **128**: 72–82.

Hooft L, Bossuyt PM. Prospective registration of marker evaluation studies: time to act. *Clinical Chemistry* 2011; **57**: 1684–1686.

Hopewell S, Clarke M, Mallett S. Grey literature and systematic reviews. In: Rothstein HR, Sutton AJ, Borenstein M, editors. *Publication bias in meta-analysis: Prevention, assessment and adjustments*. Chichester (UK): John Wiley & Sons; 2005.

Hopewell S, McDonald S, Clarke MJ, Egger M. Grey literature in meta-analyses of randomized trials of health care interventions. *Cochrane Database of Systematic Reviews* 2007; **2**: MR000010.

Horsley T, Dingwall O, Sampson M. Checking reference lists to find additional studies for systematic reviews. *Cochrane Database of Systematic Reviews* 2011; **8**: MR000026.

Janssens ACJW, Gwinn M. Novel citation-based search method for scientific literature: application to meta-analyses. *BMC Medical Research Methodology* 2015; **15**: 84.

Janssens ACJW, Gwinn M, Brockman JE, Powell K, Goodman M. Novel citation-based search method for scientific literature: a validation study. *BMC Medical Research Methodology* 2020; **20**: 25.

Jiang Y, Lin C, Meng W, Yu C, Cohen AM, Smalheiser NR. Rule-based deduplication of article records from bibliographic databases. *Database: The Journal of Biological Databases and Curation* 2014; **2014**: bat086.

Kaizik MA, Hancock MJ, Herbert RD. DiTA: a database of diagnostic test accuracy studies for physiotherapists. *Journal of Physiotherapy* 2019; **65**: 119–120.

Kaizik MA, Hancock MJ, Herbert RD. A description of the primary studies of diagnostic test accuracy indexed on the DiTA database. *Physiotherapy Research International* 2020; **25**: e1871.

Korevaar DA, Ochodo EA, Bossuyt PM, Hooft L. Publication and reporting of test accuracy studies registered in ClinicalTrials.gov. *Clinical Chemistry* 2014a; **60**: 651–659.

Korevaar DA, van Enst WA, Spijker R, Bossuyt PM, Hooft L. Reporting quality of diagnostic accuracy studies: a systematic review and meta-analysis of investigations on adherence to STARD. *Evidence-Based Medicine* 2014b; **19**: 47–54.

Korevaar DA, Wang J, van Enst WA, Leeflang MM, Hooft L, Smidt N, Bossuyt PM. Reporting diagnostic accuracy studies: some improvements after 10 years of STARD. *Radiology* 2015; **274**: 781–789.

Korevaar DA, Cohen JF, Spijker R, Saldanha IJ, Dickersin K, Virgili G, Hooft L, Bossuyt PM. Reported estimates of diagnostic accuracy in ophthalmology conference abstracts were not associated with full-text publication. *Journal of Clinical Epidemiology* 2016; **79**: 96–103.

Korevaar DA, Hooft L, Askie LM, Barbour V, Faure H, Gatsonis CA, Hunter KE, Kressel HY, Lippman H, McInnes MDF, Moher D, Rifai N, Cohen JF, Bossuyt PMM. Facilitating prospective registration of diagnostic accuracy studies: a STARD Initiative. *Clinical Chemistry* 2017; **63**: 1331–1341.

Korevaar DA, Salameh JP, Vali Y, Cohen JF, McInnes MDF, Spijker R, Bossuyt PM. Searching practices and inclusion of unpublished studies in systematic reviews of diagnostic accuracy. *Research Synthesis Methods* 2020; **11**: 343–353.

Lange T, Schwarzer G, Datzmann T, Binder H. Machine learning for identifying relevant publications in updates of systematic reviews of diagnostic test studies. *Research Synthesis Methods* 2021; **12**: 506–515.

Leeflang MM, Scholten RJ, Rutjes AW, Reitsma JB, Bossuyt PM. Use of methodological search filters to identify diagnostic accuracy studies can lead to the omission of relevant studies. *Journal of Clinical Epidemiology* 2006; **59**: 234–240.

Lefebvre C, Glanville J, Wieland LS, Coles B, Weightman AL. Methodological developments in searching for studies for systematic reviews: past, present and future? *Systematic Reviews* 2013; **2**: 78.

Lefebvre C, Glanville J, Briscoe S, Littlewood A, Marshall C, Metzendorf M-I, Noel-Storr A, Rader T, Shokraneh F, Thomas J, Wieland L. Technical Supplement to Chapter 4: Searching for and selecting studies. In: Higgins J, Thomas J, Chandler J, Cumpston M, Li T, Page M, Welch V, editors. *Cochrane Handbook for Systematic Reviews of Interventions* Version 6.2 (updated February 2021). Cochrane, 2021. Available from www.training.cochrane.org/handbook.

Mallett S, Hopewell S, Clarke M. Grey literature in systematic reviews: the first 1000 Cochrane systematic reviews. *Cochrane Collaboration Methods Groups Newsletter* 2002; **6**.

Marshall IJ, Wallace BC. Toward systematic review automation: a practical guide to using machine learning tools in research synthesis. *Systematic Reviews* 2019; **8**: 163.

McAuley L, Pham B, Tugwell P, Moher D. Does the inclusion of grey literature influence estimates of intervention effectiveness reported in meta-analyses? *Lancet* 2000; **356**: 1228–1231.

McInnes MDF, Moher D, Thombs BD, McGrath TA, Bossuyt PM, Clifford T, Cohen JF, Deeks JJ, Gatsonis C, Hooft L, Hunt HA, Hyde CJ, Korevaar DA, Leeflang MMG, Macaskill P, Reitsma JB, Rodin R, Rutjes AWS, Salameh JP, Stevens A, Takwoingi Y, Tonelli M, Weeks L, Whiting P, Willis BH. Preferred Reporting Items for a Systematic Review and Meta-analysis of Diagnostic Test Accuracy Studies: The PRISMA-DTA Statement. *JAMA* 2018; **319**: 388–396.

Meert D, Torabi N, Costella J. Impact of librarians on reporting of the literature searching component of pediatric systematic reviews. *Journal of the Medical Library Association: JMLA* 2016; **104**: 267–277.

Metzendorf M. Why medical information specialists should routinely form part of teams producing high quality systematic reviews – a Cochrane perspective. *Journal of the European Association for Health Information and Libraries* 2016; **12**: 6–9.

Mitchell R, Rinaldi F, Craig J. Performance of published search strategies for studies of diagnostic test accuracy (SDTAs) in MEDLINE and EMBASE [abstract]. XIII Cochrane Colloquium; 2005; Melbourne, Australia. Available at www.Cochrane.org/colloquia/abstracts/melbourne/O-01.htm.

Niederstadt C, Droste S. Reporting and presenting information retrieval processes: the need for optimizing common practice in health technology assessment. *International Journal of Technology Assessment in Health Care* 2010; **26**: 450–457.

Noel-Storr A, Dooley G, Elliott J, Steele E, Shemilt I, Mavergames C, Wisniewski S, McDonald S, Murano M, Glanville J, Foxlee R, Beecher D, Ware J, Thomas J. An evaluation of Cochrane Crowd found that crowdsourcing produced accurate results in identifying randomized trials. *Journal of Clinical Epidemiology* 2021; **133**: 130–139.

Noel-Storr AH, McCleery JM, Richard E, Ritchie CW, Flicker L, Cullum SJ, Davis D, Quinn TJ, Hyde C, Rutjes AW, Smailagic N, Marcus S, Black S, Blennow K, Brayne C, Fiorivanti M, Johnson JK, Köpke S, Schneider LS, Simmons A, Mattsson N, Zetterberg H, Bossuyt PM, Wilcock G, McShane R. Reporting standards for studies of diagnostic test accuracy in dementia: the STARDdem Initiative. *Neurology* 2014; **83**: 364–373.

Norman CR, Leeflang MMG, Porcher R, Névéol A. Measuring the impact of screening automation on meta-analyses of diagnostic test accuracy. *Systematic Reviews* 2019; **8**: 243.

Ogilvie D, Hamilton V, Egan M, Petticrew M. Systematic reviews of health effects of social interventions: 1. Finding the evidence: how far should you go? *Journal of Epidemiology and Community Health* 2005; **59**: 804–808.

Pereira RA, Puga MEdS, Atallah ÁN, Macedo EC, Macedo CR. lilacs search strategy for systematic reviews of diagnostic test accuracy studies. *Health Information and Libraries Journal* 2019; **36**: 223–243.

Petersen H, Poon J, Poon SK, Loy C. Increased workload for systematic review literature searches of diagnostic tests compared with treatments: challenges and opportunities. *JMIR Medical Informatics* 2014; **2**: e11.

Preston L, Carroll C, Gardois P, Paisley S, Kaltenthaler E. Improving search efficiency for systematic reviews of diagnostic test accuracy: an exploratory study to assess the viability of limiting to MEDLINE, EMBASE and reference checking. *Systematic Reviews* 2015; **4**: 82.

Quinn TJ, Fearon P, Noel-Storr AH, Young C, McShane R, Stott DJ. Informant Questionnaire on Cognitive Decline in the Elderly (IQCODE) for the detection of dementia within community dwelling populations. *Cochrane Database of Systematic Reviews* 2021; **7**: CD010079.

Rathbone J, Carter M, Hoffmann T, Glasziou P. Better duplicate detection for systematic reviewers: evaluation of Systematic Review Assistant-Deduplication Module. *Systematic Reviews* 2015; **4**: 6.

Rethlefsen ML, Farrell AM, Osterhaus Trzasko LC, Brigham TJ. Librarian co-authors correlated with higher quality reported search strategies in general internal medicine systematic reviews. *Journal of Clinical Epidemiology* 2015; **68**: 617–626.

Rethlefsen ML, Kirtley S, Waffenschmidt S, Ayala AP, Moher D, Page MJ, Koffel JB, Blunt H, Brigham T, Chang S, Clark J, Conway A, Couban R, de Kock S, Farrah K, Fehrmann P, Foster M, Fowler SA, Glanville J, Harris E, Hoffecker L, Isojarvi J, Kaunelis D, Ket H, Levay P, Lyon J, McGowan J, Murad MH, Nicholson J, Pannabecker V, Paynter R, Pinotti R, Ross-White A, Sampson M, Shields T, Stevens A, Sutton A, Weinfurter E, Wright K, Young S, PRISMA-S Group. PRISMA-S: an extension to the PRISMA Statement for Reporting Literature Searches in Systematic Reviews. *Systematic Reviews* 2021; **10**: 39.

Reveiz L, Cardona AF, Ospina EG, de Agular S. An e-mail survey identified unpublished studies for systematic reviews. *Journal of Clinical Epidemiology* 2006; **59**: 755–758.

Rice DB, Kloda LA, Levis B, Qi B, Kingsland E, Thombs BD. Are MEDLINE searches sufficient for systematic reviews and meta-analyses of the diagnostic accuracy of depression screening tools? A review of meta-analyses. *Journal of Psychosomatic Research* 2016; **87**: 7–13.

Rifai N, Altman DG, Bossuyt PM. Reporting bias in diagnostic and prognostic studies: time for action. *Clinical Chemistry* 2008; **54**: 1101–1103.

Ritchie G, Glanville J, Lefebvre C. Do published search filters to identify diagnostic test accuracy studies perform adequately? *Health Information and Libraries Journal* 2007; **24**: 188–192.

Roundtree AK, Kallen MA, Lopez-Olivo MA, Kimmel B, Skidmore B, Ortiz Z, Cox V, Suarez-Almazor ME. Poor reporting of search strategy and conflict of interest in over 250 narrative and systematic reviews of two biologic agents in arthritis: a systematic review. *Journal of Clinical Epidemiology* 2009; **62**: 128–137.

Salameh J-P, Bossuyt PM, McGrath TA, Thombs BD, Hyde CJ, Macaskill P, Deeks JJ, Leeflang M, Korevaar DA, Whiting P, Takwoingi Y, Reitsma JB, Cohen JF, Frank RA, Hunt HA, Hooft

L, Rutjes AWS, Willis BH, Gatsonis C, Levis B, Moher D, McInnes MDF. Preferred reporting items for systematic review and meta-analysis of diagnostic test accuracy studies (PRISMA-DTA): explanation, elaboration, and checklist. *BMJ* 2020; **370**: m2632.

Salameh JP, McInnes MDF, Moher D, Thombs BD, McGrath TA, Frank R, Dehmoobad Sharifabadi A, Kraaijpoel N, Levis B, Bossuyt PM. Completeness of reporting of systematic reviews of diagnostic test accuracy based on the PRISMA-DTA reporting guideline. *Clinical Chemistry* 2019; **65**: 291–301.

Sampson M, Barrowman NJ, Moher D, Klassen TP, Pham B, Platt R, St John PD, Viola R, Raina P. Should meta-analysts search Embase in addition to Medline? *Journal of Clinical Epidemiology* 2003; **56**: 943–955.

Sampson M, Shojania KG, McGowan J, Daniel R, Rader T, Iansavichene AE, Ji J, Ansari MT, Moher D. Surveillance search techniques identified the need to update systematic reviews. *Journal of Clinical Epidemiology* 2008; **61**: 755–762.

Shemilt I, Noel-Storr A, Thomas J, Featherstone R, Mavergames C. Machine learning reduced workload for the Cochrane COVID-19 Study Register: development and evaluation of the Cochrane COVID-19 Study Classifier. *Systematic Reviews* 2022; **11**: 15.

Smart RG. The importance of negative results in psychological research. *Canadian Psychologist* 1964; **5**: 225–232.

Smith ML. Sex bias in counseling and psychotherapy. *Psychological Bulletin* 1980; **87**: 392–407.

Song F, Eastwood A, Gilbody S, Duley L, Sutton A. Publication and related biases. *Health Technology Assessment* 2000; **4**.

Sounderajah V, Ashrafian H, Golub RM, Shetty S, De Fauw J, Hooft L, Moons K, Collins G, Moher D, Bossuyt PM, Darzi A, Karthikesalingam A, Denniston AK, Mateen BA, Ting D, Treanor D, King D, Greaves F, Godwin J, Pearson-Stuttard J, Harling L, McInnes M, Rifai N, Tomasev N, Normahani P, Whiting P, Aggarwal R, Vollmer S, Markar SR, Panch T, Liu X. Developing a reporting guideline for artificial intelligence-centred diagnostic test accuracy studies: the STARD-AI protocol. *BMJ Open* 2021; **11**: e047709.

Stansfield C, Brunton G, Rees R. Search wide, dig deep: literature searching for qualitative research. An analysis of the publication formats and information sources used for four systematic reviews in public health. *Research Synthesis Methods* 2014; **5**: 142–151.

Thomas J, McDonald S, Noel-Storr A, Shemilt I, Elliott J, Mavergames C, Marshall IJ. Machine learning reduced workload with minimal risk of missing studies: development and evaluation of a randomized controlled trial classifier for Cochrane Reviews. *Journal of Clinical Epidemiology* 2021; **133**: 140–151.

Treanor LM, Frank RA, Atyani A, Dehmoobad Sharifabadi A, Hallgrimson Z, Fabiano N, Salameh JP, McGrath TA, Korevaar DA, Bossuyt P, McInnes MDF. Reporting bias in imaging diagnostic test accuracy studies: are studies with positive conclusions or titles submitted and published faster? *AJR: American Journal of Roentgenology* 2021; **216**: 225–232.

Tsujimoto H, Tsujimoto Y, Nakata Y, Akazawa M, Kataoka Y. Ultrasonography for confirmation of gastric tube placement. *Cochrane Database of Systematic Reviews* 2017; **4**: CD012083.

van der Weijden T, CJ IJ, Dinant GJ, van Duijn NP, de Vet R, Buntinx F. Identifying relevant diagnostic studies in MEDLINE. The diagnostic value of the erythrocyte sedimentation rate (ESR) and dipstick as an example. *Family Practice* 1997; **14**: 204–208.

van der Windt DA, Simons E, Riphagen, II, Ammendolia C, Verhagen AP, Laslett M, Devillé W, Deyo RA, Bouter LM, de Vet HC, Aertgeerts B. Physical examination for lumbar radiculopathy due to disc herniation in patients with low-back pain. *Cochrane Database of Systematic Reviews* 2010; **2**: CD007431.

van Enst WA, Scholten RJPM, Whiting P, Zwinderman AH, Hooft L. Meta-epidemiologic analysis indicates that MEDLINE searches are sufficient for diagnostic test accuracy systematic reviews. *Journal of Clinical Epidemiology* 2014; **67**: 1192–1199.

van Enst WA, Naaktgeboren CA, Ochodo EA, de Groot JAH, Leeflang MM, Reitsma JB, Scholten RJPM, Moons KGM, Zwinderman AH, Bossuyt PMM, Hooft L. Small-study effects and time trends in diagnostic test accuracy meta-analyses: a meta-epidemiological study. *Systematic Reviews* 2015; **4**: 66.

Vincent S, Greenley S, Beaven O. Clinical evidence diagnosis: developing a sensitive search strategy to retrieve diagnostic studies on deep vein thrombosis: a pragmatic approach. *Health Information and Libraries Journal* 2003; **20**: 150–159.

Vogel U, Windeler J. [Factors modifying frequency of publications of clinical research results exemplified by medical dissertations]. *Deutsche Medizinische Wochenschrift* 2000; **125**: 110–113.

Whiting P, Westwood M, Bojke L, Palmer S, Richardson G, Cooper J, Watt I, Glanville J, Sculpher M, Kleijnen J. Clinical effectiveness and cost-effectiveness of tests for the diagnosis and investigation of urinary tract infection in children: a systematic review and economic model. *Health Technology Assessment* 2006; **10**: iii–iv, xi-xiii, 1-154.

Whiting P, Westwood M, Burke M, Sterne J, Glanville J. Systematic reviews of test accuracy should search a range of databases to identify primary studies. *Journal of Clinical Epidemiology* 2008; **61**: 357–364.

Wilczynski NL, Walker CJ, McKibbon KA, Haynes RB. Reasons for the loss of sensitivity and specificity of methodologic MeSH terms and textwords in MEDLINE. *Proceedings Symposium on Computer Applications in Medical Care* 1995: 436–440.

Wilson C, Kerr D, Noel-Storr A, Quinn TJ. Associations with publication and assessing publication bias in dementia diagnostic test accuracy studies. *International Journal of Geriatric Psychiatry* 2015; **30**: 1250–1256.

Zarei F, Zeinali-Rafsanjani B. Assessment of adherence of diagnostic accuracy studies published in radiology journals to STARD statement indexed in Web of Science, PubMed & Scopus in 2015. *Journal of Biomedical Physics and Engineering* 2018; **8**: 311–324.

Zimpel T, Windeler J. [Publications of dissertations on unconventional medical therapy and diagnosis procedures—a contribution to 'publication bias']. *Forschende Komplementarmedizin und Klassische Naturheilkunde/Research in Complementary and Natural Classical Medicine* 2000; **7**: 71–74.

7

Collecting data

Jacqueline Dinnes, Jonathan J. Deeks, Mariska M. Leeflang and Tianjing Li

---

KEY POINTS

- Systematic reviews have studies, rather than reports, as the unit of interest. Multiple reports of the same study need to be identified and linked together, and multiple studies in the same report need to be separated.
- Studies may be published or unpublished, available as pre-prints or in trial registers, regulatory documents or clinical study reports. Where studies are reported in multiple sources, plans are needed to resolve discrepancies if information is inconsistent.
- Data extraction includes collection of study characteristics, methodological detail needed to assess study quality, as well as study findings. The key to successful data collection is to construct easy-to-use forms and collect sufficient and unambiguous data that faithfully represent the source in a structured and organized manner.
- Review authors are encouraged to develop outlines of tables and figures that will appear in the review to facilitate the design of data collection forms.
- Effort should be made to identify and structure data needed for meta-analyses, including 2×2 data and relevant covariates for heterogeneity investigations or sensitivity analyses. Study data may need to be calculated or converted from data reported in diverse formats.
- Review authors should choose a data collection tool that is suited to the review type, team size and resources available.
- Duplicate independent data extraction is recommended for critical data items, such as study findings and where subjective judgement is involved. Double-checking of all data extraction and data entry is strongly recommended.
- Data should be collected and archived in a form that allows future access and data sharing.

This chapter should be cited as: Dinnes J, Deeks JJ, Leeflang MM, Li T. Chapter 7: Collecting data. In: Deeks JJ, Bossuyt PM, Leeflang MM, Takwoingi Y, editors. *Cochrane Handbook for Systematic Reviews of Diagnostic Test Accuracy*. 1st edition. Chichester (UK): John Wiley & Sons, 2023: 131–168.

> This chapter re-uses and builds on material included in the following chapter of the *Cochrane Handbook for Systematic Reviews of Interventions* to ensure consistency in guidance for authors of Cochrane Reviews.
> Li T, Higgins JPT, Deeks JJ (editors). Chapter 5: Collecting data. In: Higgins JPT, Thomas J, Chandler J, Cumpston M, Li T, Page MJ, Welch VA (editors). *Cochrane Handbook for Systematic Reviews of Interventions* version 6.1 (updated September 2020). Cochrane, 2020.

7.1 Introduction

The findings of a systematic review depend critically on decisions relating to which data from the included studies are presented and analysed. Data collected for systematic reviews should be accurate, complete and accessible for future updates of the review and for data sharing. Methods used for these decisions should be transparent; they should be chosen to minimize biases and human error. This chapter describes approaches that should be used in systematic reviews of test accuracy for collecting data, including extraction of data directly from journal articles and other study reports.

7.2 Sources of data

Journal articles are the source of the majority of data included in systematic reviews of test accuracy (Korevaar 2020). They are relatively easy to identify, provide useful information about study methods and results, and data can be extracted quickly. A study can be reported in multiple journal articles, each selecting different subgroups of the population or reporting the results of different tests or testing thresholds. It is therefore important to link together multiple reports of the same study.

Preprints and online publications are early versions of articles that may subsequently be accepted and published in journals. These publications may be found in open access repositories, such as medRxiv or F1000, or in preprint repositories belonging to a journal or scientific publisher. The status of these publications varies from first drafts, to yet to be peer-reviewed final drafts, to peer-reviewed pre-publication versions. This means that data quality varies and that versions may follow each other quickly. Preprints therefore may require extra checks to ensure that the extracted data are accurate, and subsequent checking when final peer-reviewed publications are available.

Conference abstracts are commonly available and can provide a means of identifying unpublished studies. However, they provide limited information on study methods and can be highly variable in reliability, accuracy and level of detail (Li 2017).

Errata and **letters** can be important sources of information about studies, including critical weaknesses and retractions, and review authors should examine these if they are identified. Letters may also report additional test accuracy data from the correspondents' own institution, for example in response to a primary study previously published in the same journal. Furthermore, some journals publish short reports of studies as a research letter.

Trials registers (e.g. ClinicalTrials.gov) catalogue trials that have been planned, started or completed, and have become an important data source for identifying trials, for comparing published outcomes and results with those planned, and for obtaining efficacy and safety data that are not available elsewhere. Trials registers can also include records for test accuracy studies, although most are not registered before their initiation (Korevaar 2014, Korevaar 2017).

Clinical study reports (CSRs) contain unabridged and comprehensive descriptions of the clinical problem, design, conduct and results of clinical trials, following a structure and content guidance prescribed by the International Conference on Harmonisation (ICH 1995). CSRs must be submitted by pharmaceutical companies to regulatory authorities in order to obtain marketing approval of drugs and biologics for a specific indication. CSRs are less likely to exist or will be difficult to obtain for the majority of medical tests or devices, as the same detailed documentation is not required by regulators as for drug trials. Manufacturers of in vitro diagnostics (IVDs) often provide some information on clinical performance characteristics in the package inserts or 'instructions for use' for tests. Limited detail is usually reported in regard to study methods and participant characteristics. Caution should be taken to clearly identify the source of such data if used in a systematic review.

Regulatory reviews such as those available from the US Food and Drug Administration, the World Health Organization (WHO), the European Medicines Agency, Centers for Disease Control and Prevention or independent public health organizations such as national reference laboratories may provide useful information about general medical devices (including software-based devices) and IVD medical devices that has been submitted by manufacturers for marketing approval (www.fda.gov/medical-devices/ivd-regulatory-assistance/overview-ivd-regulation). These documents are summaries of submitted evidence, prepared by agency staff as part of the process of approving the products for marketing. In the EU the evidence required to be submitted in support of a device varies according to the device class or perceived risk. For most tests, there is no minimum performance standard.

Individual participant data (IPD) are usually sought directly from the researchers responsible for the study, or may be identified from open data repositories (e.g. www.clinicalstudydatarequest.com). Access to IPD has the advantage of allowing review authors to reanalyse the data flexibly, in accordance with the preferred analysis methods outlined in the protocol, and can reduce the variation in analysis methods across studies included in the review (Riley 2008, Stewart 2015). Although IPD analyses for systematic reviews of test accuracy are available (e.g. Hooper 2015), they are less common than for intervention reviews.

7.2.1 Studies (not reports) as the unit of interest

In a systematic review, *studies* rather than *reports* of studies are the principal unit of interest. Often, data for series of participants from an individual institution, or who were recruited to a particular study, are published multiple times with slight differences in periods of recruitment or eligibility criteria and limited cross-referencing between study reports. Since a study may have been reported in several sources, a comprehensive search for studies for the review may identify several reports from a potentially relevant study (Mayo-Wilson 2017a, Mayo-Wilson 2018). Conversely, a report (e.g. Smith 2020) may describe more than one study, in which case several study iden-tifiers (e.g. Smith 2020a and Smith 2020b) may need to be created to uniquely identify them in the review, with a separate data extraction completed for each. Similarly, a report may separately describe data for participants from more than one centre. If there is a suspicion of systematic differences in participants between centres despite the use of the same eligibility criteria (e.g. due to endemicity of infection, or centre specialization affecting the underlying spectrum of participants between centres), then review authors may choose to consider data from each centre as a separate 'study' in the review. The extraction of data from multiple reports of the same study is considered further in Section 7.5.4.

Multiple reports of the same study should be linked together. Some review authors prefer to link reports before they collect data and collect data from across the reports onto a single form. Other review authors prefer to collect data from each report and then link together the collected data across reports. Either strategy may be appropriate, depending on the nature of the reports. It may not be clear that two reports relate to the same study until data collection has commenced. Although sometimes there is a single report for each study, it should never be assumed that this is the case.

It can be difficult to link multiple reports from the same study, and review authors may need to do some 'detective work'. Multiple sources about the same study may not reference each other, may not share common authors (Gøtzsche 1989, Tramèr 1997) or report discrepant information about the study design, characteristics and results (von Elm 2004, Mayo-Wilson 2017a).

Some of the most useful criteria for linking reports are:

- authors' names;
- study location and setting (particularly if institutions, such as hospitals, are named);
- date and duration of the study (which also can clarify whether different sample sizes are due to different periods of recruitment), length of follow-up or subgroups selected to address secondary objectives;
- numbers of participants and participant characteristics; and
- specific details of the tests, thresholds and timing of tests.

Other criteria to consider include:

- sponsor for the study and sponsor identifiers (e.g. grant or contract numbers); and
- study registration numbers.

Review authors should use as many study characteristics as possible to link multiple reports. When uncertainties remain after considering these and other factors, it may be necessary to correspond with the study authors or sponsors for confirmation.

7.2.2   Correspondence with investigators

Review authors often find that they are unable to obtain all the information they seek from available reports about the details of the study design, eligibility criteria, index tests or reference standards, or key pieces of data needed to construct 2×2 contingency tables may be missing. Missing information frequently affects review authors' assessments of the methodological quality of included studies and reduces the potential to conduct informative heterogeneity investigations. In such circumstances, review authors are strongly encouraged to contact the original investigators. Contact details of study authors, when not available from the study reports, can be obtained from more recent publications, from university or institutional staff listings, from membership directories of professional societies or by a general search of the internet. If the contact author named in the study report cannot be contacted or does not respond, it is worthwhile attempting to contact other authors. Response rates from study authors vary (from 43% (Cooper 2019) to 68% (Selph 2014) in published case studies). A number of strategies have been investigated to try to increase the number of successful contacts, including short emails with attachments compared to long emails without attachments (Godolphin 2019), the use of reminder emails (Cooper 2019) or the use of phone calls to supplement email contact (Danko 2019).

In the absence of a clear consensus regarding the optimal approach, review authors should consider the nature of the information they require and make their request accordingly. For descriptive information about the conduct of the study, it may be most appropriate to ask open-ended questions (e.g. how were participants recruited, or what threshold was used to define a positive test result?). If particular numerical data are required, it may be more helpful to request them specifically, possibly providing a short data collection form with a 2×2 contingency table indicating test and threshold (either blank for the study author to complete or partially completed with blank fields for missing data), or to offer to run the analyses on the original data.

Similar strategies may be used to identify additional unpublished studies or to access full reports of studies available only as conference abstracts.

It is good practice for review authors to keep a record of author contact, to acknowledge authors who have taken the time to respond and, importantly, for data included in a review as a result of author contact to be clearly identified.

7.3   What data to collect

7.3.1   What are data?

For the purposes of this chapter, we define 'data' to be any information about (or derived from) a study, including details of methods, participants, setting, context, index tests, target condition and reference standards, results, publications and investigators. Review authors should plan in advance what data will be required for their systematic review and develop a strategy for obtaining them. The data to be sought should be described in the protocol with an explanation of the relevance of the data where needed.

The data collected for a review should be displayed for each included study in a table of 'Characteristics of included studies'. Important study characteristics should be collected that adequately describe the included studies and that support review author judgements of methodological quality (see Chapter 8). Data collection should also support the construction of summary tables and figures, and enable syntheses and meta-analyses, including the investigation of potential sources of heterogeneity. It is advisable to develop outlines of tables and figures that will appear in the review prior to commencing data extraction so that sufficient data items are extracted, and to avoid extracting information that will not appear in the final review. Review authors should familiarize themselves with reporting guidelines for systematic reviews (see PRISMA extension for Diagnostic Test Accuracy studies (McInnes 2018)) to ensure that relevant elements and sections are incorporated.

Chapter 8 details the information needed to inform the assessment of risk of bias and applicability of study results. The following sections review the types of information that should be sought, and these are summarized in Table 7.3.a (Li 2015). Review authors may need to request missing information from study authors.

Table 7.3.a Checklist of items to consider in data collection

---

Information about data extraction from reports

Name of data extractors, date of data extraction, and identification features of each report from which data are being extracted

Eligibility criteria

Confirm eligibility of the study for the review

Reason for exclusion

Study methods (participant sampling)

Study design (see Chapter 3)

Recruitment (how were eligible participants identified) and sampling procedures used[*]

Single or multicentre study; if multicentre, number of recruiting centres

Enrolment start and end dates

Source(s) of funding or other material support for the study

Authors' financial relationship and other potential conflicts of interest

Participant characteristics and setting

Setting

Region(s) and country/countries from which study participants were recruited

Study eligibility criteria, including any prior testing or treatment

Sample size (participants and unit of analysis, if different), distinguishing number recruited, if reported, from number analysed

Number of participants with the target condition

Characteristics of participants (e.g. age, sex, comorbidity, socio-economic status)

Index test(s)

Describe the index test(s), ideally with sufficient detail for replication:

- Technical aspects of each index test, including full test name, test manufacturer, version numbers and catalogue number if relevant
- Threshold(s) for test positivity (and any rationale for selection[*])
- Details of who performed the test (if different from test interpreter)
- Factors relevant to test interpretation (e.g. staff qualifications, timing of interpretation, number of observers and method of interpretation (single, consensus, mean etc.))
- Any attempts at blinding of test assessors to final diagnosis and to additional clinical information or other test results[*]

Table 7.3.a (Continued)

Target condition and reference standard(s)

Describe target condition and reference standard, including:

- Severity of disease in participants with the target condition
- Differential diagnoses of participants without the target condition

Describe reference standard(s) used to establish presence of target condition, including details of:

- Tests (single test, combination of tests, expert panel etc.)
- Threshold for defining presence of the target condition, if relevant
- Observers
- Any attempts at blinding of assessors to index test results[*]

Flow and timing

Time interval between index tests, if more than one test evaluated[*]

Timing of reference standard in relation to application of index tests[*]

If more than one reference standard, report number of participants (with and without the target condition) per reference standard

Report any study investigator exclusion of participants from analysis, with reasons (e.g. lost to follow-up, missing data, index test failures, etc.)

Report any review team exclusion of participants from analysis, with reasons (e.g. if data for only a subgroup of participants in the study are eligible for the review)

Results

Report 2×2 contingency table data for each relevant combination of index test, threshold and reference standard or target condition (i.e. true positives (TP), false positives (FP), false negatives (FN), true negatives (TN)) and indicate if data were back-calculated from published data or if data were obtained from investigators

Report covariates to be coded for each 2×2 contingency table, including any categorization of data

If subgroup analysis is planned, the same information would need to be extracted for each participant subgroup

Miscellaneous (optional)

Reference to other relevant studies

Correspondence required and information received following author contact

Miscellaneous comments from the study authors or by the review authors

[*] Full description required for assessments of risk of bias (see Chapter 8).

7.3.2   Study methods (participant recruitment and sampling)

Poor research methods can influence study findings and introduce biases into results. For detailed guidance on study designs for estimating test accuracy, refer to Chapter 3.

Test accuracy can be estimated in any study where participants receive one or more index test(s) and at least one reference standard. Designs can recruit participants and obtain index test results in different ways. Some studies may start recruiting newly identified participants. Others may obtain index test results in previously collected samples or acquired images. Details of sampling methods (consecutive, random, 'convenience') and recruitment dates should be collected.

Additional information on study design characteristics that may affect the rigour of the study's conduct but may not lead directly to risk of bias may also be collected; for example, the funding source of the study, potential conflicts of interest of the study authors, whether ethical approval was obtained, and whether a sample size calculation was performed a priori.

7.3.3 Participant characteristics and setting

Details of participants are collected to enable assessment of the comparability of participants between included studies, and to allow assessment of how directly and completely the participants in the included studies reflect the original review question. Data need to be identified that allow assessment of whether the test is being used in the participants for whom it is intended.

Typically, aspects that should be collected are those that could (or are believed to) affect test accuracy and those that could help review users assess applicability, including to populations beyond the direct review question. For example, if the test is considered for use in symptomatic and asymptomatic people, this information should be collected and consideration should be given to separate analysis by symptom status. Care should be taken to avoid extracting information that is not thought to affect test accuracy, nor to help apply results.

Age and sex are standard characteristics to report, and summary information about these should always be collected unless they are clearly obvious from the context. These characteristics are likely to be presented in different formats (e.g. ages as means or medians, with standard deviations or ranges; sex as percentages or counts for the whole study or for participants with and without the target condition). Review authors should seek consistent quantities where possible, and indicate whether summary characteristics apply to the study as a whole (before or after any exclusions) or to those with and without the target condition separately. It may not be possible to select the most consistent statistics until data collection is complete across all or most included studies.

It is critical to collect information that characterizes why participants were selected for testing. This may relate to the symptoms they present with, their clinical history or results of previous tests. For some tests and target conditions, the presence of certain comorbid conditions may also be important to record. Clinical characteristics relevant to the review question (e.g. glucose level for reviews on diabetes) are also important for understanding the severity or stage of the disease. It may be important to obtain expert clinical input to identify aspects that are regarded as critical to collect and report to ensure that a review will be useful.

Criteria that were used to define eligible participants can be a particularly important source of diversity across studies. For example, in a review of a test for skin cancer it is important to know what type of skin lesions were eligible for inclusion (e.g. melanocytic only, any pigmented lesion, or any pigmented or non-pigmented lesion).

If the setting of studies may influence test accuracy or the applicability of results, then information on these should be collected. Typical settings include specialist diagnostic centres, tertiary care hospitals, acute care hospitals, emergency facilities, general practice or community settings. Sometimes studies are conducted in different geographical regions with important differences that could affect the prevalence or severity of the target condition, for example endemicity of an infectious disease. Timing of the study may be associated with important technology differences or trends in accuracy over time. If such information is important for the interpretation of the review, it should be collected.

Important characteristics of the participants in each included study should be summarized for the reader in the table of 'Characteristics of included studies'. It is recommended that a structure for this text is set up when planning the data extraction, identifying which items will be reported and in what format. This will ensure that data extraction and creation of this table entry can be performed efficiently.

7.3.4 Index test(s)

Details of index tests should be collected. Again, details are required for aspects that could affect test accuracy or that could help review users assess applicability both for the intended use of the test and for allowing judgement by review readers in relation to other circumstances. Where feasible, information should be sought (and presented in the review) that is sufficient for replication of the index test. This includes any additional testing procedures or the initiation of any therapeutic interventions.

A full description of index test characteristics could include some or all of the following:

- Technical aspects of each index test and test manufacturer if applicable, e.g.:
  - biomarker assay, method of analysis (ELISA, PCR, other), batch specifications, sample collection and storage;
  - imaging test, type of test, frequency or magnet strength, use of contrast, scan coverage; or
  - instructions followed when using the test (e.g. manuals and 'instructions for use' documents, also called 'product inserts').
- Classification system or algorithm used, e.g. for clinical assessment or image interpretation, including details of the version used, if more than one available.
- Threshold(s) for test positivity (and rationale for selection).
- Who performed the test (if different from the test interpreter).
- Factors relevant to test interpretation, e.g. staff qualifications or expertise, number of assessors or observers, method of interpretation (single, consensus, mean or other), and availability of additional clinical information.
- Timing of test interpretation in relation to reference standard.

It is important to identify where a test is being used in a clinical pathway in each study. Where the index test is likely to be an add on to other available tests (Chapter 3), a description of other tests that may be carried out concurrently or within the time frame of testing should be provided. For evaluations of complex testing strategies that involve the application of more than one test according to some predefined rule, the degree to which specified procedures or components of the strategy were implemented as planned may need to be reported.

Comparisons of variations on the delivery of a test, for example whether it was undertaken in accordance with the manufacturer's instructions for use, may be important secondary objectives and sensitivity analyses to consider in a review. It is important that data are extracted and coded in a way that enables such analyses to be completed.

Important characteristics of the index tests in each included study should be summarized for the reader in the table of 'Characteristics of included studies'. Additional tables or diagrams depicting the testing pathway can assist descriptions of multi-component testing strategies so that review users can better assess review applicability to their context.

7.3.5 Target condition and reference standard

The definition of the target condition and the reference standard used to identify the presence or absence of the target condition should be collected. It is important to report both differences between studies as to how the target condition is defined and the use of different reference standards for confirming the presence and/or absence of the target condition, and to investigate if they lead to variations in test accuracy or affect the applicability of a study beyond the review question.

The target condition, proportion of participants with the target condition and severity of disease in participants with the target condition should be provided. The differential diagnoses of participants without the target condition can also affect test performance and should be recorded.

The reference standard may be a single test (e.g. histology), may be composed of a number of individual tests (composite reference standard, e.g. an imaging test plus participant follow-up to identify false positive or false negative results) or could be based on a consensus diagnosis by an expert group of clinicians (e.g. based on one-year follow-up and all available information). Details of all tests and assessors and the definition of the threshold for defining presence of the target condition should be recorded along with any rules for combining individual test results. If a disease classification system is used, details of the specific version or versions used should be specified. For example, the Liver Imaging Reporting and Data System (LI-RADS) has a number of iterations (van der Pol 2019), as does the American College of Rheumatology classification criteria for rheumatoid arthritis (Cader 2011). The availability of additional clinical information that might influence the reference standard should also be recorded. Where feasible, information should be sought (and presented in the review) that is sufficient for replication of the reference standard. Review authors may need to request missing information from study authors.

There may be more than one eligible reference standard for the review question. If possible, these should be ranked prior to data extraction, so that priority can be given to extracting data according to the preferred reference standard in studies presenting data according to more than one reference standard.

Important characteristics of the target condition and reference standards used in each included study should be summarized for the reader in the table of 'Characteristics of included studies'.

7.3.6 Flow and timing

Participants' flow through a study and the timing of tests and reference standards should be recorded in order to identify any missing data, the completeness and approach to verification by the reference standard, and timings of tests to investigate possible changes to disease status between application of the index test and the reference standard (due to progression of disease or to any therapeutic intervention received during the time interval between tests). Information on the timing of the reference standard in relation to the application of index tests and the number of participants receiving each reference standard should be collected. Missing data can result from participants not undergoing the index test(s) or reference standards as planned, or from failure of the index test or reference standard.

Each review is likely to present its own unique issues, and review authors should be alert to particular aspects of the way in which studies are undertaken and reported. For example, some studies discuss 'samples' rather than 'participants' and it is not always clear whether they are analysing multiple samples from individual patients.

Relevant details related to flow and timing in each included study should be summarized for the reader in the table of 'Characteristics of included studies'.

7.3.7 Extracting study results and converting to the desired format

Results data arise from the cross-classification of the results of the index test for individual participants in a study against the reference standard result. For most reviews, results are summarized at study level as paired data by the reference standard (sensitivity and specificity) or by index test results (positive and negative predictive values).

Reports of studies can include several results for a single index test according to different test thresholds, different scoring systems used or different reference standards. For example, a number of different imaging characteristics can be observed for the same image, different numerical thresholds can be applied to test results reported as continuous data, or categorical variables can be grouped in different ways. Review protocols should be as specific as possible about relevant test thresholds and a framework should be pre-specified in the protocol to facilitate making choices between multiple eligible measures or results. For instance, a hierarchy of preferred thresholds or approaches to scoring or interpretation of images might be created. Any additional decisions or changes to this framework made once the data are collected should be reported in the review as changes to the protocol.

The unit of analysis (e.g. participant, or body part, or site) should be recorded for each result when it is not obvious (see Chapter 4). For many tests simple 2×2 tables will be available; for others with multiple categories for index and/or reference standard results, 3×2, 3×3 or even larger contingency tables can potentially be extracted and decisions will be required about how to extract these into a 2×2 format.

In most cases, it is desirable to collect contingency table data for each combination of index test, threshold, reference standard and other variables of relevance to the review question. Sometimes studies will report accuracy results in a 2×2 table format, but more often the numbers required for meta-analysis are not reported in this way. Other statistics can be collected and converted into the required format. For example, reports of sample size, the proportion of participants with the target condition and sensitivity and specificity can be used to reconstruct 2×2 tables. Details of recalculation are provided below. When insufficient information is presented in a study report, author contact should be considered (see Section 7.2.2).

7.3.7.1 Obtaining 2×2 data from accuracy measures
The data needed to populate a 2×2 table can be calculated from reported accuracy measures if the sample size for the table is known (this is not always the same as the total sample size for the study) and at least one additional piece of information is provided. The calculations can be straightforward and easily calculated using a hand

calculator. The calculator in Cochrane's primary review authoring tool, Review Manager (RevMan; training.cochrane.org/online-learning/core-software-cochrane-reviews/revman), is useful for less straightforward combinations of accuracy measures.

If the total number tested is known and the proportion with the target condition is reported, the 2×2 data can be derived from the reported sensitivity and specificity in six simple steps described in Table 7.3.b. At Step 1, the number of people with the target condition can be calculated from the total tested multiplied by 29.7% (proportion with the target condition). The number without the target condition is obtained by subtracting the number with the target condition from the total tested (Step 2). At Step 3, the number of true positives is derived by calculating 40.8% (sensitivity) of the number with the target condition, and the number of true negatives derived by calculating 97.8% (specificity) of the number without the target condition (Step 4). The number of false negatives and false positives can then be calculated by subtracting the number of true positives and true negatives from the column totals (Step 5 and Step 6).

A similar procedure can be followed for reported positive predictive value (PPV) and negative predictive value (NPV) if the total number tested and the number of participants with a positive index test result are known, as described in Table 7.3.c. At Step 1 the number testing positive in the study is entered or derived from the reported percentage testing positive (in this case 13.6%), and the number testing negative calculated by subtraction of test positives from the total number tested (Step 2). The number

Table 7.3.b Estimating 2×2 contingency table data from reported sensitivity and specificity

Example of reported data →	Sensitivity 40.8%	Specificity 97.8%	Sample size 330 Target condition present 29.7%
Estimation of 2×2 data	People with target condition	People without target condition	Row totals
Index test positive	(Step 3) **TP = 98 × 0.408 = 40**	(Step 6) **FP = 232 – 227 = 5**	TP+FP
Index test negative	(Step 5) **FN = 98 – 40 = 58**	(Step 4) **TN = 232 × 0.978 = 227**	FN+TN
Column totals	(Step 1) 330 × 0.297 = **98**	(Step 2) 330 – 98 = **232**	**330**

Table 7.3.c Estimating 2×2 contingency table data from reported PPV and NPV

Example of reported data →	PPV 88.9%	NPV 79.6%	Sample size 330 Index test positive 13.6%
Estimation of 2×2 data	People with target condition	People without target condition	Row totals
Index test positive	(Step 3) **TP = 45 × 0.889 = 40**	(Step 5) **FP = 45 – 40 = 5**	(Step 1) 330 × 0.136 = **45**
Index test negative	(Step 6) **FN = 285 – 227 = 58**	(Step 4) **TN = 285 × 0.796 = 227**	(Step 2) 330 – 45 = **285**
Column totals	TP+FN	FP+TN	**330**

Table 7.3.d Estimating 2×2 contingency table data from reported specificity and NPV

Example of reported data →	Specificity 97.8%	NPV 79.6%	Sample size 330 Target condition present 29.7%
Estimation of 2×2 data	People with target condition	People without target condition	Row totals
Index test positive	(Step 7) **TP** = 98 − 58 = **40**	(Step 4) FP = 232 − 227 = **5**	TP+FP
Index test negative	(Step 6) **FN** = 285 − 227 = **58**	(Step 3) TN = 232 × 0.978 = **227**	(Step 5)* 227/0.796 = **285**
Column totals	(Step 1) 330 × 0.297 = **98**	(Step 2) 330 − 98 = **232**	**330**

* Based on formula NPV × Index test negative = TN → Index test negative = TN/NPV

of true positives is 88.9% (PPV) of the number testing positive (Step 3) and the number of true negatives is 79.6% (NPV) of the number testing negative (Step 4). The rest of the 2×2 table can be completed by subtraction of true positives and true negatives from the row totals (Steps 5 and 6).

Contingency tables can also be calculated from studies that report the total number tested with a combination of either sensitivity or specificity and either PPV or NPV, as long as the number with the target condition or number testing positive on the index test is also known. Table 7.3.d shows that once the column totals are known (Step 1 and Step 2), the number of true negatives and false positives can be calculated from reported specificity in the same way as previously described for Table 7.3.b (Step 3 and Step 4). The number of true negatives and reported NPV can then be entered into a rearranged formula for calculation of NPV to calculate the total number testing negative (row total in Step 5). The number of false negatives can be completed by subtraction of true negatives from the row total (Step 6) and the number of true positives completed by subtraction of false negatives from the column total (Step 7).

Although the formulae are more complicated, the 2×2 contingency table data can also be hand calculated from reported positive and negative likelihood ratios or using sensitivity (or specificity) and the positive (or negative) likelihood ratio. Box 7.3.a shows the formulae for calculating sensitivity and specificity from reported positive likelihood ratios (LRP) and negative likelihood ratios (LRN).

Once sensitivity and specificity are known, the steps laid out in Table 7.3.b can be followed to calculate the 2×2 data. Alternatively, the RevMan calculator can be used. It is also possible to use sample size and reported sensitivity and specificity with 95% confidence intervals to calculate 2×2 tables. However, due to the possibility for error, this should only be carried out by those familiar with the underlying equations for estimation of confidence intervals and access to software for the appropriate methods.

Whenever 2×2 tables are calculated from reported results, it is helpful to cross-check the results against any other reported accuracy measures. For example, if a 2×2 table is derived from reported sensitivity and specificity, the PPV and NPV from the resulting 2×2 table can be checked against the PPV and NPV reported in the study, if available. If there are any discrepancies between the derived results based on the 2×2 table and the data in the study report, review authors should consider whether the difference could

---

Box 7.3.a Estimating sensitivity or specificity from likelihood ratios

To calculate sensitivity and specificity:

$$\text{Sensitivity} = \frac{LRP - (LRP \times LRN)}{(LRP - LRN)}$$

$$\text{Specificity} = \frac{(LRP - 1)}{(LRP - LRN)}$$

Recalculate LRP to double-check calculations:

$$LRP = \frac{sensitivity}{(1 - specificity)}$$

$$LRN = \frac{(1 - sensitivity)}{specificity}$$

LRN, negative likelihood ratio; LRP, positive likelihood ratio.

---

be due to a typographical or calculation error. If no error is suspected, then contacting the study authors should be attempted. If the difference is large and the numbers cannot be resolved satisfactorily, then the study should be considered for exclusion on the basis of being internally inconsistent.

Some reviews will include studies where estimation of test accuracy was not the primary objective, but data are presented in such a way that 2×2 tables can still be extracted. For example, reviews of tests used in standard clinical practice, such as routine laboratory markers or imaging tests, could include studies where participant characteristics, including the results of the index test of interest, are tabulated according to the presence or absence of the target condition according to the reference standard, providing the required numbers of true-positive and false positive results, respectively.

The information required to calculate 2×2 tables from accuracy measures is usually provided in study tables; however, if one or more pieces of information needed is missing it is important also to check the Abstract and any available (online) supplementary information. Sometimes the data needed can even be provided in the Discussion section of an article, where study authors may discuss or present their results in a different way from the main Results section.

Any 2×2 tables that have been derived from reported accuracy measures should be clearly identified on the data extraction form.

7.3.7.2 Using global measures

In some studies, global measures of test accuracy such as the diagnostic odds ratio (DOR) or, more commonly, the area under the receiver operating characteristic (ROC) curve or c-statistic may be reported instead of paired sensitivities and specificities. These global measures cannot be used to derive 2×2 contingency table data. Where indicated, these global measures of test accuracy should always be extracted with their respective 95% confidence intervals or standard errors.

7.3.7.3 Challenges defining reference standard positive and negative: strategies when there are more than two categories

There are a number of situations where accuracy data may not be presented as a simple 2×2 contingency table, including the case of multiple reference categories where the target condition is not classed as present or absent but, for example, as present, possible or absent.

An example is provided in a review of galactomannan for the diagnosis of invasive aspergillosis (Leeflang 2015), where a composite reference standard classifies the target condition as proven, probable, possible or absent (Table 7.3.e). In order to calculate sensitivity and specificity, the reference standard results have to be dichotomized into two categories, representing those with the target condition and those without the target condition. For this review, the reference standard classification was guided by the anticipated treatment decision for each group; the 'proven' and 'probable' categories would likely be treated with antimycotics and were considered to have the target condition, and 'possible' or 'absent' would not be treated and were considered not to have the target condition.

There is a further challenge if some studies in a review do not report their results according to all possible reference standard categories. Continuing the aspergillosis example, studies could report results in three categories, e.g. 'proven', 'probable or possible' and 'absent', or in some other format, in which case a decision has to be made regarding how to dichotomize results to allow extraction and how to deal with any variation in the definition of the target condition in subsequent analysis.

Any 2×2 tables that have been derived by combining reference standard categories should be clearly identified on the data extraction form, and the original data presented by the study authors should also be extracted.

7.3.7.4 Challenges defining index test positive and negative: inconclusive results

The other situation where accuracy data may not be presented as a simple 2×2 contingency table is if not all index test results are classified as positive or negative but, for example, as positive, indeterminate or negative, or when a continuous test result is categorized into separate ranges of results with the middle group considered 'borderline' (see Chapter 4).

Table 7.3.e Estimating 2×2 contingency table data when there are multiple reference standard categories, invasive aspergillosis example

	Reported categories of invasive aspergillosis				
	Proven	Probable	Possible	None	Total
Galactomannan positive	1	3	8	2	14
Galactomannan negative	0	2	13	54	69
Estimation of 2×2 data	**People with invasive aspergillosis**		**People without invasive aspergillosis**		
Galactomannan positive	4		10		14
Galactomannan negative	2		67		69
Column totals	**6**		**77**		**83**

In order to calculate sensitivity and specificity, inconclusive results are usually considered as either positive or negative results. This decision should be guided by what the clinical decision would be for people with inconclusive results (Shinkins 2013), and it is important for review authors to be guided by clinical expert opinion, especially if the review authors are not content experts. If some intervention is likely to be initiated, then inconclusive results should be considered positive, but if invasive further investigations are indicated, for example, then inconclusive results might be considered negative unless there is strong clinical evidence to support their interpretation as positive. If the clinical pathway for inconclusive results is not clear, or is not definitive, then data can be extracted considering inconclusive results as positive and as negative and sensitivity analysis can be used to explore the effect on accuracy.

In the example of an interferon-gamma release assay for diagnosing active tuberculosis in Table 7.3.f, study authors excluded borderline results in the main analysis but included them as index test positive in a sensitivity analysis. It is important that the decision is applied consistently across all studies and is agreed within the review author team at the outset. In most cases borderline test results should not be excluded, as that would either over-estimate sensitivity or over-estimate specificity compared to the situation of borderline results being considered negative or positive, as shown in Table 7.3.f.

Table 7.3.f Estimating 2×2 contingency table data when there are multiple index test categories, example of interferon-gamma release assay (IGRA) for diagnosis of active tuberculosis (TB)

(1) Borderline results excluded	People with active TB	People with no active TB	Row totals
IGRA positive	253	51	304
IGRA negative	58	319	377
IGRA borderline	(17)	(16)	(33)
Column totals	**311**	**370**	681
Accuracy measures	**Sensitivity** 253/311 = 81%	**Specificity** 319/370 = 86%	

(2) Borderline results considered positive			
IGRA positive + borderline	270	67	337
IGRA negative	58	319	377
Column totals	**328**	**386**	714
Accuracy measures	**Sensitivity** 270/328 = 82%	**Specificity** 319/386 = 83%	

(3) Borderline results considered negative			
IGRA positive	253	51	304
IGRA negative + borderline	75	335	410
Column totals	**328**	**386**	714
Accuracy measures	**Sensitivity** 253/328 = 77%	**Specificity** 335/386 = 87%	

Adapted from Whitworth 2019.

Any 2×2 tables that have been calculated by combining index test categories should be clearly identified on the data extraction form, and the original data presented by the study authors should also be extracted.

In some reports, the study authors may have excluded intermediate results from the calculation of sensitivity and specificity, or sensitivity may have been calculated based on one cut-off and specificity based on a second cut-off. In those cases it is necessary to reconstruct the 2×2 tables, including all tested study participants with a test result, using a single cut-off for all, and calculate sensitivity and specificity based on that reconstructed 2×2 table, not on the reported results.

7.3.7.5 Challenges defining index test positive and negative: test failures

Failed index test procedures are distinct from inconclusive results in that there is no valid test result, i.e. they represent some kind of failure of the index test (Shinkins 2013). Test failure could be due to the test not being conducted to a sufficient standard (e.g. inadequate sampling or some technical error with the test) or could be for clinical reasons (e.g. concurrent infection masking true results or lack of fasting affecting a blood glucose result). In this case, repeating the test under more optimal conditions is likely to lead to a positive or negative result.

Unlike inconclusive results, it is reasonable for test failures to be excluded from analysis if they cannot be considered as either positive or negative. The proportion of test failures should always be extracted and reported in a review, as an indicator of how often the test is likely to fail (Shinkins 2013).

7.3.7.6 Challenges defining index test positive and negative: dealing with multiple thresholds and extracting data from ROC curves or other graphics

Studies of index tests that report results on a continuous scale can report accuracy data at multiple thresholds that may not all be relevant to the review question. Where this situation is anticipated, review authors should set out a strategy in the protocol for selecting the datasets that should be extracted. Possible strategies include selecting:

- the 'standard' threshold currently used in practice;
- the threshold recommended by the manufacturer;
- the most commonly reported threshold;
- a randomly selected threshold; or
- all thresholds.

Data can be extracted from a ROC curve if the thresholds associated with each point on the ROC curve are reported, and if the number with and without the target condition is known. This is not a very precise method of identifying sensitivity and specificity and should be used with caution.

Dot plots can be used to represent the results of biomarker tests. The plots can show the test result for each participant according to the value of the test result (y-axis) and the presence of the target condition or other differential diagnosis on the x-axis. The number of participants with a test result above or below the cut-off value of choice can be counted for each category of participants. Dot plots are often used to represent biomarker results from studies using multi-gate designs, as depicted in Figure 7.3.a.

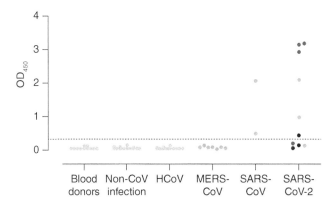

Figure 7.3.a **Example of a dot plot for estimation of sensitivity and specificity**. Source: **Okba 2020** / U.S Department of Health and Human Services / Public domain

Any 2×2 tables that have been calculated by extracting data from graphics should be clearly identified on the data extraction form.

7.3.7.7   Extracting data from figures with software
Numerous tools for extracting data from figures are available, many of which are free. Those available at the time of writing include Plot Digitizer, WebPlotDigitizer, Engauge, Dexter, ycasd and GetData Graph Digitizer. The software works by taking an image of a figure and then digitizing the data points off the figure using the axes and scales set by the users. The numbers exported can be used for systematic reviews, although additional calculations may be needed to obtain or validate accuracy measures.

It has been demonstrated that software is more convenient and accurate than visual estimation or use of a ruler (Gross 2014, Jelicic Kadic 2016). Review authors should consider using software for extracting numerical data from figures when the data are not available elsewhere.

7.3.7.8   Corrections for missing data: adjusting for partial verification bias
Partial verification, whereby some participants eligible for a test accuracy study do not receive the reference standard, can occur for a number of reasons, for example due to the invasive nature of the reference standard, or because there is no practical way of confirming the absence of the target condition in an index test negative participant. It is also an approach used when the condition is rare, only sampling a random subset of those who test negative. Study authors may use statistical approaches to correct for the bias introduced by missing data (de Groot 2011), such as inverse sampling probability weighting. Direct inclusion of the original 2×2 table in a systematic review where corrections have been made will re-introduce the bias that has been corrected for by the analysis. Rather, a new 2×2 table should be created that provides equal estimates of sensitivity and specificity with the same uncertainty as from the weighted analysis.

7.3.7.9   Multiple index tests from the same study
Studies that report the use of different index tests in different participants can be considered as different studies, with study naming as suggested in Section 7.2.1. More

often, studies evaluate and report accuracy data for multiple eligible index tests in the same participants.

The same data extraction considerations apply to each index test and threshold. Any differences in the selection criteria for participants undergoing each test should be documented and any differences in the number of participants undergoing each index test, or any resulting differences in the number with the target condition, should be accounted for in the 2×2 tables.

Studies that report accuracy data for multiple eligible index tests could also present data for combinations of different test results. For example, a study of anti-CCP and rheumatoid factor for the diagnosis of rheumatoid arthritis could present results for either test positive or for both tests positive. A worked example is provided in Table 7.3.g.

The choice of 2×2 tables to extract should always be guided by the review question and should be specified prior to commencing data extraction.

Table 7.3.g Calculating 2×2 contingency table data from a cross-tabulation of two index tests against a reference standard

Results of the anti-CCP assays in relation to the presence or absence of RF (reported data Luis Caro-Oleas 2007)

Anti-CCP assay	RA patients (n = 124)		Other groups (n = 158)		Total
	n	%	n	%	n
QUANTA Lite™ CCP2					
Anti-CCP2 positive	67	54.0	3	1.9	70
RF positive	56	45.1	3	1.9	59
RF negative	11	8.9	0	0.0	11
Anti-CCP2 negative	57	46.0	155	98.1	207
RF positive	14	11.3	4	2.5	18
RF negative	43	34.7	151	95.6	194

	People with RA	People with no RA	Total
Estimation of 2×2 data for anti-CCP2			
anti-CCP2 positive	56 + 11 = 67	3 + 0 = 3	70
anti-CCP2 negative	14 + 43 = 57	4 + 151 = 155	212
Column totals	**124**	**158**	**282**
Estimation of 2×2 data for RF			
RF positive	56 + 14 = 70	3 + 4 = 7	77
RF negative	11 + 43 = 54	0 + 151 = 151	205
Column totals	**124**	**158**	**282**

(Continued)

Table 7.3.g (Continued)

Estimation of 2×2 data for both tests positive			
Both tests positive	56	3	59
Either test negative	11 + 14 + 43 = 68	0 + 4 + 151 = 155	223
Column totals	**124**	**158**	**282**
Estimation of 2×2 data for either test positive			
Either test positive	56 + 11 + 14 = 81	3 + 0 + 4 = 7	88
Both tests negative	43	151	194
Column totals	**124**	**158**	**282**

RA, rheumatoid arthritis; RF, rheumatoid factor.

Most software for conducting meta-analysis or plotting data allows only one 2×2 table from each study to be included in a single analysis. Where studies compare different tests in the same participants and review authors wish to include all 2×2 tables for each test in the same analysis, special consideration is needed. For example, a review of commercially available point-of-care biomarker assays for an infectious disease such as tuberculosis or malaria may include studies that compare tests produced by different manufacturers in the same study participants. Studies that evaluate imaging tests often report separate 2×2 tables for different observer interpretations of the same images. Unless it is decided a priori that results for only one observer will be reported, for example for the most experienced observer, it is usual to extract all available 2×2 tables, clearly labelled by observer experience.

7.3.7.10 Subgroups of patients
Accuracy data for subgroups of study participants should be extracted only if there is a stated a priori interest in that subgroup. There is no obligation to extract all possible 2×2 contingency tables from any individual study.

7.3.7.11 Individual patient data
Some reviews (Hooper 2015, Manzotti 2019) present individual patient data (IPD). For example, in case of continuous tests it may be helpful to have all data from all participants, so that ROC plots of individual studies can be reconstructed and alternative thresholds applied. Alternatively, IPD could allow review authors to restrict data to participants meeting the review question, for example in regard to age or underlying health conditions. If a review looks at a test strategy that combines results from several tests, IPD may allow results for strategies to be obtained where they have not been investigated in the original report. If review authors plan to use IPD, this should be specified in the protocol, along with a description of the methods to be used to elicit those data from study authors or, where available, to extract from study reports. The success, or otherwise, of contacting study authors should be documented in the review.

7.3.7.12 Extracting covariates

Covariates that are relevant to the analysis of study data, or that could be displayed on forest plots of sensitivity and specificity, could be related to study design, participant, index test or reference standard characteristics. Detailed information on each of these should be extracted as described in sections 7.3.2 to 7.3.5. For analysis or display purposes, however, a separate field for each covariate can be useful, especially as covariates can apply to all 2×2 data extracted from an individual study ('study' level) or can vary between different 2×2 tables extracted from the same study ('test' level).

The decision as to whether a covariate applies at study level or at test level will vary between reviews. For example, a covariate related to participant age would apply at study level if all studies reported data either for children, adults or mixed age groups, or would apply at test level if individual studies reported data for a mixed age group as well as for either adults or children separately. Similarly, if accuracy results are expected to vary according to the experience of the assessor interpreting the test, then 2×2 data could be presented for all assessors combined and separately according to the experience level of the assessor, for example high, intermediate or low.

Covariates can be either categorical (with a finite number of categories) or continuous (with an infinite number of values between any two values) variables. Categorical variables are easier for the analysis of test accuracy data, but categorization of continuous variables before data analysis is discouraged, as information will be lost. Categorical covariates are required in order to display results per subgroup on a SROC plot, but either categorical or continuous covariates can be displayed on a forest plot of sensitivities and specificities.

Covariates that will be investigated in heterogeneity analyses should be pre-specified whenever possible, and any categories to be used should be standardized. In the same way that the number of covariates defined for a review should be guided by the expected number of data sets for the review, the number of categories defined for each covariate should be kept to a minimum in order to maximize the number of data sets in each category and thereby increase the power of the heterogeneity investigation (see Chapter 9, Section 9.4.6).

7.3.8 Other information to collect

Collection of information about the harmful effects of testing may be desirable depending on the nature of the test. In test accuracy studies, adverse events can be collected either systematically or non-systematically. Systematic collection refers to collecting adverse events in the same manner for each participant using defined methods such as a questionnaire or a laboratory test. Non-systematic collection refers to collection of information on adverse events using methods such as open-ended questions (e.g. 'Have you noticed any symptoms since your last visit?') or reported by participants spontaneously. In either case, adverse events may be selectively reported based on their severity, and whether the participant suspected that the effect may have been caused by the test, which could lead to bias in the available data.

Further comments by the study authors, for example any explanations they provide for unexpected findings, may be noted; however, it is not necessary to report these in the data extraction. References to other studies that are cited in the study report may be useful, although review authors should be aware of the possibility of citation bias (see Chapter 6). Documentation of any correspondence with the study authors is important for review transparency.

7.4 Data collection tools

7.4.1 Rationale for data collection forms

Data collection for systematic reviews should be performed using structured data collection forms. These can be paper forms, electronic forms (e.g. Excel or Google Form), or commercially available (e.g. Covidence or EPPI-Reviewer) or custom-built data systems that allow online form building, data entry by several users, data sharing and efficient data management (Li 2015). At the time of writing, most commercially available data systems do not have standard extraction form templates for reviews of test accuracy and, although some modification is possible, 2×2 contingency table data cannot be extracted. All different means of data collection require data collection forms.

The data collection form is a bridge between what is reported by the original investigators (e.g. in journal articles, abstracts, personal correspondence) and what is ultimately reported by the review authors. The data collection form serves several important functions (Meade 1997). First, the form is linked directly to the review question and criteria for assessing eligibility of studies, and provides a clear summary of these that can be used to identify and structure the data to be extracted from study reports. Second, the data collection form is the historical record of the provenance of the data used in the review, as well as the multitude of decisions (and changes to decisions) that occur throughout the review process. Third, the form is the source of data for inclusion in an analysis and provides support for judgements related to quality assessment.

Given the important functions of data collection forms, ample time and thought should be invested in their design. Because each review is different, data collection forms will vary across reviews. However, there are many similarities in the types of information that are important. Thus, forms can be adapted from one review to the next. Although we use the term 'data collection form' in the singular, in practice it may be a series of forms used for different purposes; for example, a separate form could be used to assess the eligibility of studies for inclusion in the review to assist in the quick identification of studies to be excluded from or included in the review.

7.4.2 Considerations in selecting data collection tools

The choice of data collection tool is largely dependent on review authors' preferences, the size of the review and resources available to the review author team. Potential advantages and considerations of selecting one data collection tool over another are outlined in Table 7.4.a (Li 2015). A significant advantage that data systems have is in data management (Chapter 1, Section 1.2.4) and re-use, and in their accessibility to multiple author review teams. They make review updates more efficient and facilitate methodological research across reviews. Numerous 'meta-epidemiological' studies have been carried out using Cochrane Review data, resulting in methodological advances that would not have been possible if thousands of studies had not all been described using the same data structures in the same system.

Table 7.4.a Considerations in selecting data collection tools

	Paper forms	Electronic forms	Data systems
Examples	Forms developed using word processing software	Microsoft Access Microsoft Excel Google Forms Forms developed using word processing software (Microsoft Word, Google Docs, Zoho Writer, etc.)	Covidence EPPI-Reviewer Systematic Review Data Repository (SRDR) DistillerSR (Evidence Partners) REDCap
Suitable review type and team sizes	Small-scale reviews (<10 included studies) Small team with 2 to 3 data extractors in the same physical location	Small- to medium-scale reviews (10 to 20 studies) Small to moderate-sized team with 4 to 6 data extractors	For small-, medium- and especially large-scale reviews (>20 studies), as well as reviews that need constant updating All team sizes, especially large teams (i.e. >6 data extractors)
Resource needs	Low	Low to medium (most if not all institutions provide access and free word processing software is increasingly available online)	Low to medium (open-access tools such as SRDR, or tools for which authors have institutional licences or, for Cochrane Reviews, tools for which Cochrane has obtained licences on behalf of review authors) High (commercial data systems with no access via an institutional licence)
Advantages	Do not rely on access to computer and network or internet connectivity Can record notes and explanations easily Require minimal software skills	Allow extracted data to be processed electronically for editing and analysis Allow electronic data storage, sharing and collation Easy to expand or edit forms as required Can automate data comparison with additional programming Can copy data to analysis software without manual re-entry, reducing errors	Specifically designed for data collection for systematic reviews Allow online data storage, linking and sharing Easy to expand or edit forms as required Can be integrated with title/abstract, full-text screening and other functions Can link data items to locations in the report to facilitate checking Can readily automate data comparison between independent data collection for the same study Allow easy monitoring of progress and performance of the author team

(Continued)

Table 7.4.a (Continued)

	Paper forms	Electronic forms	Data systems
			Facilitate coordination among data collectors such as allocation of studies for collection and monitoring team progress
			Allow simultaneous data entry by multiple authors
			Can export data directly to analysis software
			Can import included and excluded studies, with reasons for exclusion, directly into RevMan (Cochrane Reviews only)
			In some cases, improve public accessibility through open data sharing
Disadvantages	Inefficient and potentially unreliable because data must be entered into software for analysis and reporting Susceptible to errors Data collected by multiple authors must be manually collated Difficult to amend as the review progresses If the papers are lost, all data will need to be recreated	Require familiarity with software packages to design and use forms Carry risk of introducing mistakes in data entering or copy-pasting between versions Possible data security issue if files are not encrypted or securely backed up (especially relevant for IPD)	Up-front and considerable investment of resources to set up and adapt the form for studies of test accuracy Requires training of data extractors Cannot extract 2×2 contingency tables for accuracy data Structured templates may not be as flexible as electronic forms Cost of commercial data systems Require familiarity with data systems Susceptible to changes in software versions

7.4.3 Design of a data collection form

Regardless of whether data are collected using a paper or electronic form or a data system, the key to successful data collection is to construct easy-to-use forms and collect sufficient and unambiguous data that faithfully represent the source in a structured and organized manner (Li 2015). In most cases, a document format should be developed for the form before building an electronic form or a data system. This can be distributed to others, including programmers and data analysts, and used as a guide for creating an electronic form and any guidance or codebook to be used by data extractors. Review authors also should consider the compatibility of any electronic form or data system with analytical software, as well as mechanisms for recording, assessing and correcting data entry errors.

Data described in multiple reports (or even within a single report) of a study may not be consistent. Review authors will need to describe how they will work with multiple reports in the protocol, for example by pre-specifying which report will be used when sources contain conflicting data that cannot be resolved by contacting the investigators. Likewise, when there is only one report identified for a study, review authors should specify the section within the report (e.g. abstract, methods, results, tables and figures) for use in case of inconsistent information.

A good data collection form should minimize the need to go back to the source documents. When designing a data collection form, review authors should involve all members of the team; that is, content area experts, authors with experience in systematic review methods and data collection form design, statisticians and persons who will perform data extraction. Here are suggested steps and some tips for designing a data collection form, based on the informal collation of experiences from numerous review authors (Li 2015).

Step 1. Develop outlines of tables and figures expected to appear in the systematic review, considering the comparisons to be made between index tests within the review, and whether different definitions of the target condition or multiple reference standards are to be included. This step will help review authors decide the right amount of data to collect (not too much or too little). Collecting too much information can lead to forms that are longer than original study reports, and can be very wasteful of time. Collection of too little information, or omission of key data, can lead to the need to return to study reports later in the review process.

Step 2. Assemble and group data elements to facilitate form development. Review authors should consult Table 7.3.a, in which the data elements are grouped to facilitate form development and data collection. It may be more efficient to group data elements in the order in which they are usually found in study reports (e.g. starting with reference information, followed by eligibility criteria, description of index test, description of reference standard, baseline characteristics and results).

Step 3. Identify the optimal way of framing the data items. Much has been written about how to frame data items for developing robust data collection forms in primary research studies. We summarize a few key points and highlight issues that are pertinent to systematic reviews.

- Ask closed-ended questions (i.e. questions that define a list of permissible responses) as much as possible. Closed-ended questions do not require post hoc coding and provide better control over data quality than open-ended questions. When setting up a closed-ended question, one should anticipate and structure possible responses and include an 'other, specify' category, because the anticipated list may not be exhaustive. Avoid asking data extractors to summarize data into uncoded text, no matter how short it is.

- Avoid asking a question in such a way that the response may be left blank. Include 'not applicable', 'not reported' and 'cannot tell' options as needed. The 'cannot tell' option tags uncertain items that may promote review authors to contact study authors for clarification, especially on data items critical to reach conclusions.
- Remember that the form will focus on what is reported in the report rather than what has been done in the study. The study report may not fully reflect how the study was actually conducted. For example, a question 'Did the study report whether the reference standard results were interpreted without knowledge of the results of the index test?' is more appropriate than 'Were assessors blinded?'
- Where a judgement is required, record the raw data (i.e. quote directly from the source document) used to make the judgement. This can be particularly important for any data that will support review author judgements of study quality. It is also important to record the source of information collected, including where it was found in a report or whether information was obtained from unpublished sources or personal communications. As much as possible, questions should be asked in a way that minimizes subjective interpretation and judgement to facilitate data comparison and adjudication.
- Incorporate flexibility to allow for variation in how data are reported. It is strongly recommended that outcome data be collected in the format in which they were reported and transformed in a subsequent step if required. Review authors also should consider the software they will use for analysis and for publishing the review.

Step 4. Develop and pilot-test data collection forms, ensuring that they provide data in the right format and structure for subsequent analysis. In addition to data items described in Step 2, data collection forms should record the title of the review as well as the person who is completing the form and the date of completion. Forms occasionally need revision; forms should therefore include the version number and version date to reduce the chances of using an outdated form by mistake. Because a study may be associated with multiple reports, it is important to record the study ID as well as the report ID. Definitions and instructions helpful for answering a question should appear next to the question to improve quality and consistency across data extractors (Stock 1994). Provide space for notes, regardless of whether paper or electronic forms are used.

All data collection forms and data systems should be thoroughly pilot-tested before launch. Testing should involve several people extracting data from at least a few reports. The initial testing focuses on the clarity and completeness of questions. Users of the form may provide feedback that certain coding instructions are confusing or incomplete (e.g. a list of options may not cover all situations). The testing may identify data that are missing from the form, or likely to be superfluous. After initial testing, accuracy of the extracted data should be checked against the source document or verified data to identify problematic areas. It is wise to draft entries for the table of 'Characteristics of included studies' and complete a risk-of-bias assessment (Chapter 8) using these pilot reports to ensure that all necessary information is collected. A consensus between review authors may be required before the form is modified to avoid any misunderstandings or later disagreements. It may be necessary to repeat the pilot testing on a new set of reports if major changes are needed after the first pilot test.

Problems with the data collection form may surface after pilot testing has been completed, and the form may need to be revised after data extraction has started. When changes are made to the form or coding instructions, it may be necessary to return to reports that have already undergone data extraction. In some situations, it may be necessary to clarify only coding instructions without modifying the actual data collection form.

7.5 Extracting data from reports

7.5.1 Introduction

In most systematic reviews, the primary source of information about each study is published in reports of studies, usually in the form of journal articles. Despite recent developments in machine learning models to automate data extraction in systematic reviews (see Chapter 6), data extraction is still largely a manual process. Electronic searches for text can provide a useful aid to locating information within a report. Examples include using search facilities in PDF viewers, internet browsers and word processing software. However, text searching should not be considered a replacement for reading the report, since information may be presented using variable terminology and presented in multiple formats.

7.5.2 Who should extract data?

Data extractors should have at least a basic understanding of the topic and have knowledge of study design, data analysis and statistics. They should pay attention to detail while following instructions on the forms. Because errors that occur at the data extraction stage are rarely detected by peer reviewers, editors or users of systematic reviews, it is recommended that more than one person extract data from every report to minimize errors and reduce introduction of potential biases by review authors. As a minimum, information that involves subjective interpretation (e.g. related to quality judgements) and information that is critical to the interpretation of results (e.g. accuracy data) should be extracted independently by at least two people. In common with implementation of the selection process (see Chapter 6), it is preferable that data extractors are from complementary disciplines, for example a methodologist and a topic area specialist. It is important that everyone involved in data extraction has practice using the form and, if the form was designed by someone else, receives appropriate training.

Evidence in support of duplicate data extraction for at least some data extraction items comes from a number of indirect sources. One study observed that independent data extraction by two review authors resulted in fewer errors than data extraction by a single review author followed by verification by a second (Buscemi 2006). A second study showed similar odds of errors for independent data extraction compared to extraction by a less experienced review author with verification by a more experienced data abstractor for items related to study characteristics, but suggested higher odds of errors for items related to outcomes and results (Li 2019). A further study suggested that more experienced extractors made fewer errors in regard to outcomes and results, but more errors in baseline characteristics (Jian-Yu 2020).

7.5.3 Training data extractors

Training of data extractors is intended to familiarize them with the review topic and methods, the data collection form or data system, and issues that may arise during data extraction. Results of the pilot testing of the form should prompt discussion among review authors and extractors of ambiguous questions or responses to establish consistency. Training should take place at the onset of the data extraction process and periodically over the course of the project (Li 2015). For example, when data related to a single item on the form are present in multiple locations within a report (e.g. abstract, main body of text, tables and figures) or in several publications, the development and documentation of instructions to follow an agreed algorithm are critical and should be reinforced during the training sessions.

Some researchers have proposed that some information in a report, such as its authors, be blinded to the review author prior to data extraction and assessment of risk of bias (Jadad 1996). However, blinding of review authors to aspects of study reports generally is not recommended for Cochrane Reviews, as there is little evidence that it alters the decisions made (Berlin 1997).

7.5.4 Extracting data from multiple reports of the same study

Studies can be reported in more than one publication or in more than one source (Tramèr 1997, von Elm 2004). In systematic reviews of test accuracy, a single source often provides complete information about a study, but some studies do have multiple associated reports, which may contain conflicting information (Mayo-Wilson 2017a, Mayo-Wilson 2017b, Mayo-Wilson 2018). Alternatively, multiple publications may arise from the same participant cohort, with detailed testing methods or participant eligibility criteria provided only in the earliest publications rather than described in the eligible publication of interest.

Because the unit of interest in a systematic review is the study and not the report, information from multiple reports often needs to be collated and reconciled. It is not appropriate to discard any report of an included study without careful examination, since it may contain valuable information not included in the primary report. Review authors will need to decide between two strategies:

- extract data from each report separately, then combine information across multiple data collection forms; or
- extract data from all reports directly into a single data collection form.

The choice of which strategy to use will depend on the nature of the reports and may vary across studies and across reports. For example, when a full journal article and multiple conference abstracts are available, it is likely that the majority of information will be obtained from the journal article; completing a new data collection form for each conference abstract may be a waste of time. Conversely, when there are two or more detailed journal articles, perhaps relating to different recruitment periods for the same cohort or to different index tests for the same cohort, then it is likely to be easier to perform data extraction separately for these articles and collate information from the data collection forms afterwards. When data from all reports are extracted into a single data collection form, review authors should identify the 'main' data source for each study when sources include conflicting data and these differences cannot be resolved by contacting study authors (Mayo-Wilson 2018). Flow diagrams such as those modified from the PRISMA statement can be particularly helpful when collating and documenting information from multiple reports (Mayo-Wilson 2018).

7.5.5 Reliability and reaching consensus

When more than one review author extracts data from the same reports, there is potential for disagreement. After data have been extracted independently by two or more extractors, responses should be compared to ensure agreement or to identify discrepancies. An explicit procedure or decision rule should be specified in the protocol for identifying and resolving disagreements. The source of the disagreement may be an error by one of the extractors, which can be easily resolved. Thus, discussion among the review authors is a sensible first step. A disagreement may also require arbitration by another person. Disagreements that cannot be resolved could be addressed by contacting the study authors.

Agreement of coded items before reaching consensus can be quantified, for example using kappa statistics (Orwin 1994), although this is not routinely done in Cochrane Reviews. Regardless, the presence and resolution of disagreements should be carefully recorded. Maintaining a copy of the data 'as extracted' (in addition to the consensus data) allows assessment of the reliability of coding. Examples of ways in which this can be achieved include the following.

- Use one review author's (paper) data collection form and record changes after consensus in a different ink colour.
- Enter consensus data onto an electronic form.
- Record original data extracted and consensus data in separate forms (some online tools do this automatically).

If agreement is assessed, this should be done only for the most important data (e.g. key risk of bias assessments, or availability of key outcomes).

Throughout the review process informal consideration should be given to the reliability of data extraction. For example, if after reaching consensus on the first few studies the review authors note a frequent disagreement for specific data, then coding instructions may need modification. Furthermore, a review author's coding strategy may change over time as the coding rules are forgotten, indicating a need for retraining and, possibly, some recoding.

7.5.6 Suspicions of scientific misconduct

Systematic review authors can uncover suspected misconduct in the published literature. Misconduct includes fabrication or falsification of data or results, plagiarism and research that does not adhere to ethical norms. Review authors need to be aware of scientific misconduct, because the inclusion of fraudulent material could undermine the reliability of a review's findings. Plagiarism of results data in the form of duplicated publication (either by the same or by different authors) may, if undetected, lead to study participants being double-counted in a synthesis. If plagiarism is suspected, text-matching software and systems such as CrossCheck may be helpful, but they can detect only matching text, so data tables or figures need to be inspected by hand or using other systems (e.g. to detect image manipulation). The comparison of extracted 2×2 tables could also provide a useful means of detecting duplicated studies. Section 7.2.1 lists a number of different strategies for identifying multiple reports of the same study.

If misconduct is suspected, Cochrane Review authors are advised to consult with their Cochrane editors. Searching for comments, letters or retractions may uncover additional information. Sensitivity analyses can be used to determine whether the studies arousing suspicion are influential in the conclusions of the review. Guidance for editors for addressing suspected misconduct will be available from Cochrane's Editorial Publishing and Policy Resource (see community.cochrane.org). Further information is available from the Committee on Publication Ethics (COPE; publicationethics.org), including a series of flowcharts on how to proceed if various types of misconduct are suspected. Cases should be followed up, typically including an approach to the editors of the journals in which suspect reports were published. It may be useful to write first to the primary investigators to request clarification of apparent inconsistencies or unusual observations.

Because investigations may take time and institutions may not always be responsive (Wager 2011), studies suspected of being fraudulent should be classified as 'awaiting assessment'. If a misconduct investigation indicates that the publication is unreliable, or if a publication is retracted, it should not be included in the systematic review, and the reason should be noted in the 'excluded studies' section.

7.5.7 Key points in planning and reporting data extraction

In summary, the methods section of both the protocol and the review should detail:

- the data categories that are to be extracted;
- how extracted data from each report will be verified (e.g. extraction by two review authors, independently);
- whether data extraction is undertaken by content area experts, methodologists or both;
- pilot testing, training and existence of coding instructions for the data collection form;
- how data are extracted from multiple reports from the same study;
- how data should be handled for multiple index tests or multiple reference standards from the same study; and
- how disagreements are handled when more than one review author extracts data from each report.

7.6 Managing and sharing data and tools

When data have been collected for each individual study, it is helpful to organize them into a comprehensive electronic format, such as a database or spreadsheet, before such data can be used for a meta-analysis or other synthesis. When data are collated electronically, all or a subset of them can easily be exported for cleaning, consistency checks and analysis.

Table 7.6.a Example of a simple review with a single 'test'

Study	Test	TP	FP	FN	TN	Analysis
Basile 2015	Ultrasound	17	10	17	2	1
Brun 2012	Ultrasound	80	0	8	8	1
Brun 2014	Ultrasound	27	0	1	4	1
Chenaitia 2012	Ultrasound	116	0	2	12	1
Gok 2015	Ultrasound	52	0	4	0	1
Kim 2012	Ultrasound	38	1	6	2	1
Lock 2003	Ultrasound	43	0	15	2	1
Nikandros 2006	Ultrasound	15	0	1	0	1
Radulescu 2015	Ultrasound	28	0	2	2	1
Vigneau 2005	Ultrasound	34	0	1	0	1

Tabulation of collected information about studies can facilitate classification of study data sets into appropriate groups. It is important through this process to retain clear information on the provenance of the data, with a clear distinction between data from a source document and data obtained through calculations.

Although RevMan cannot be used for meta-analysis of test accuracy data (see Chapter 9), we recommend that all extracted and checked 2×2 data and covariates are copied to RevMan before exporting them for analysis. This ensures as far as possible that the data used to create forest plots of sensitivity and specificity and any SROC plots are the same as those used for meta-analysis.

An example of a simple review is provided in Table 7.6.a. This review of ultrasonography for confirmation of gastric tube placement in people who are unable to swallow included 10 studies contributing 2×2 data to a single RevMan 'test' (Tsujimoto 2017).

An example of a more complex review is provided in Table 7.6.b. This review of second-trimester serum tests for screening for Down syndrome included 59 studies with 2×2 tables organized into 89 different RevMan 'tests' (Alldred 2012). A number of different assays were reported at varying thresholds and data were therefore organized according to test and threshold. The 'Analysis' column shows how data sets might be coded for analysis purposes.

Another example of a complex review is shown in Table 7.6.c. This review of rapid tests for diagnosing malaria (Abba 2014) included studies of tests to detect two different types of malaria (non-falciparum or *Plasmodium vivax*) using multiple different assays (e.g. Falcifax or Onsite Pf/Pv) against different reference standards (microscopy or polymerase chain reaction (PCR)) that are likely to significantly affect observed accuracy.

Although the collation and reconciliation of information from multiple reports is recommended (Section 7.5.4), sometimes more than one 2×2 table from a study will be eligible for the same analysis. For example, a study can report accuracy data for the same test in more than one participant cohort from different centres. In the review of rapid tests for diagnosing malaria, one study contributed data to the same analysis from 10 different health centres (Table 7.6.d).

Table 7.6.b Example of a more complex review with multiple 'tests'

Study	Test	TP	FP	FN	TN	Analysis
Bartels 1990	SP1 at mixed cut-points	4	0	39	282	4
Bartels 1990	SP1 at 2.5 MoM	7	4	36	278	5
Haddow 1998	Inhibin A at mixed cut-points	27	21	25	235	1
Haddow 1998	Inhibin A at 2 MoM	27	21	25	235	3
Pandian 2004	Inhibin A at mixed cut-points	5	4	11	80	1
Pandian 2004	Inhibin A at 5% FPR	5	4	11	80	2
Pandian 2004	SP1 at mixed cut-points	13	4	3	80	4
Pandian 2004	SP1 at 5% FPR	13	4	3	80	6
Van Lith 1992	Inhibin A at mixed cut-points	5	8	5	72	1
Van Lith 1992	Inhibin A at 2 MoM	5	8	5	72	3
Wald 2003a	Inhibin A at mixed cut-points	48	51	34	959	1
Wald 2003a	Inhibin A at 5% FPR	48	51	34	959	2

FPR, false positive rate; MoM, multiples of the median.

Table 7.6.c Example of a more complex review with multiple 'tests' and reference standards

Study	Test	TP	FP	FN	TN	Target condition	Reference standard	Analysis
Alam 2011	OnSite Pf/pv	20	3	6	309	*P. vivax*	PCR	4
Chanie 2011	Carestart Pf/Pv	25	4	0	1063	*P. vivax*	Microscopy	3
Mekonnen 2010	Carestart Pf/Pv	61	0	3	176	*P. vivax*	Microscopy	3
Rakotonirina 2008	PALUTOP	19	0	2	292	*P. vivax*	PCR	4
Rakotonirina 2008	OptiMAL	15	6	2	290	Non-falciparum	PCR	5
Sharew 2009	Carestart Pf/Pv	155	9	1	503	*P. vivax*	Microscopy	3
Singh 2010	Parascreen	44	6	13	309	Non-falciparum	Microscopy	1
Xiaodon 2013	Carestart Pf/Pan	59	0	6	115	Non-falciparum	Microscopy	1
Xiaodon 2013	Carestart Pf/Pan	59	0	6	113	Non-falciparum	PCR	2
Yan 2013	One Step Malaria Pf/Pan	51	5	22	528	Non-falciparum	Microscopy	1
Yan 2013	One Step Malaria Pf/Pan	51	15	20	520	Non-falciparum	PCR	2
Yan 2013	Pf/Pv Malaria Device	43	7	30	270	*P. vivax*	PCR	4

Table 7.6.d Example of a review with a study with multiple centres

Study	Test	TP	FP	FN	TN	Target condition	Reference standard
Ashton 2010	Parascreen	203	96	43	2041	Non-falciparum	Microscopy
Bendezu 2010	Parascreen	64	6	19	243	Non-falciparum	Microscopy
Elahi 2013	Parascreen	49	3	5	270	Non-falciparum	Microscopy
Endeshaw 2012(a)	Parascreen	3	4	3	190	Non-falciparum	Microscopy
Endeshaw 2012(b)	Parascreen	32	4	4	160	Non-falciparum	Microscopy
Endeshaw 2012(c)	Parascreen	6	3	5	184	Non-falciparum	Microscopy
Endeshaw 2012(d)	Parascreen	2	1	2	195	Non-falciparum	Microscopy
Endeshaw 2012(e)	Parascreen	5	7	0	185	Non-falciparum	Microscopy
Endeshaw 2012(f)	Parascreen	8	0	0	192	Non-falciparum	Microscopy
Endeshaw 2012(g)	Parascreen	3	1	2	192	Non-falciparum	Microscopy
Endeshaw 2012(h)	Parascreen	14	0	2	184	Non-falciparum	Microscopy
Endeshaw 2012(i)	Parascreen	10	4	0	186	Non-falciparum	Microscopy
Endeshaw 2012(j)	Parascreen	4	3	12	181	Non-falciparum	Microscopy
Singh 2010	Parascreen	44	6	13	309	Non-falciparum	Microscopy

Ideally, data only need to be extracted once and should be stored in a secure and stable location for future updates of the review, regardless of whether the original review authors or a different group of authors update the review (Ip 2012).

Standardizing and sharing data collection tools as well as data management systems among review authors working in similar topic areas can streamline systematic review production. Review authors have the opportunity to work with study investigators, journal editors, funders, regulators and other stakeholders to make study data publicly available, increasing the transparency of research. When legal and ethical to do so, we encourage review authors to share the data and the tools used in their systematic reviews to reduce waste and to allow verification and reanalysis, because data will not have to be extracted again for future use (Mayo-Wilson 2018).

7.7 Chapter information

Authors: Jacqueline Dinnes (*Institute of Applied Health Research, University of Birmingham, UK*), Jonathan J. Deeks (*Institute of Applied Health Research, University of Birmingham, UK*), Mariska M. Leeflang (*Department of Epidemiology and Data Science, University of Amsterdam, The Netherlands*), Tianjing Li (*Department of Ophthalmology, University of Colorado Anschutz Medical Campus, USA*)

Sources of support: Jonathan J. Deeks is a UK National Institute for Health Research (NIHR) Senior Investigator Emeritus. Jonathan J. Deeks and Jacqueline Dinnes are supported by the NIHR Birmingham Biomedical Research Centre at the University Hospitals

Birmingham NHS Foundation Trust and the University of Birmingham. The views expressed are those of the authors and not necessarily those of the NHS, the NIHR or the Department of Health and Social Care. No other authors declare sources of support for writing this chapter.

Declarations of interest: Jacqueline Dinnes, Jonathan J. Deeks and Mariska M. Leeflang are members of Cochrane's Diagnostic Test Accuracy Editorial Team. Mariska M. Leeflang is co-convenor of the Cochrane Screening and Diagnostic Tests Methods Group. Tianjing Li is co-convenor of the Cochrane Comparing Multiple Interventions Methods Group and a member of the Cochrane Methods Executive. The authors declare no other potential conflicts of interest relevant to the topic of this chapter.

Acknowledgements: This chapter re-uses and builds on material included in the following chapter of the *Cochrane Handbook for Systematic Reviews of Interventions* to ensure consistency in guidance for authors of Cochrane Reviews: Li T, Higgins JPT, Deeks JJ (editors). Chapter 5: Collecting data. In: Higgins JPT, Thomas J, Chandler J, Cumpston M, Li T, Page MJ, Welch VA (editors). *Cochrane Handbook for Systematic Reviews of Interventions* version 6.1 (updated September 2020). Cochrane, 2020.

The authors would like to thank Jérémie Cohen, Eleanor Ochodo and Jean-Paul Salameh for useful peer review comments.

7.8 References

Abba K, Kirkham AJ, Olliaro PL, Deeks JJ, Donegan S, Garner P, Takwoingi Y. Rapid diagnostic tests for diagnosing uncomplicated non-falciparum or Plasmodium vivax malaria in endemic countries. *Cochrane Database of Systematic Reviews* 2014; **12**: CD011431.

Alldred SK, Deeks JJ, Guo B, Neilson JP, Alfirevic Z. Second trimester serum tests for Down's Syndrome screening. *Cochrane Database of Systematic Reviews* 2012; **6**: CD009925.

Berlin JA. Does blinding of readers affect the results of meta-analyses? University of Pennsylvania Meta-analysis Blinding Study Group. *Lancet* 1997; **350**: 185–186.

Buscemi N, Hartling L, Vandermeer B, Tjosvold L, Klassen TP. Single data extraction generated more errors than double data extraction in systematic reviews. *Journal of Clinical Epidemiology* 2006; **59**: 697–703.

Cader MZ, Filer A, Hazlehurst J, de Pablo P, Buckley CD, Raza K. Performance of the 2010 ACR/EULAR criteria for rheumatoid arthritis: comparison with 1987 ACR criteria in a very early synovitis cohort. *Annals of the Rheumatic Diseases* 2011; **70**: 949.

Cooper C, Bou JT, Varley-Campbell J. Evaluating the effectiveness, efficiency, cost and value of contacting study authors in a systematic review: a case study and worked example. *BMC Medical Research Methodology* 2019; **19**: 45.

Danko KJ, Dahabreh IJ, Ivers NM, Moher D, Grimshaw JM. Contacting authors by telephone increased response proportions compared with emailing: results of a randomized study. *Journal of Clinical Epidemiology* 2019; **115**: 150–159.

de Groot JA, Janssen KJ, Zwinderman AH, Bossuyt PM, Reitsma JB, Moons KG. Correcting for partial verification bias: a comparison of methods. *Annals of Epidemiology* 2011; **21**: 139–148.

Godolphin PJ, Bath PM, Montgomery AA. Short email with attachment versus long email without attachment when contacting authors to request unpublished data for a systematic review: a nested randomised trial. *BMJ Open* 2019; **9**: e025273.

Gøtzsche PC. Multiple publication of reports of drug trials. *European Journal of Clinical Pharmacology* 1989; **36**: 429–432.

Gross A, Schirm S, Scholz M. Ycasd – a tool for capturing and scaling data from graphical representations. *BMC Bioinformatics* 2014; **15**: 219.

Hooper L, Abdelhamid A, Attreed NJ, Campbell WW, Channell AM, Chassagne P, Culp KR, Fletcher SJ, Fortes MB, Fuller N, Gaspar PM, Gilbert DJ, Heathcote AC, Kafri MW, Kajii F, Lindner G, Mack GW, Mentes JC, Merlani P, Needham RA, Olde Rikkert MG, Perren A, Powers J, Ranson SC, Ritz P, Rowat AM, Sjöstrand F, Smith AC, Stookey JJ, Stotts NA, Thomas DR, Vivanti A, Wakefield BJ, Waldréus N, Walsh NP, Ward S, Potter JF, Hunter P. Clinical symptoms, signs and tests for identification of impending and current water-loss dehydration in older people. *Cochrane Database of Systematic Reviews* 2015; **4**: CD009647.

ICH. ICH Harmonised tripartite guideline: Struture and content of clinical study reports E31995. ICH1995. www.ich.org/fileadmin/Public_Web_Site/ICH_Products/Guidelines/Efficacy/E3/E3_Guideline.pdf.

Ip S, Hadar N, Keefe S, Parkin C, Iovin R, Balk EM, Lau J. A web-based archive of systematic review data. *Systematic Reviews* 2012; **1**: 15.

Jadad AR, Moore RA, Carroll D, Jenkinson C, Reynolds DJM, Gavaghan DJ, McQuay H. Assessing the quality of reports of randomized clinical trials: is blinding necessary? *Controlled Clinical Trials* 1996; **17**: 1–12.

Jelicic Kadic A, Vucic K, Dosenovic S, Sapunar D, Puljak L. Extracting data from figures with software was faster, with higher interrater reliability than manual extraction. *Journal of Clinical Epidemiology* 2016; **74**: 119–123.

Jian-Yu E, Saldanha I, Canner J, Schmid C, Le J, Li T. Adjudication rather than experience of data abstraction matters more in reducing errors in abstracting data in systematic reviews. *Research Synthesis Methods* 2020; **11**: 354–362.

Korevaar DA, Bossuyt PM, Hooft L. Infrequent and incomplete registration of test accuracy studies: analysis of recent study reports. *BMJ Open* 2014; **4**: e004596.

Korevaar DA, Hooft L, Askie LM, Barbour V, Faure H, Gatsonis CA, Hunter KE, Kressel HY, Lippman H, McInnes MDF, Moher D, Rifai N, Cohen JF, Bossuyt PMM. Facilitating prospective registration of diagnostic accuracy studies: a STARD initiative. *Clinical Chemistry* 2017; **63**: 1331–1341.

Korevaar DA, Salameh JP, Vali Y, Cohen JF, McInnes MDF, Spijker R, Bossuyt PM. Searching practices and inclusion of unpublished studies in systematic reviews of diagnostic accuracy. *Research Synthesis Methods* 2020; **11**: 343–353.

Leeflang MM, Debets-Ossenkopp YJ, Wang J, Visser CE, Scholten RJ, Hooft L, Bijlmer HA, Reitsma JB, Zhang M, Bossuyt PM, Vandenbroucke-Grauls CM. Galactomannan detection for invasive aspergillosis in immunocompromised patients. *Cochrane Database of Systematic Reviews* 2015; **12**: CD007394.

Li G, Abbade LPF, Nwosu I, Jin Y, Leenus A, Maaz M, Wang M, Bhatt M, Zielinski L, Sanger N, Bantoto B, Luo C, Shams I, Shahid H, Chang Y, Sun G, Mbuagbaw L, Samaan Z, Levine MAH, Adachi JD, Thabane L. A scoping review of comparisons between abstracts and full reports in primary biomedical research. *BMC Medical Research Methodology* 2017; **17**: 181.

Li TJ, Vedula SS, Hadar N, Parkin C, Lau J, Dickersin K. Innovations in data collection, management, and archiving for systematic reviews. *Annals of Internal Medicine* 2015; **162**: 287–294.

Li T, Saldanha IJ, Jap J, Smith BT, Canner J, Hutfless SM, Branch V, Carini S, Chan W, de Bruijn B, Wallace BC, Walsh SA, Whamond EJ, Murad MH, Sim I, Berlin JA, Lau J, Dickersin K, Schmid CH. A randomized trial provided new evidence on the accuracy and efficiency of traditional vs. electronically annotated abstraction approaches in systematic reviews. *Journal of Clinical Epidemiology* 2019; **115**: 77–89.

Luis Caro-Oleas J, Fernández-Suárez A, Reneses Cesteros S, Porrino C, Núñez-Roldán A, Wichmann Schlipf I. Diagnostic usefulness of a third-generation anti-cyclic citrulline antibody test in patients with recent-onset polyarthritis. *Clinical Chemistry and Laboratory Medicine* 2007; **45**: 1396–1401.

Manzotti C, Casazza G, Stimac T, Nikolova D, Gluud C. Total serum bile acids or serum bile acid profile, or both, for the diagnosis of intrahepatic cholestasis of pregnancy. *Cochrane Database of Systematic Reviews* 2019; **7**: CD012546.

Mayo-Wilson E, Li TJ, Fusco N, Bertizzolo L, Canner JK, Cowley T, Doshi P, Ehmsen J, Gresham G, Guo N, Haythomthwaite JA, Heyward J, Hong H, Pham D, Payne JL, Rosman L, Stuart EA, Suarez-Cuervo C, Tolbert E, Twose C, Vedula S, Dickersin K. Cherry-picking by trialists and meta-analysts can drive conclusions about intervention efficacy. *Journal of Clinical Epidemiology* 2017a; **91**: 95–110.

Mayo-Wilson E, Fusco N, Li TJ, Hong H, Canner JK, Dickersin K, MUDS Investigators. Multiple outcomes and analyses in clinical trials create challenges for interpretation and research synthesis. *Journal of Clinical Epidemiology* 2017b; **86**: 39–50.

Mayo-Wilson E, Li T, Fusco N, Dickersin K. Practical guidance for using multiple data sources in systematic reviews and meta-analyses (with examples from the MUDS study). *Research Synthesis Methods* 2018; **9**: 2–12.

McInnes MDF, Moher D, Thombs BD, McGrath TA, Bossuyt PM, Clifford T, Cohen JF, Deeks JJ, Gatsonis C, Hooft L, Hunt HA, Hyde CJ, Korevaar DA, Leeflang MMG, Macaskill P, Reitsma JB, Rodin R, Rutjes AWS, Salameh JP, Stevens A, Takwoingi Y, Tonelli M, Weeks L, Whiting P, Willis BH. Preferred Reporting Items for a Systematic Review and Meta-analysis of Diagnostic Test Accuracy Studies: The PRISMA-DTA Statement. *JAMA* 2018; **319**: 388–396.

Meade MO, Richardson WS. Selecting and appraising studies for a systematic review. *Annals of Internal Medicine* 1997; **127**: 531–537.

Okba NMA, Müller MA, Li W, Wang C, GeurtsvanKessel CH, Corman VM, Lamers MM, Sikkema RS, de Bruin E, Chandler FD, Yazdanpanah Y, Le Hingrat Q, Descamps D, Houhou-Fidouh N, Reusken C, Bosch BJ, Drosten C, Koopmans MPG, Haagmans BL. Severe Acute Respiratory Syndrome Coronavirus 2-specific antibody responses in coronavirus disease patients. *Emerging Infectious Diseases* 2020; **26**: 1478–1488.

Orwin R. Evaluating coding decisions. In: Cooper H, Hedges L, editors. *Handbook of Research Synthesis*. New York (NY): Russell Sage Foundation; 1994.

Riley RD, Dodd SR, Craig JV, Thompson JR, Williamson PR. Meta-analysis of diagnostic test studies using individual patient data and aggregate data. *Statistics in Medicine* 2008; **27**: 6111–6136.

Selph SS, Ginsburg AD, Chou R. Impact of contacting study authors to obtain additional data for systematic reviews: diagnostic accuracy studies for hepatic fibrosis. *Systematic Reviews* 2014; **3**: 107.

Shinkins B, Thompson M, Mallett S, Perera R. Diagnostic accuracy studies: how to report and analyse inconclusive test results. *BMJ* 2013; **346**: f2778.

Stewart LA, Clarke M, Rovers M, Riley RD, Simmonds M, Stewart G, Tierney JF, PRISMA-IPD Development Group. Preferred reporting items for a systematic review and meta-analysis of individual participant data: the PRISMA-IPD statement. *JAMA* 2015; **313**: 1657–1665.

Stock WA. Systematic coding for research synthesis. In: Cooper H, Hedges L, editors. *Handbook of Research Synthesis*. New York (NY): Russell Sage Foundation; 1994.

Tramèr MR, Reynolds DJ, Moore RA, McQuay HJ. Impact of covert duplicate publication on meta-analysis: a case study. *BMJ* 1997; **315**: 635–640.

Tsujimoto H, Tsujimoto Y, Nakata Y, Akazawa M, Kataoka Y. Ultrasonography for confirmation of gastric tube placement. *Cochrane Database of Systematic Reviews* 2017; **4**: CD012083.

van der Pol CB, Lim CS, Sirlin CB, McGrath TA, Salameh J-P, Bashir MR, Tang A, Singal AG, Costa AF, Fowler K, McInnes MDF. Accuracy of the liver imaging reporting and data system in computed tomography and magnetic resonance image analysis of hepatocellular carcinoma or overall malignancy – a systematic review. *Gastroenterology* 2019; **156**: 976–986.

von Elm E, Poglia G, Walder B, Tramèr MR. Different patterns of duplicate publication: an analysis of articles used in systematic reviews. *JAMA* 2004; **291**: 974–980.

Wager E. Coping with scientific misconduct. *BMJ* 2011; **343**: d6586.

Whitworth HS, Badhan A, Boakye AA, Takwoingi Y, Rees-Roberts M, Partlett C, Lambie H, Innes J, Cooke G, Lipman M, Conlon C, Macallan D, Chua F, Post FA, Wiselka M, Woltmann G, Deeks JJ, Kon OM, Lalvani A, Abdoyeku D, Davidson R, Dedicoat M, Kunst H, Loebingher MR, Lynn W, Nathani N, O'Connell R, Pozniak A, Menzies S. Clinical utility of existing and second-generation interferon-gamma release assays for diagnostic evaluation of tuberculosis: an observational cohort study. *Lancet Infectious Diseases* 2019; **19**: 193–202.

8

Assessing risk of bias and applicability

Johannes B. Reitsma, Anne W. Rutjes, Penny Whiting, Bada Yang, Mariska M. Leeflang, Patrick M. Bossuyt and Jonathan J. Deeks

---

KEY POINTS

- Shortcomings in the design and conduct of test accuracy studies can lead to biased estimates of test accuracy. This is supported by empirical evidence for studies of the accuracy of single tests.
- Cochrane recommends using the QUADAS-2 tool to evaluate the risk of bias and applicability of test accuracy studies.
- QUADAS-2 assesses the risk of bias of a study across four domains: participant selection, index test, reference standard, and flow and timing, as well as an overall assessment of risk of bias. Applicability of the findings to the review question is evaluated for participant selection, index test and reference standard.
- In studies evaluating the accuracy of two or more index tests, an assessment of risk of bias and applicability should be performed for each index test included in the review.
- If the accuracy of different tests will be compared in the review, corresponding comparisons of accuracy in primary studies should also be assessed for risk of bias using QUADAS-C, an extension of QUADAS-2 for comparative accuracy studies.
- Review authors need to provide guidance in both the protocol and the final review on how to answer each signalling question and how to arrive at the judgement of risk of bias for each QUADAS-2 domain.
- Assessments should preferentially be undertaken in parallel by two or more review authors, and there should be an explicit procedure to resolve disagreements.

This chapter should be cited as: Reitsma JB, Rutjes AW., Whiting P, Yang B, Leeflang MM, Bossuyt PM, Deeks JJ. Chapter 8: Assessing risk of bias and applicability. In: Deeks JJ, Bossuyt PM, Leeflang MM, Takwoingi Y, editors. *Cochrane Handbook for Systematic Reviews of Diagnostic Test Accuracy*. 1st edition. Chichester (UK): John Wiley & Sons, 2023: 169–202.

8.1   Introduction

The findings of the assessment of risk of bias and applicability play an important role in the systematic review process, in particular in the analysis and interpretation of results. Whether a systematic review of test accuracy studies allows conclusions about the accuracy of a test, or differences in accuracy between two or more tests, will depend on having available studies at low risk of bias that directly apply to the review question.

Certain flaws in the design and conduct of test accuracy studies can produce incorrect or biased results. These flaws put the corresponding study at 'risk of bias', meaning that its internal validity is threatened. Examples of potential issues include the use of an imperfect reference standard, omitting results from the analyses, or interpreting index test results with knowledge of the result of the reference standard.

Even in the absence of such flaws, a test accuracy study may generate results that do not help answer the review question. Study participants may not be similar to those defined by the review question, the test may be used at a different point in the clinical pathway, or the test may be used in a different way than intended in the review question. Such a mismatch may lead to concerns regarding the applicability of the results from a particular study to the review question. In systematic reviews of test accuracy, both the risk of bias and applicability are assessed.

Risk of bias and concerns regarding applicability can be considered at different points in the systematic review process. First, eligibility criteria are defined to ensure that the included studies meet some minimum criteria. For example, a review may include only studies that use a particular reference standard, or include only studies in which a third-generation computed tomography (CT) scanner has been compared to more recent CT scanners. The use of eligibility criteria is discussed in Chapter 5. Detailed assessment of risk of bias and applicability of all studies included in the review is then undertaken and the results reported. This process is addressed in this chapter.

In the analysis phase, studies may be grouped according to characteristics related to risk of bias or concerns regarding applicability. This can be done both in investigations of heterogeneity, which investigate differences in results attributable to identifiable study features, and in sensitivity analyses, which limit the impact of studies of questionable rigour on study estimates, as described in Chapter 9.

The strength of evidence supporting a review's conclusions depends on the overall assessment of risk of bias and applicability of the evidence base. Recommendations for future research are made, noting particular methodological deficiencies in the existing studies, as outlined in Chapter 12. If the results of individual studies are biased and they are synthesized without consideration of this bias, then the conclusions of the review cannot be trusted.

The focus of this chapter is on assessing risk of bias and applicability for individual studies in a review. These studies may have assessed the accuracy of one index test, of multiple tests, or they may have compared the accuracy of two or more tests.

Specific issues arise for individual studies making a comparison between two or more index tests. For example, a head-to-head comparison between two index tests made within a study where all individuals receive both tests under evaluation will be regarded as more valid than comparisons made between studies where the two tests are evaluated in different studies (see Chapter 3). This chapter also provides guidance on assessing comparative accuracy studies (Yang 2021a).

8.2   Understanding bias and applicability

8.2.1   Bias and imprecision

Bias is a systematic error or deviation from the truth, either in the results of a study or in inference based on these results. Biases can act in either direction, leading to over-estimation or under-estimation of the true test accuracy.

It is difficult to evaluate whether the results of a single study are biased, and often impossible to predict the magnitude of a bias. However, when weaknesses or short-comings are identified, judgements can be made of the risk of bias in an individual study, and sometimes its likely direction and size can be hypothesized.

Bias should not be confused with imprecision, which arises when an estimate is based on a small sample. Imprecision results from random error, whereas bias reflects a systematic error. Statistical analysis can appropriately describe the uncertainty in an estimate caused by random error, by using confidence intervals for example, but the confidence interval provides no information about the presence or absence of systematic error. In a systematic review we assess the risk of bias by examining the design and conduct of included studies.

8.2.2   Bias versus applicability

Traditionally the broader phrase 'assessment of methodological quality' was used (Moher 1996, Ioannidis 1998, Verhagen 2001), but in 2008 this was replaced by 'assessment of risk of bias' in Cochrane Reviews of interventions. Risk of bias focuses on whether the results of an individual study are valid and should be believed (Higgins 2008). Assessments focused on judging whether the methods used could introduce a risk of systematic error (i.e. bias) rather than on assessing the broader concept of methodological quality.

In addition to the assessment of risk of bias, a separate concept is considered in systematic reviews of test accuracy: the applicability of the results of individual studies to the review question (see Box 8.2.a). In test accuracy research the applicability of study findings to the review question matters, because estimates of accuracy can differ depending on population and setting characteristics (Ransohoff 1978, Mulherin 2002, Whiting 2013).

Box 8.2.a Bias and applicability

Bias: the degree to which estimates of diagnostic accuracy deviate from the truth. Risk of bias occurs if systematic flaws or limitations in the design or conduct of a test accuracy study produce study results that do not reflect the true accuracy of the test(s), as evaluated in the study.

Applicability: the extent to which findings from a primary study apply to the review question. Concerns regarding applicability may arise if the index test was evaluated in conditions that differ from those in the review question: if the index test was applied or interpreted differently, in a study group with different demographic or clinical features, or with a different definition of the target condition.

Concerns regarding applicability address partial or potential mismatches between the question addressed in an individual study and the question addressed in the systematic review. A study of a rapid antigen detection test in children, for example, may be done without serious limitations in design and conduct, and therefore be classified as at low risk of producing biased results. Yet if the review question addressed the performance of that same test in adults, the study findings may not directly answer the question of the systematic review, and review authors can express concerns regarding the applicability of the results of that study to their review.

A single diagnostic test can be applied in different ways and in different positions in the clinical pathway. For example, positron emission tomography–computed tomography (PET-CT) could be used as an add-on test after conventional staging to detect additional metastases in colorectal cancer patients with negative findings on earlier tests. In contrast, PET-CT could also be used as the first test in persons just diagnosed with colorectal cancer. Both are relevant uses of the test (potential review questions), but diagnostic accuracy may vary depending on the intended use of PET-CT. A study of PET-CT without methodological shortcomings, at low risk of producing biased results, may receive different applicability judgements, depending on the specific review question being addressed.

Poor and incomplete reporting of test accuracy studies frequently hampers the assessment of key features of design or conduct, making it difficult to judge the risk of bias or applicability (Reid 1995, Bossuyt 2003a, Lumbreras-Lacarra 2004, Smidt 2005, Korevaar 2015). When aspects of study design or execution are not reported, it is impossible for the reader to differentiate between poorly reported studies that used robust methodology, and studies applying poor methods that are likely to produce biased results. There are signs that the publication of the STARD statement (STAndards for the Reporting of Diagnostic accuracy studies) in 2003 (Bossuyt 2003a, Bossuyt 2003b) has improved the reporting of test accuracy studies, and it is hoped that this trend will continue (Korevaar 2014, Korevaar 2015). The STARD statement was updated in 2015 to STARD 2015 (Cohen 2016).

8.2.3 Biases in test accuracy studies: empirical evidence

The bias associated with particular study features can be examined in a field known as meta-epidemiology (Naylor 1997, Sterne 2002). A meta-epidemiological study starts with one or more sets of primary test accuracy studies. Each set examines a similar test accuracy question, but diagnostic tests and questions can differ across sets. Within each set, accuracy estimates of studies with and without a specific design feature are compared to get an empirical estimate of the bias associated with that feature. In the case of multiple sets of studies, estimates from each set can be included in meta-analysis, to obtain a more precise estimate of the bias.

While estimation and detection of the impact of certain design features have been well studied for randomized controlled trials in meta-epidemiology, only a few such projects have been undertaken for test accuracy studies (Lijmer 1999, Rutjes 2006). For many aspects of study methodology, conclusions about the existence or the magnitude of bias are based on case studies or on theoretical reasoning (Whiting 2013). Where meta-epidemiological evidence of bias for particular design items exists, we profile both empirical and theoretical evidence when discussing and illustrating specific issues within each domain.

8.3 QUADAS-2

8.3.1 Background

A large number of methodological quality assessment tools are available for test accuracy studies. A review of such tools in 2005 identified over 90 instruments (Whiting 2005). Because of the lack of a universal tool that can be used for test accuracy studies across all clinical domains and types of index tests, an initiative was started to develop a generic tool named QUADAS (Whiting 2003).

QUADAS-2 is a revision of the original QUADAS tool (Whiting 2011). QUADAS was formally revised and redesigned based on feedback from review authors, developments in the risk-of-bias tool for intervention reviews and new evidence about sources of bias and variation in test accuracy studies (Whiting 2013).

The QUADAS-2 tool has been widely accepted and is now the most frequently used tool for the assessment of risk of bias and applicability of primary studies in a systematic review of test accuracy; it is recommended by Cochrane for Cochrane Reviews of diagnostic test accuracy. The latest version of the tool, a template and background information can be found at www.quadas.org.

Key characteristics of the QUADAS-2 tool are:

- It evaluates the risk of bias of a study in four key domains:
  - participant selection (Section 8.4);
  - index test (Section 8.5);
  - reference standard (Section 8.6); and
  - flow and timing (Section 8.7).
- Signalling questions are included to facilitate judgements of the risk of bias.
- The first three domains are also assessed to identify concerns regarding applicability.
- For each domain, studies are rated as 'low', 'high' or 'unclear' for risk of bias; and 'low', 'high' or 'unclear' for concerns regarding applicability.

QUADAS-C, an extension of QUADAS-2 designed to assess risk of bias in primary studies comparing the accuracy of two or more tests, was published in 2021 (Yang 2021a). Later, we discuss QUADAS-2 as a starting point and explain where in the process the assessment should be modified for comparative accuracy studies, as recommended by QUADAS-C.

8.3.2 Risk-of-bias assessment

Signalling questions have been included to facilitate the process of reaching a judgement on the risk of bias for each domain. These questions are mainly factual questions that flag the potential for bias. Signalling questions are answered 'Yes', 'No' or 'Unclear', and are phrased such that 'Yes' indicates low risk of bias. If all signalling questions for a domain are answered 'Yes', then risk of bias for this domain can be judged as 'low'. If any signalling question is answered 'No', this flags the potential for bias.

It is possible that one or more signalling questions are answered 'No' while the domain-level judgement is still 'low risk of bias'. A 'No' answer should lead to a closer examination of the potential effect of design deficiencies, in terms of bias. If the shortcoming exists but is relatively minor, the final judgement could still be that the study is at low risk of producing biased results.

Review authors should rely on judgement to decide whether the potential source of bias flagged by the signalling question puts the study at risk of bias for that domain. The 'unclear' category should be used only when insufficient data are reported to permit a judgement.

When assessing risk of bias in a comparative accuracy study, the same structure and the same domains are assessed. The domains are first evaluated for each index test and then, with additional signalling questions, for the comparison. In Section 8.4 to Section 8.7, specific guidance for comparative accuracy will be discussed in addition to the guidance for single test accuracy.

8.3.3 Applicability assessment

Review authors are expected to record the information on which the judgement of applicability is based and then to rate their concern that the study does not match the review question. Concerns regarding applicability are judged as 'low', 'high' or 'unclear'. Applicability judgements depend on precise formulations of review questions. Here also, the 'unclear' category should only be used when insufficient data are reported. The specific sections on each domain provide a more detailed explanation on how to judge the concerns regarding applicability in all relevant domains.

In comparative accuracy studies, concerns regarding applicability are captured by the QUADAS-2 assessments for each of the index tests in the comparison. Therefore, QUADAS-C does not include questions on applicability.

8.3.4 Using and tailoring QUADAS-2

Detailed information on how to answer the signalling questions and how to arrive at a risk-of-bias judgement for each domain are provided in Section 8.4. To make the process as transparent and objective as possible, review authors should produce guidance specifically for their review on how to answer each signalling question and how to use the answers to signalling questions to reach a judgement of risk of bias for each domain. Providing clear instructions on how to answer the signalling questions will improve consistency of interpretation between assessors. This should be done at the protocol stage, prior to conducting the QUADAS-2 assessment.

Review authors also have the option of adding specific signalling questions within a domain if particular issues relevant to their review are not fully covered by the standard QUADAS-2 tool. If review authors decide to add their own questions to the tool, they should phrase these in the same way as the questions in the main tool, to facilitate standardized reporting and interpretation of risk of bias and applicability in the review. Signalling questions should always be phrased so that a 'Yes' answer indicates no or limited risk of bias, and care should be taken that each question only covers one potential aspect of bias. For many reviews, the need to add questions will be limited.

8.3.5 Flow diagram

A flow diagram depicts the method of recruiting participants (for example, using a consecutive series of participants with specific symptoms suspected of having the target condition or separate groups of participants, one with and one without the target condition), the number of participants receiving which index test(s), which reference standard(s) and in which order. For a comparative accuracy study, drawing a flow diagram may help differentiate different study designs, e.g. (1) studies in which all eligible participants were given all index tests from (2) studies in which participants were given either one or both index tests, but of which only the fully paired subset was analysed. A good flow diagram will facilitate the answering of signalling questions and lead to better judgements of the risk of bias in a test accuracy study.

Review authors should draw a flow diagram for each included primary study if none is reported in the publication or if the published flow diagram is inadequate.

No single flow diagram structure can apply to all test accuracy designs; review authors will need to construct carefully the diagram for the study under evaluation. An example of a flow diagram, representing the recruitment of participants and the flow of participants, is given in Figure 8.3.a. Additional examples of flow diagrams can be found in the online supplementary material (8.S1 Example study flow diagrams).

8.3.6 Performing the QUADAS-2 assessment

Once the tool has been adapted to the review question and a final version with accompanying guidance has been produced, the next step is to develop a form to record the risk-of-bias and applicability assessment. On this form the review authors can record the answers to the signalling questions, and the judgement of risk of bias and applicability for each domain. This form should also contain space to record support for the judgement, a

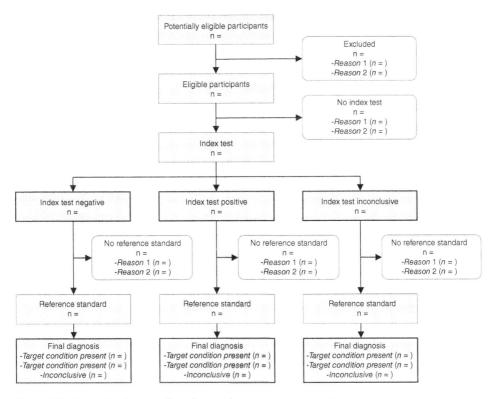

Figure 8.3.a Example of a study flow diagram for a test accuracy study

succinct summary of the stated facts given in the study report upon which the judgement is based. Review authors may find it useful to note where the description is taken from (e.g. the exact location within a report) for their own reference purposes.

A period of testing and training is essential to improve the quality of forms and to calibrate answers between review authors, thereby lowering the number of future disagreements. It is usually a good idea for review authors to pilot the form on a diverse sample of at least five reports included in the review and then to meet and discuss any discrepancies in ratings.

Poor reporting is a major obstacle to risk-of-bias assessment because it obscures whether a design feature was correctly applied but not reported, or was inappropriately applied, potentially introducing bias. Contacting study authors for further information is one method of dealing with poor reporting (Pai 2003) (see Chapter 7, Section 7.2.2). This process may provide useful information and so is a worthwhile undertaking. To reduce the risk of overly positive answers, caution should be exercised in ensuring that study authors are not asked leading questions. For example, it is better to ask the study authors to describe their processes, such as 'How did the physicians in the study decide whether an individual underwent biopsy?' or 'What information was the radiologist given about a patient?', rather than directly asking them to make a judgement as to whether their study was at risk of producing biased results.

Preferably, at least two review authors should perform the assessment independently. The review authors should have relevant knowledge of both the methodological issues of test accuracy studies and the clinical topic area. There should be an explicit procedure for resolving disagreements among review authors. This may involve discussion between review authors or referral to a third author if agreement cannot be reached.

Blinding for journal, and/or names of study authors, is not recommended, as it can be difficult to achieve in practice, is time consuming and its benefit is uncertain (Jadad 1996, Berlin 1997, Kjaergard 2001, Gluud 2008).

Review authors are encouraged to clarify, for each question, why they assigned a judgement for the corresponding domain, in light of potential problems being present.

8.4 Domain 1: Participant selection

The first domain relates to participant selection: how study participants were identified, contacted and included in the study, and whether this could have introduced bias. Applicability refers to the match, or the lack thereof, between study participants and the target population, as defined in the review question.

8.4.1 Participant selection: risk-of-bias signalling questions (QUADAS-2)

The key issue to address here is whether the selection of participants could have introduced bias. QUADAS-2 includes three signalling questions to flag the risk of bias for the participant selection domain.

Signalling question 1: Was a consecutive or random sample of participants enrolled?
A test accuracy study should ideally enrol a consecutive series of participants suspected of having the target condition, or a random sample thereof. Studies that recruit

participants in a different way may produce estimates of test accuracy that do not reflect the performance of the test in clinical practice.

Enrolling a consecutive series of participants, or a random sample thereof, ensures that study participants are likely to be representative of those undergoing testing in practice. It guarantees that persons more difficult to diagnose are not purposefully excluded from a study, or that persons for whom there is a strong suspicion of the target condition are not preferentially selected for inclusion in the study. Review authors should note that the term 'consecutive' is used liberally by authors in primary study reports, and does not always indicate a truly consecutive series of participants suspected of having the target condition.

A large number of studies reporting on the accuracy of a test have included a study group that does not form a consecutive series of participants suspected of having the target condition. Instead, they have recruited what can best be described as convenience samples: they used results at hand or recruited study participants in a non-systematic way, for example.

Examples are studies that searched hospital records for patients who, in the past, had undergone both the index test and the reference standard, or comparative accuracy studies enrolling only participants in whom a second index test was deemed necessary. Such situations should be flagged as having non-consecutive series (signalling question), but when judging the risk of bias for this domain, review authors need to consider whether the sampling strategy is likely to have introduced bias.

Critical in this judgement is whether the included group of participants can still be considered representative of the target population. This judgement can be difficult, as many studies do not explicitly report on the processes for identifying, selecting and inviting potentially eligible study participants.

Signalling question 2: Was a case-control design avoided?
Some studies use one selection process to recruit participants already known to have the target condition and a different one to recruit participants known not to have the target condition (see 'multiple groups' in Chapter 3) (Rutjes 2005). This used to be referred to as a 'case-control design'. The selection of 'cases' (those with the target condition) and 'controls' (those without the target condition) then becomes a critical issue, as estimates of sensitivity and specificity will be biased if cases and/or controls systematically differ from individuals with and without the target condition within the target population.

A clear example is a study including one group of participants with the target condition and a second group of healthy controls (Lijmer 1999, Pai 2003). Including healthy, asymptomatic controls, such as blood donors, can be expected to lead to fewer false positive test results compared to the inclusion of participants with symptoms suggesting the presence of the target condition. As a consequence, estimates of specificity are likely to be inflated.

Accuracy studies with multiple groups of participants, each recruited in a different way, often also include more typical or more extreme phenotypes of the target condition. These typical cases are more likely to receive true-positive test results, compared to a group of participants that represents the full spectrum of the target condition, from less severe to more severe.

A design in which those with the target condition and those without are each randomly sampled from one consecutive series of participants suspected of having the target condition will not lead to biased estimates (Biesheuvel 2008, Pepe 2008). Such a study bears similarities with what is known as a nested case-control study in aetiological research. This is an example of a situation in which a signalling question will be answered with 'No' (red flag), without assigning a high risk of bias for this domain.

Signalling question 3: Did the study avoid inappropriate selection criteria?

This signalling question draws attention to whether a study excluded persons at the point of enrolment, even though such persons are or will be evaluated with the index test in clinical practice. This may influence estimates of test accuracy for that study, which then no longer reflects the accuracy of the test in clinical practice.

This question about inappropriate selection criteria relates only to the eligibility criteria and the recruitment process, i.e. how participants were invited for the study; exclusion of study participants after enrolment is covered in the flow and timing domain (domain 4).

Examples include the exclusion of patients with high body mass index (BMI) in ultrasound studies for abdominal pain, or the exclusion of patients with pre-existing lung disease in studies examining the accuracy of CT in patients with suspected pulmonary embolism. In both situations, patients who potentially were more difficult to diagnose were not enrolled in the study, which may lead to inflated estimates of diagnostic accuracy.

It is possible that a study did not have explicit exclusion criteria, but specific subgroups undergoing the test in practice are notably absent from the study group. This can sometimes be deduced from a table with baseline characteristics. In that case, study-specific accuracy estimates may also be biased, if the risk of false positive test results, or the risk of false negative test results, is known to vary depending on patient characteristics. For example, the specificity of D-dimer, a test for pulmonary embolism, is known to be lower in higher age groups. A study to estimate its accuracy in an emergency department may produce biased estimates if that study failed to include elderly patients.

Given the complexity of the problem underlying this signalling question, review authors are encouraged to generate detailed guidance on how to answer this signalling question for their review.

8.4.2 Participant selection: additional signalling questions for comparative accuracy studies (QUADAS-C)

Informative comparisons of the accuracy of tests should reflect the performance of these tests in the same target population. If one test is evaluated in one group of participants and the other tests in different groups, any difference in accuracy may be due, in part or in full, to differences between these groups, rather than to the tests evaluated. QUADAS-C contains four additional signalling questions for the participant selection domain to cover specific sources of bias that are relevant for comparative accuracy studies.

Additional signalling question 1: Was the risk of bias for each index test judged 'low' for this domain?

We first consider whether the risk-of-bias judgement in QUADAS-2 for the participant selection domain was judged as 'low' for all index tests in the comparison. If not, the study group or combination of study groups may not be representative of the target population. This may be the case, for example, if participants difficult to evaluate with one of the index tests were excluded.

This question should be answered with 'No' if at least one of the index tests was judged to be at 'unclear' or 'high' risk of bias for this domain.

Additional signalling question 2: Was a fully paired or randomized design used?
This question addresses whether an appropriate design was used to compare multiple index tests. The preferred option for comparing multiple tests is to perform all index tests in all participants (fully paired design); an alternative is random allocation to one index test or to another (randomized design).

If neither a fully paired nor randomized design was used, those receiving one index test and those receiving another may not be comparable in terms of factors that affect test accuracy. An example is allocation of study participants to one specific index test based on presenting features, and allocation of all other participants, without such features, to a different index test.

It may be challenging to distinguish a fully paired design with missing index test results from a 'partially paired' design, in which some participants receive all index tests while others receive only one of the tests. Examining the study protocol (if available) or careful examination of the Methods section of the study report may clarify if this partially paired design was the design intended by the study investigators (Yang 2021b).

Additional signalling question 3: Was the allocation sequence random? (only applicable to randomized designs)
The allocation sequence in a randomized comparative accuracy study should be generated by a truly random process. This could be achieved by computer-based random number generators, drawing lots, random number tables, or other methods that involve a truly random component. Assigning tests to a person based on admission date or date of birth is not a fully random process. Details about the randomization process may often be poorly reported in studies and it may be necessary to contact the study authors for further details.

Additional signalling question 4: Was the allocation sequence concealed until participants were enrolled and assigned to index tests? (only applicable to randomized designs)
A failure to conceal the allocation when deciding about the eligibility of a potential study participant may lead to selective enrolment of participants. If so, the groups assigned to the respective tests may no longer be comparable and estimates of relative accuracy may be biased.

Concealment of allocation may be achieved, for example, by assigning the randomly generated number only after the participant was enrolled, by allocating participants by means of a central randomization procedure, or by keeping random numbers in sequentially numbered opaque and sealed envelopes.

Table 8.4.a summarizes the signalling questions used in the risk-of-bias assessment for the participant selection domain. Additional signalling questions are listed in Table 8.4.b.

Table 8.4.a Summary of risk-of-bias assessment for Domain 1: Participant selection

Signalling question 1: Was a consecutive or random sample of participants enrolled?	
Yes	If the method of recruitment was consecutive or a random sample was taken from a consecutive series
No	If there is evidence for non-consecutive or non-random inclusion of eligible participants
Unclear	If the method of participant sampling is unclear
Signalling question 2: Was a case-control design avoided?	
Yes	If a single group of participants suspected of having the target condition was recruited
No	If two or more groups of participants were separately recruited, with one group consisting of participants already known to have the target condition, and a second group consisting of healthy controls, or a group of participants with a specific alternative condition
Unclear	If the selection of participants is unclear
Signalling question 3: Did the study avoid inappropriate selection criteria?	
Yes	If all patients who would undergo the test in practice were eligible for the study
No	If selection criteria were defined such that specific subgroups within the target population were ineligible, or if such patients were not invited to the study
Unclear	If it is unclear whether inappropriate selection criteria were used
Risk-of-bias assessment: Could the selection of participants have introduced bias?	
Low	If the answer to all signalling questions is 'Yes' then risk of bias can be considered low
High	If the answer to any of the signalling questions is 'No', there is a potential for bias. If one or more of the answers is 'No', the judgement could still be low risk of bias, but specific reasons why the risk of bias can be considered low should be provided
Unclear	If relevant information is missing for all or some of the signalling questions, and none of the answers to signalling questions is judged to put the study at high risk of bias

Table 8.4.b Comparative accuracy, additional signalling questions for the participant selection domain (QUADAS-C)

Additional question 1: Was risk of bias for this domain judged 'low' for all index tests?	
Yes	if risk of bias in QUADAS-2 was judged 'low' for all index tests
No	if risk of bias in QUADAS-2 was judged to be 'high' or 'unclear' for one or more index tests
Additional question 2: Was a fully paired or randomized design used?	
Yes	If it is clear from the study report or from the study protocol that, by design, all participants would receive all tests (fully paired design) or that participants would be randomly allocated to one of the tests (randomized design)
No	Neither a fully paired nor randomized design was used to allocate participants to index tests

Table 8.4.b (Continued)

Unclear	If it was unclear how participants were allocated to the tests being compared

Additional question 3: Was the allocation sequence random? (only applicable to randomized designs)

Yes	If authors used a truly random process to generate the allocation sequence
No	If authors generated an allocation sequence that was not the result of a truly random process
Unclear	If authors only stated that the study was randomized without further information

Additional question 4: Was the allocation sequence concealed until participants were enrolled and assigned to index tests? (only applicable to randomized designs)

Yes	If authors report an appropriate method to conceal allocation
No	If authors did not conceal the allocation at the time of enrolment
Unclear	If it is unclear whether allocation was concealed

Risk-of-bias judgement:

Low	If the answer to all additional questions is 'Yes', then risk of bias can be considered low
High	If the answer to any of the signalling questions is 'No', there is a potential for bias. If one or more of the answers is 'No', the judgement could still be low risk of bias, but specific reasons why the risk of bias can be considered low should be provided
Unclear	If relevant information is missing for all or some of the signalling questions, and none of the answers to signalling questions is judged to put the study at high risk of bias

8.4.3   Participant selection: concerns regarding applicability

The question to be answered is whether there are concerns that the included participants and setting do not match the review question. It is possible that the primary study was designed to answer a research question that differs from the review question. For that reason, the group of participants in a study may not match the population that is targeted by the review question.

Concerns regarding applicability may arise if study participants differ from those targeted by the review question in terms of severity of the target condition, demographic features, presence of alternative conditions or comorbidity, setting of the study, or previous tests. For example, larger tumours are more easily detected on imaging than smaller ones, and larger myocardial infarctions lead to higher levels of cardiac enzymes than small infarctions, making them easier to detect and so increasing estimates of sensitivity. A D-dimer test may be evaluated in an emergency department setting, while the review addresses the question of its accuracy when performed by general practitioners.

If a test accuracy study recruits one group of patients with known severe disease and a second group of healthy controls, it will be flagged here, but also assessed as being at high risk of bias in the participant selection domain, because such a study will produce inflated estimates of sensitivity and specificity.

Table 8.4.c Summary of main issues when evaluating applicability for the participant selection domain

Domain 1: Participant selection	Concerns regarding applicability
Are there concerns that the included participants and setting do not match the review question?	
Low	If the spectrum of participants (inclusion and exclusion criteria, setting, prior testing) matches the pre-stated requirements in the review question
High	If the spectrum of participants does not fully match the pre-stated requirements in the review question
Unclear	If there is insufficient information available to make a judgement about applicability

Table 8.4.c summarizes the main issues when evaluating applicability for the participant selection domain.

8.5   Domain 2: Index test

This domain relates to the index test: whether conduct or interpretation of the index test could have introduced bias, and whether the index test, as used in the study, reflects the one in the review question (applicability).

8.5.1   Index test: risk-of-bias signalling questions (QUADAS-2)

The key issue to answer is whether the conduct or interpretation of the index test could have introduced bias. Two signalling questions are included to flag potential issues within a study that could lead to bias.

Signalling question 1: Were the index test results interpreted without knowledge of the results of the reference standard?
Interpretation of index test results may be influenced by knowledge of the reference standard, thereby artificially increasing concordance between them, leading to higher estimates of accuracy (Whiting 2013). The potential for bias is related to the degree of subjectivity involved in interpreting the index test. When an index test requires an interpretation, interpreters are more likely to be influenced by the results of the reference standard than with a fully automated or objective test. It therefore matters whether the unblinded interpretation of the index test could have led to bias.

Whether or not blinding was undertaken in a study may not be stated explicitly in the study report or protocol; if index tests and reference standard are undertaken and interpreted in a specified order, the first test will have been performed without access to the results of the second.

Where the index test and reference standard were undertaken by different individuals, a degree of ambiguity may exist about what information was available for each test. In some instances, knowledge of standard laboratory practices may allow reasonable assumptions to be made, but confirmation from the study authors is always desirable.

Signalling question 2: If a threshold was used, was it pre-specified?
For index tests that give ordered categories, counts or continuous measurements, a threshold is applied to classify test results as positive or negative (see Chapter 4). Selecting a positivity threshold in a study during data analysis, instead of during study design or protocol development, can lead to inflated estimates of test accuracy. This is especially the case when the selection is based on calculations of accuracy. In many studies, for example, authors select the positivity threshold that maximizes the sum of sensitivity and specificity (Youden index, see Chapter 4) in the data they have collected.

The reason post-hoc selection of the positivity threshold causes bias is that the observed ROC curve will fluctuate considerably around the true underlying ROC curve, especially in small studies. A data-driven selection of a threshold is likely to result in selecting a point estimate that is by chance further away from the true underlying ROC curve. Subsequently using that same threshold in an independent sample of patients is likely to lead to lower estimates of accuracy (Leeflang 2008). Pre-specifying the threshold before collecting or analysing will prevent this bias.

The following should be considered when judging whether a data-driven threshold is likely to produce a biased result. First, the magnitude of the bias is inversely related to sample size (Leeflang 2008). In a large study the observed ROC curve will be closer to the true underlying curve. Bias due to data-driven selection of thresholds is therefore smaller in studies with at least 100 participants with and, at the same time, 100 without the target condition (Leeflang 2008). Second, researchers may have used more robust methods for selecting a threshold, for example by first fitting smooth ROC curves based on parametric or non-parametric assumptions. Such methods generally reduce bias, but their performance depends on whether underlying assumptions are met (Leeflang 2008).

Ideally, study authors should use a positivity threshold that was predefined in the study protocol, or one that is specified by the manufacturer of the test. In the case of truly dichotomous index test results, this signalling question can be answered 'Yes', because there is no risk of bias due to selection of thresholds.

8.5.2   Index test: additional signalling questions for comparative accuracy studies (QUADAS-C)

For comparative accuracy studies, the signalling questions should first be answered for each index test separately. There are four additional questions to consider for the index test domain when dealing with comparative accuracy studies.

Additional signalling question 1: Was the risk of bias for each index test judged 'low' for this domain?
If the risk-of-bias judgement in QUADAS-2 for the index test domain was judged as 'high' for one or more index tests, then the comparison between these index tests would likely be biased as well. For example, if index test A was interpreted with knowledge of the results of the reference standard, then not only is the estimated accuracy of A possibly biased, but also the estimate of the difference in accuracy between A and another index test B. If estimates of both test A and test B are judged to be at high risk of bias, the comparison between them will still be at high risk of bias, as the direction and magnitude of bias affecting each index test may not be the same.

Additional signalling question 2: Were the index test results interpreted without knowledge of the results of the other index test(s)? (only applicable if participants received multiple index tests)

Interpreting an index test while knowing the results of another may artificially increase concordance between the results of these index tests and could therefore bias the comparison. Such a bias could be mitigated by blinding the index test interpreter from the results of the other index test(s).

When answering this signalling question, similar considerations from the QUADAS-2 question 'Were the index test results interpreted without knowledge of the results of the reference standard?' apply: the potential for bias depends on the degree of subjectivity involved in test interpretation. The order in which the tests were performed and interpreted may suggest whether or not the interpretation was blinded.

In addition, authors of systematic reviews comparing the accuracy of one index test versus a combination of that test with another should note that blinding is not always necessary. For example, in a comparative accuracy study of ultrasound versus ultrasound followed by CT, CT readers do not need to be blinded to the results of ultrasound if ultrasound results are also available to the CT interpreter in practice. In this example, only the ultrasound interpreter needs to be blinded to the results of CT.

Additional signalling question 3: Is undergoing one index test unlikely to affect the performance of the other index test(s)? (only applicable if participants received multiple index tests)

It is possible for an index test to influence or interfere with the performance of subsequent index tests. Possible reasons for interference include patient or investigator fatigue (if performing the index tests requires mental or physical effort) and contrast agents or relaxants used for the first imaging test that may also affect the performance of the second test. If so, accuracy estimates for the second index test may not reflect its accuracy when performed as a first test.

Randomizing the order of index tests is sometimes done with the intention of preventing this bias, but a random order is expected to prevent bias only under the following circumstances: (1) the first test interferes with the performance of the second test and the other way round, if the order is reversed; and (2) the bias affecting each test has the same direction and magnitude on the scale of interest (absolute or relative difference in accuracy).

Additional signalling question 4: Were the index tests conducted and interpreted without advantaging one of the tests?

There may be ways of handling or interpreting the index tests that may advantage one test over the other. An example is when one index test is interpreted by an experienced reader whereas the competing index test is interpreted by a less experienced reader. One index test may be performed in a specialized clinic whereas the other is performed in a busy general practice. One index test may be performed on fresh samples while frozen samples are used for the other test. Differences between the index tests that reflect differences in clinical practice should not be considered to be a source of bias.

Table 8.5.a summarizes the signalling questions and how these should be answered to assess the risk of bias for the index test domain. Additional signalling questions are listed in Table 8.5.b.

Table 8.5.a Summary of risk-of-bias assessment for Domain 2: Index test

Signalling question 1: Were the index test results interpreted without knowledge of the results of the reference standard?	
Yes	If the index tests were interpreted without access to the results of the reference standard (explicitly stated or assumed from typical practice)
No	If the index tests were clearly interpreted with access to the results of the reference standard
Unclear	If it is unclear whether index tests were interpreted without access to the results of the reference standard
Signalling question 2: If a threshold was used, was it pre-specified?	
Yes	If the positivity threshold was pre-specified during protocol development
No	If the positivity threshold was based on an analysis of data collected in the study itself
Unclear	If it is unclear how the positivity threshold for the index test was selected
Risk-of-bias judgement: Could the conduct or interpretation of the index test have introduced bias?	
Low	If the answer to all signalling questions is 'Yes', then risk of bias can be considered low
High	If the answer to any of the signalling questions is 'No', there is a potential for bias. If one or more of the answers is 'No', one could still assign a low risk of bias but specific reasons for doing so should be provided. For example, if information on reference standard results was available to the person interpreting the index test, but the index test results were generated by a device, then this is unlikely to have introduced bias
Unclear	If relevant information is missing for all or some of the signalling questions, and none of the answers to signalling questions is judged to put the study at high risk of bias

Table 8.5.b Comparative accuracy, additional signalling questions for the index test domain (QUADAS-C)

Additional question 1: Was the risk of bias for each index test judged 'low' for this domain?	
Yes	If risk of bias in QUADAS-2 was judged 'low' for both or all index tests
No	If risk of bias in QUADAS-2 was judged to be 'high' or 'unclear' for one or more index tests
Additional question 2: Were the index test results interpreted without knowledge of the results of the other index test(s)? (only applicable if participants received multiple index tests)	
Yes	If it is likely that the interpretation of each index test was done without knowledge of the results of the other index test(s) in the study
No	If it is likely that the interpreter of any one of the index tests was aware of the results of any of the other index tests
Unclear	If it is unclear whether the interpreters of the index tests were aware of the results of the other index tests
Additional question 3: Is undergoing one index test unlikely to affect the performance of the other index test(s)? (only applicable if participants received multiple index tests)	
Yes	If the conduct of the index tests could not have influenced the performance of any of the other index tests

(Continued)

Table 8.5.b (Continued)

No	If it is likely that the conduct of one index test influenced the performance of subsequent index test(s)
Unclear	If it is unclear whether an index test could have influenced the performance of subsequent index test(s)

Additional question 4: Were the index tests conducted and interpreted without advantaging one of the tests?

Yes	If all index tests were performed and interpreted under similar circumstances
No	If there are substantial differences in how the index tests were performed or interpreted, and these differences are likely to affect the accuracy of one of the tests more favourably relative to the other test(s)
Unclear	If the study provides insufficient information to judge whether the index tests were done under similar circumstances

Risk-of-bias assessment: Could the conduct or interpretation of the index tests have introduced bias in the comparison?

Low	If the answer to all additional questions is 'Yes', then risk of bias can be considered low
High	If the answer to any of the signalling questions is 'No', there is a potential for bias. If one or more of the answers is 'No', the judgement could still be low risk of bias, but specific reasons why the risk of bias can be considered low should be provided
Unclear	If relevant information is missing for all or some of the signalling questions, and none of the answers to signalling questions is judged to put the study at high risk of bias

Table 8.5.c Summary of the main issues when evaluating applicability for the index test domain

Domain 2: Index test	Concerns regarding applicability
Are there concerns that the index test, its conduct or its interpretation differ from the review question?	
Low	If the index test technology and the way the test has been applied and interpreted in the study match the pre-stated requirements in the review question
High	If there are differences in index test technology, execution and interpretation between the study and the review question
Unclear	If there is insufficient information available to make a judgement about applicability for this domain

8.5.3 Index test: concerns regarding applicability

Variations in test technology, execution or interpretation may affect test accuracy. If index test methods vary from those specified in the review question, there may be concerns regarding applicability (Stengel 2005). An accuracy study of an imaging modality, for example, may use a consensus read by three radiologists, whereas in clinical practice such images would be read by only one person.

Table 8.5.c summarizes the main issues when evaluating applicability for the index test domain.

8.6   Domain 3: Reference standard

The central issue in this domain is whether the reference standard, its conduct or interpretation could have introduced bias, and whether the target condition, as detected by the reference standard, reflects the review question.

8.6.1   Reference standard: risk-of-bias signalling questions (QUADAS-2)

Two signalling questions in QUADAS-2 flag potential issues within a study that could lead to bias.

Signalling question 1: Is the reference standard likely to correctly classify the target condition?
Measures of test accuracy are calculated by assuming that the reference standard is error free; any disagreement between the index test and the reference standard results will be classified as either a false positive or false negative index test result.

Bias in estimates of accuracy is likely if the reference standard does not correctly classify study participants. If there are misclassifications by the reference standard, an index test result that is classified as a false positive may in fact be a true positive, and a false negative index test result may be a true negative. As a consequence, imperfect reference standards can bias estimates of the accuracy of an index test (Boyko 1988).

The net effect of misclassification by the reference standard can be an upward or downward bias in estimates of test accuracy, depending on the frequency of the misclassification and the type of misclassification. Under-estimation can occur when the index test and the reference standard measure different aspects of the target condition, such that errors in the reference standard are unrelated to errors in the index test. Accuracy may be overestimated when the index test and reference standard measure similar aspects of the target condition, such that errors in the reference standard are likely to occur together with errors in the index test (van Rijkom 1995, Biesheuvel 2007).

Knowledge about imperfections in the reference standard cannot be obtained from a study in which the accuracy of one or more index tests is evaluated. Evidence about the likelihood of reference standard misclassifications will have to be found in other studies or systematic reviews of such studies, for example studies that assessed the reproducibility and repeatability of the reference standard. An example are tandem colonoscopy studies, in which consenting participants undergo two same-day colonoscopies with polypectomy (Zhao 2019). Another example is a study in which liver biopsies are evaluated by not one but a team of hepatopathologists, who are invited to read these biopsies independently, blinded from one another's judgement (Davison 2020).

A perfect reference standard – a gold standard – will rarely be available; most reference standards have imperfections. Some degree of imperfection may still be acceptable, if the frequency of misclassification errors from the reference standard is low. At the protocol stage, review authors will define the preferred reference standard. Many reviews will then restrict inclusion of studies based on the acceptability of the reference standard in light of the target condition. In addition, the criteria for scoring this signalling question as 'Yes' for included studies will be defined at the protocol stage.

If one expects the index test to outperform the reference standard, assessing the accuracy of such a test by assessing index test results against this reference standard will not be helpful (see Chapter 3). Reviews of test accuracy should not be undertaken in these circumstances without careful consideration of the methodological issues (Glasziou 2008, Reitsma 2009).

Signalling question 2: Were the reference standard results interpreted without knowledge of the results of the index test?
The results of the reference standard are ideally obtained without knowledge of the results of the index test(s). Knowledge of the index test results can influence the interpretation of the reference standard (Whiting 2013). The danger is that this may artificially increase agreement between the index test and the reference standard results, leading to inflated estimates of test accuracy. This is also known as test-review bias (Ransohoff 1978).

The potential for bias is related to the degree of subjectivity involved in interpreting the results of the reference standard. When a reference standard requires a more subjective reading, interpreters are more likely to be influenced by the results of the index test than for a fully automated reference standard or a reference standard with explicit criteria.

An example is the use of an expert panel as the reference standard, where the expert panel has access to the index test results (Bertens 2013). In a study examining the accuracy of magnetic resonance imaging (MRI) in detecting multiple sclerosis, the reference standard was a panel-based assignment of a final diagnosis, based on all available information, including MRI results, cerebrospinal fluid analysis and clinical follow-up of participants. To avoid bias, studies using an expert panel may decide not to present the results of the index test to the panel, to prevent giving these results too much weight when deciding whether the target condition is present or not.

An extreme form occurs if index test results are a formal component of the reference standard; i.e. when the result of the index test is incorporated into the evidence used to conclude that the target condition is present or absent. The resulting bias is known as incorporation bias (Ransohoff 1978, Worster 2008).

8.6.2   Reference standard: additional signalling questions for comparative accuracy studies (QUADAS-C)

For comparative accuracy studies, the signalling questions should first be answered for each index test separately. There are two additional questions to consider for the reference standard domain when dealing with comparative accuracy studies.

Additional signalling question 1: Was the risk of bias for each index test judged 'low' for this domain?
Similar to the previous domains, we first ask whether the risk of bias in QUADAS-2 for the reference standard domain was judged as 'low' for the index tests being compared. If that is not the case, the comparison between these index tests could be biased. The use of an imperfect reference standard in all study participants would not only affect accuracy estimates for each index test, but could also bias estimates of comparative accuracy.

Table 8.6.a Summary of risk-of-bias assessment for Domain 3: Reference standard

Signalling question 1: Is the reference standard likely to correctly classify the target condition?	
Yes	If a reference standard has been used that is considered by clinical experts to be error free for the target condition
No	If a reference standard has been used that is known to lead to misclassifications
Unclear	If it is unclear exactly what reference standard was used
Signalling question 2: Were the reference standard results interpreted without knowledge of the results of the index test?	
Yes	If it is clear that the index test results were not available to those interpreting the reference standard results
No	If it is clear that the index test results were available to those interpreting the reference standard results
Unclear	If it is unclear whether the results of the index test were available to those interpreting the reference standard results
Risk-of-bias judgement: Could the reference standard, its conduct or its interpretation have introduced bias?	
Low	If the answer to all signalling questions is 'Yes', then risk of bias can be considered low
High	If the answer to any of the signalling questions is 'No', there is a potential for bias. If one or more of the answers is 'No', the judgement could still be low risk of bias, but specific reasons why the risk of bias can be considered low should be provided
Unclear	If relevant information is missing for all or some of the signalling questions, and none of the answers to signalling questions is judged to put the study at high risk of bias

Additional signalling question 2: Did the reference standard avoid incorporating any of the index tests?

The second signalling question in this domain is whether one or more index tests were part of the reference standard, i.e. used to decide on the presence or absence of the target condition. If this was the case for one index test (A) and not for another index test (B), the accuracy of A will be over-estimated, leading to a biased estimate of the difference in accuracy between the index tests. If both index tests A and B are part of the reference standard, there is still risk of a biased comparison, as the two index tests may not contribute equally to the final diagnosis.

Table 8.6.a summarizes the signalling questions and how these should be answered to assess the risk of bias for the reference standard domain. Additional signalling questions are listed in Table 8.6.b.

8.6.3 Reference standard: concerns regarding applicability

The question to be answered is whether there are concerns that the target condition as detected by the reference standard does not match the review question.

Many diseases and conditions are not dichotomous; instead they present as a spectrum, ranging from less to more severe. When specifying the review question(s), review authors should be specific about the definition of the target condition in their review, and should reflect on what reference standard is best able to detect that target

Table 8.6.b Comparative accuracy, additional signalling questions for the reference standard domain (QUADAS-C)

Additional question 1: Was the risk of bias for each index test judged 'low' for this domain?	
Yes	if risk of bias in QUADAS-2 was judged 'low' for both or all index tests
No	if risk of bias in QUADAS-2 was judged to be 'high' or 'unclear' for one or more index tests
Additional question 2: Did the reference standard avoid incorporating any of the index tests?	
Yes	If none of the index tests was part of the reference standard
No	If one or more of the index tests were used to decide on presence or absence of the target condition
Unclear	If it is unclear whether any of the index tests were part of the reference standard
Risk-of-bias assessment: Could the reference standard, its conduct or its interpretation have introduced bias in the comparison?	
Low risk of bias	If the answer to all additional questions is 'Yes', then risk of bias can be considered low
High risk of bias	If the answer to any of the signalling questions is 'No', there is a potential for bias. If one or more of the answers is 'No', the judgement could still be low risk of bias, but specific reasons why the risk of bias can be considered low should be provided
Unclear risk of bias	If relevant information is missing for all or some of the signalling questions, and none of the answers to signalling questions is judged to put the study at high risk of bias

Table 8.6.c Summary of the main issues when judging applicability for the reference standard domain

Domain 3: Reference standard	Concerns regarding applicability
Are there concerns that the target condition as detected by the reference standard does not match the review question?	
Low	If the reference standard, as used in the study, detects the target condition defined in the review question
High	If the reference standard, as used in the study, does not detect the same (form of) target condition as defined in the review question
Unclear	If there is insufficient information available to make a judgement about applicability for this domain

condition. The reference standard should then be selected in light of this target condition. Different reference standards may detect different forms of the target condition.

For example, when defining urinary tract infection, the reference standard is generally based on specimen culture, but the threshold above which a result is considered positive may vary (Tullus 2019). In studies evaluating screening tests for colorectal cancer, colonoscopy is the accepted reference standard, but the definition of what the test aims to detect (referred to as 'advanced neoplasia') can vary between studies. Table 8.6.c summarizes the main issues when judging applicability for the reference standard domain.

8.7   Domain 4: Flow and timing

The fourth and final domain focuses on the flow of participants through a test accuracy study and the timing of the index test(s) and the reference standard. This domain is only assessed in terms of consequences for risk of bias. The central issue is whether the participant flow could have introduced bias.

In the ideal test accuracy study, each participant receives both the index test and the reference standard at the same point in time. Bias may be introduced if the time interval between the index test and the reference standard is not appropriate. Bias may also be introduced if not all study participants are included in the analysis.

8.7.1   Flow and timing: risk-of-bias signalling questions (QUADAS-2)

QUADAS-2 includes four signalling questions to flag potential issues within a study that could lead to bias in this domain.

Signalling question 1: Was there an appropriate interval between the index test and reference standard?
Ideally, the index test and reference standard are performed in the same participant at the same time. If there is a delay, natural disease progression and/or treatment between index test and reference standard can lead to changes in the target condition: it may be present at the time of testing with the index test, but resolved by the time the reference standard is performed, or the other way around. If the target condition resolved during the time interval, a true positive index test result may be erroneously classified as a false positive. A delay is therefore a potential cause of bias. The potential for changes in the target condition because of a delay, and the potential for bias, will vary between conditions.

Conversely, when the reference standard is based on observations during follow-up, a minimum length may be required to capture the symptoms or signs indicating that the target condition was present when the index test was performed. For example, for the evaluation of MRI for the early diagnosis of multiple sclerosis, a minimum follow-up period of around 10 years is required to be confident that all participants who will go on to fulfil the diagnostic criteria for multiple sclerosis will have done so (Whiting 2006). If there are concerns that (effective) treatments may have been applied during the time interval, this potential for bias may be highlighted in the flow and timing domain.

Starting treatment for the target condition before the reference standard has been performed (i.e. before the end of follow-up) can affect results, since it may lead to recovery. When judging the potential for bias, it is important to estimate the proportion of participants in whom the interval was inappropriate. The magnitude of the bias will increase if the number of participants outside the appropriate interval is larger.

The acceptable length of the interval between index test and reference standard needs to be specified in the review protocol. A delay of a few days may not be a problem for chronic conditions, while for acute infectious diseases a short delay may be influential.

Signalling question 2: Did all participants receive a reference standard?
Researchers should aim to use the preferred reference standard for identifying participants with the target condition, and they should do so in all study participants. Failure to adhere to these principles could lead to bias.

Due to practical or ethical constraints, it is sometimes impossible to ascertain disease status in all participants using the preferred reference standard. If such participants remain unverified, this is known as partial verification. The biasing effect of partial verification is difficult to predict, because it depends on whether test-positive or test-negative results are not verified, whether unverified participants are omitted from the 2×2 table, whether unverified test negatives are classified as true negatives and unverified positives as true positives, and whether unverified participants can be considered random samples of index test negatives and positives (Begg 1983, Diamond 1991).

There is no correct way of handling unverified participants in an analysis; sensitivity analysis in which they are alternately considered as different combinations of test positives and test negatives may allow an assessment of the potential magnitude of any bias to be ascertained.

Partial verification is a likely threat in studies using routine care data. It may be considered good clinical practice not to perform the preferred reference standard (which can be invasive or costly) in all participants, especially in cases where the available test results indicate that the probability of the target condition being present is very low.

Random sampling of participants for verification is sometimes undertaken for reasons of efficiency, particularly in scenarios where disease prevalence is low. If participants are randomly selected to receive the reference standard (either across the whole sample or, more commonly, as random samples from index test positives and index test negatives), unbiased estimates of overall diagnostic performance of the test can be obtained if one relies on methods that compensate for the sampling plan (Zhou 1998).

Signalling question 3: Did all participants receive the same reference standard?

Some studies use an alternative reference standard in some participants, instead of a single reference standard in all. The use of different reference standards in a test accuracy study, often guided by index test results, is known as differential verification (Naaktgeboren 2013).

One clear case is when those with positive index test results receive one reference standard and those testing negative receive a different one, often a less invasive or less expensive one. For example, a study evaluating the accuracy of the D-dimer test for the diagnosis of pulmonary embolism might use CT scanning (reference standard 1) in those testing positive, but rely on clinical follow-up to decide whether or not those testing negative had a pulmonary embolism (reference standard 2). This may result in misclassifying some of the false negatives as true negatives, as some participants with a pulmonary embolism who were index test negative may be missed by clinical follow-up and so be classified as false negatives. This misclassification will over-estimate the sensitivity and specificity of the index test, compared to a study where all participants with suspected pulmonary embolism undergo CT scanning.

The studies by Lijmer et al and Rutjes et al found that the presence of differential verification was associated with an up to 2.2-fold higher diagnostic odds ratio (Lijmer 1999, Rutjes 2006).

An assessment of the risk of bias will require an understanding of the reasons for different individuals receiving different reference standards, and the nature of the differences between the reference standards.

Signalling question 4: Were all participants included in the analysis?
All participants recruited into the study should be reported and, in some form, included in the analysis. If the number of participants in the 2×2 table, used for obtaining estimates of test accuracy, differs from the number of participants included, then there is a potential for bias. Assessors should then carefully consider the intended use, context and setting of the index test, as defined in the review question, and whether the failure to include all included participants in the 2×2 table is justified.

Participants may be excluded from the 2×2 table because they had an inconclusive reference standard result. If this is a non-random subset of all participants in the study, the estimate of sensitivity generated by that study may not reflect the true proportion of test positives among those with the target condition, and the same applies to estimates of specificity.

Participants may also be excluded from the 2×2 table because of index test failures, or inconclusive index test results. The corresponding number of participants will be relevant when judging the potential usefulness of the index test in practice. Whether exclusion of the failures is justified will depend on the type of index test and the intended use, for example whether or not the test procedure can be repeated.

Whether or not a failure to include all participants in the analysis will lead to bias is a matter of judgement. A 'No' to this signalling question will not automatically lead to a high risk-of-bias judgement. Review authors will have to consider the proportion of participants not included in the analysis, the mechanisms for these failures and the associations, or lack thereof, with the presence or absence of the target condition. There is no universally acceptable proportion of non-included participants, although review authors may define such a proportion for their specific review in the protocol.

8.7.2 Flow and timing: additional signalling questions for comparative accuracy studies (QUADAS-C)

For comparative accuracy studies, the signalling questions should first be answered for each index test separately. There are four additional questions to consider for the flow and timing domain when dealing with comparative accuracy studies.

Additional signalling question 1: Was the risk of bias for each index test judged 'low' for this domain?
As discussed in the previous domains, bias in the estimates of the accuracy of an individual test may also lead to bias in the estimates of comparative accuracy of two or more index tests. Therefore, the risk of bias of each index test should be 'low' for the flow and timing domain as well.

Additional signalling question 2: Was there an appropriate interval between the index tests?
Even if the time interval between the respective index test and the reference standard is judged to be appropriate, the time interval between the index tests may not be. If the target condition is progressive, and one index test is performed at a point later in the disease progression, the accuracy of these tests may appear different only because of disease progression, even if there is no true difference in accuracy between them. The definition of appropriate interval between the index tests will be guided by the review question.

Additional signalling question 3: Was the same reference standard used for all index tests?
Ideally, in comparative accuracy studies all study participants receive the same reference standard, irrespective of the index test used. If this is not possible or feasible, then reference standards may differ between index tests. As the reference standard is a key element in the assessment of test accuracy, this will almost always affect differences in accuracy between index tests.

Additional signalling question 4: Are the proportions and reasons for missing data similar across index tests?
Differences in the number of missing data or exclusions between index tests may lead to biased estimates of comparative accuracy if missing data do not occur completely at random. For example, one index test may generate more inconclusive test results than other index test(s) being evaluated in the study. In that case, there is potential for bias if all such test results from one index test are excluded from the analysis. This question requires careful examination of the participant flow through the study and any reasons for unavailable, or inconclusive, test results as well as exclusion of participants.

Table 8.7.a summarizes the signalling questions and how these should be answered to assess the risk of bias for the flow and timing domain. Additional signalling questions are listed in Table 8.7.b.

Table 8.7.a Summary of risk-of-bias assessment for Domain 4: Flow and timing

Signalling question 1: Was there an appropriate interval between the index test and reference standard?	
Yes	If the interval between index test and reference standard was sufficiently short to avoid changes in disease status
No	If the interval is too long or too short for valid estimates of test accuracy
Unclear	If the interval between index test and reference standard was unclear

Signalling question 2: Did all participants receive a reference standard?	
Yes	If all participants received a reference standard
No	If not all participants received a reference standard
Unclear	If it is unclear whether all participants received a reference standard

Signalling question 3: Did all participants receive the same reference standard?	
Yes	If all participants received the same reference standard
No	If some participants received a different reference standard
Unclear	If it is unclear whether all participants received the same reference standard

Signalling question 4: Were all participants included in the analysis?	
Yes	If data on all study participants were included in the analysis
No	If data on all study participants were not included in the analysis
Unclear	If it is unclear whether all study participants were included in the analysis

Table 8.7.a (Continued)

Risk-of-bias judgement: Could participant flow have introduced bias?	
Low	If the answer to all signalling questions is 'Yes', then risk of bias can be considered low
High	If the answer to any of the signalling questions is 'No', there is a potential for bias. If one or more of the answers is 'No', the judgement could still be low risk of bias, but specific reasons why the risk of bias can be considered low should be provided
Unclear	If relevant information is missing for all or some of the signalling questions, and none of the answers to signalling questions is judged to put the study at high risk of bias

Table 8.7.b Comparative accuracy, additional signalling questions for the flow and timing domain (QUADAS-C)

Additional question 1: Was the risk of bias for each index test judged 'low' for this domain?	
Yes	If risk of bias in QUADAS-2 was judged 'low' for both or all index tests
No	If risk of bias in QUADAS-2 was judged to be 'high' or 'unclear' for one or more index tests

Additional question 2: Was there an appropriate interval between the index tests?	
Yes	If the interval between index tests is sufficiently short to avoid changes in disease status
No	If the interval is too long and it is likely for disease status to change in between the index tests
Unclear	If the time interval between the index tests was unclear or not reported

Additional question 3: Was the same reference standard used for all index tests?	
Yes	A single reference standard was used or, in case of differential verification, the same reference standards were used across index tests
No	The results of one index test were verified with a reference standard different to that of the other index test(s)
Unclear	It is unclear whether different reference standards were used across index tests

Additional question 4: Are the proportions and reasons for missing data similar across index tests?	
Yes	If no or only a small proportion of participant data were missing or excluded, or if the proportions and reasons for missing data were similar between the index test groups being compared
No	If more data were clearly missing from one index test group than the other(s), or the reasons for missing data differed between the index test groups
Unclear	If it is unclear whether data were missing and the extent of missing data. If data were missing, the reasons for being missing were unclear

Risk-of-bias judgement: Could the flow of participants have introduced bias in the comparison?	
Low	If the answer to all additional questions is 'Yes', then risk of bias can be considered low
High	If the answer to any of the signalling questions is 'No', there is a potential for bias. If one or more of the answers is 'No', the judgement could still be low risk of bias, but specific reasons why the risk of bias can be considered low should be provided
Unclear	If relevant information is missing for all or some of the signalling questions, and none of the answers to signalling questions is judged to put the study at high risk of bias

8.8   Presentation of risk-of-bias and applicability assessments

The results of the assessment of risk of bias and applicability are usually presented in systematic reviews of test accuracy using graphs or tables. The following two graphical methods provide a succinct summary of the results of the assessment – one presents a summary showing individual study results (Figure 8.8.a), while the other summarizes the results across studies (Figure 8.8.b).

The risk-of-bias and applicability concerns summary in Figure 8.8.a presents, for each included study, the 'low', 'high' and 'unclear' judgements for each risk-of-bias and applicability domain. This presentation works well when there are not many included studies such that the figure fits on a page and is legible.

The risk-of-bias and applicability concerns graph in Figure 8.8.b is a stacked bar chart showing the proportion of included studies for each judgement of 'high', 'low' and 'unclear' for each risk-of-bias and applicability domain. These two graphical methods give readers a quick overview of the risk of bias and applicability of studies included in the review.

For QUADAS-C, suggested graphical methods combining QUADAS-2 and QUADAS-C assessments are available at www.quadas.org.

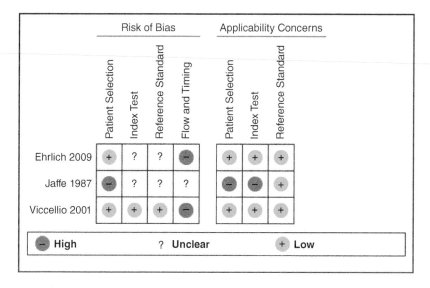

Figure 8.8.a **Risk-of-bias and applicability concerns summary table**. Source: Slaar 2017

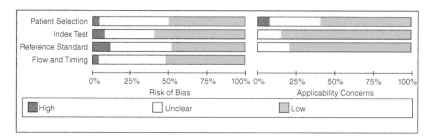

Figure 8.8.b **Risk-of-bias and applicability concerns graph**. Source: Leeflang 2015

8.9   Narrative summary of risk-of-bias and applicability assessments

In addition to presenting the results in graphs and/or tables, it is essential that a written summary of the assessment of risk of bias and applicability is included in the review. This summary should provide a narrative guide to the main potential sources of bias in the studies included in the review, and the main reasons for high risk-of-bias judgements. It may also consider the likely severity and direction of the possible biases and the nature of the applicability concerns.

In preparing a narrative summary, review authors need to incorporate:

- the frequency of 'high' and 'unclear' judgements of risk of bias and concerns regarding applicability for each domain; and
- any particular features that drive the high risk of bias and high applicability concern judgements.

For example, it is not sufficient to say that studies were at high risk of bias for participant selection; review authors should explain *why* they were at high risk of bias. This summary should facilitate a careful judgement of the degree to which the body of evidence may be compromised by bias and lack of applicability.

8.10   Chapter information

Authors: Johannes B. Reitsma (*Julius Center for Health Sciences and Primary Care, Utrecht University, The Netherlands*), Anne W. Rutjes (*Department of Medical and Surgical Sciences SMECHIMAI, University of Modena and Reggio Emilia, Italy*), Penny Whiting (*Population Health Sciences, University of Bristol, UK*), Bada Yang (*Julius Center for Health Sciences and Primary Care, Utrecht University, The Netherlands*), Mariska M. Leeflang (*Department of Epidemiology and Data Science, University of Amsterdam, The Netherlands*), Patrick M. Bossuyt (*Department of Epidemiology and Data Science, University of Amsterdam, The Netherlands*), Jonathan J. Deeks (*Institute of Applied Health Research, University of Birmingham, UK*).

Sources of support: Jonathan J. Deeks is a UK National Institute for Health Research (NIHR) Senior Investigator Emeritus. He is supported by the NIHR Birmingham Biomedical Research Centre at the University Hospitals Birmingham NHS Foundation Trust and the University of Birmingham. The views expressed are those of the authors and not necessarily those of the NHS, the NIHR or the Department of Health and Social Care. The authors declare no other sources of support for writing this chapter.

Declarations of interest: Penny Whiting is the lead author of QUADAS-2. Bada Yang is the lead author of QUADAS-C. All other authors have been involved in the development of both QUADAS-2 and QUADAS-C. Anne W. Rutjes is an Editor with Cochrane Dementia and Cognitive Improvement Group. Mariska M. Leeflang is co-convenor of the Screening and Diagnostic Test Methods Group. Mariska M. Leeflang and Jonathan J. Deeks are members of Cochrane's Diagnostic Test Accuracy Editorial Team. The authors declare no other potential conflicts of interest relevant to the topic of this chapter.

Acknowledgements: The authors thank Vasiliy Vlassov and Anne Eisinga for their contribution to previous versions of this chapter. The authors would like to thank Jacqueline Dinnes, Danielle van der Windt and Trevor McGrath for helpful peer review comments.

8.11 References

Begg CB, Greenes RA. Assessment of diagnostic tests when disease verification is subject to selection bias. *Biometrics* 1983; **39**: 207–215.

Berlin JA. Does blinding of readers affect the results of meta-analyses? University of Pennsylvania Meta-analysis Blinding Study Group. *Lancet* 1997; **350**: 185–186.

Bertens LC, Broekhuizen BD, Naaktgeboren CA, Rutten FH, Hoes AW, van Mourik Y, Moons KG, Reitsma JB. Use of expert panels to define the reference standard in diagnostic research: a systematic review of published methods and reporting. *PLoS Medicine* 2013; **10**: e1001531.

Biesheuvel C, Irwig L, Bossuyt P. Observed differences in diagnostic test accuracy between patient subgroups: is it real or due to reference standard misclassification? *Clinical Chemistry* 2007; **53**: 1725–1729.

Biesheuvel CJ, Vergouwe Y, Oudega R, Hoes AW, Grobbee DE, Moons KG. Advantages of the nested case-control design in diagnostic research. *BMC Medical Research Methodology* 2008; **8**: 48.

Bossuyt PM, Reitsma JB, Bruns DE, Gatsonis CA, Glasziou PP, Irwig LM, Lijmer JG, Moher D, Rennie D, de Vet HC. Towards complete and accurate reporting of studies of diagnostic accuracy: the STARD initiative. *BMJ* 2003a; **326**: 41–44.

Bossuyt PM, Reitsma JB, Bruns DE, Gatsonis CA, Glasziou PP, Irwig LM, Moher D, Rennie D, de Vet HC, Lijmer JG. The STARD statement for reporting studies of diagnostic accuracy: explanation and elaboration. *Annals of Internal Medicine* 2003b; **138**: W1–W12.

Boyko EJ, Alderman BW, Baron AE. Reference test errors bias the evaluation of diagnostic tests for ischemic heart disease. *Journal of General Internal Medicine* 1988; **3**: 476–481.

Cohen JF, Korevaar DA, Altman DG, Bruns DE, Gatsonis CA, Hooft L, Irwig L, Levine D, Reitsma JB, de Vet HC, Bossuyt PM. STARD 2015 guidelines for reporting diagnostic accuracy studies: explanation and elaboration. *BMJ Open* 2016; **6**: e012799.

Davison BA, Harrison SA, Cotter G, Alkhouri N, Sanyal A, Edwards C, Colca JR, Iwashita J, Koch GG, Dittrich HC. Suboptimal reliability of liver biopsy evaluation has implications for randomized clinical trials. *Journal of Hepatology* 2020; **73**: 1322–1332.

Diamond GA. Affirmative actions: can the discriminant accuracy of a test be determined in the face of selection bias? *Medical Decision Making* 1991; **11**: 48–56.

Glasziou P, Irwig L, Deeks JJ. When should a new test become the current reference standard? *Annals of Internal Medicine* 2008; **149**: 816–822.

Gluud LL, Thorlund K, Gluud C, Woods L, Harris R, Sterne JA. Correction: reported methodologic quality and discrepancies between large and small randomized trials in meta-analyses. *Annals of Internal Medicine* 2008; **149**: 219.

Higgins JPT, Altman DG. Chapter 8: Assessing risk of bias in included studies. In: Higgins JPT, Green S, editors. *Cochrane Handbook for Systematic Reviews of Interventions*. Chichester (UK): John Wiley & Sons; 2008: 187–241.

Ioannidis JP, Lau J. Can quality of clinical trials and meta-analyses be quantified? *Lancet* 1998; **352**: 590–591.

Jadad AR, Moore RA, Carroll D, Jenkinson C, Reynolds DJ, Gavaghan DJ, McQuay HJ. Assessing the quality of reports of randomized clinical trials: is blinding necessary? *Controlled Clinical Trials* 1996; **17**: 1–12.

Kjaergard LL, Villumsen J, Gluud C. Reported methodologic quality and discrepancies between large and small randomized trials in meta-analyses. *Annals of Internal Medicine* 2001; **135**: 982–989.

Korevaar DA, van Enst WA, Spijker R, Bossuyt PM, Hooft L. Reporting quality of diagnostic accuracy studies: a systematic review and meta-analysis of investigations on adherence to STARD. *Evidence-Based Medicine* 2014; **19**: 47–54.

Korevaar DA, Wang J, van Enst WA, Leeflang MM, Hooft L, Smidt N, Bossuyt PM. Reporting diagnostic accuracy studies: some improvements after 10 years of STARD. *Radiology* 2015; **274**: 781–789.

Leeflang MM, Moons KG, Reitsma JB, Zwinderman AH. Bias in sensitivity and specificity caused by data-driven selection of optimal cutoff values: mechanisms, magnitude, and solutions. *Clinical Chemistry* 2008; **54**: 729–737.

Leeflang MM, Debets-Ossenkopp YJ, Wang J, Visser CE, Scholten RJ, Hooft L, Bijlmer HA, Reitsma JB, Zhang M, Bossuyt PM, Vandenbroucke-Grauls CM. Galactomannan detection for invasive aspergillosis in immunocompromised patients. *Cochrane Database of Systematic Reviews* 2015; **12**: CD007394.

Lijmer JG, Mol BW, Heisterkamp S, Bonsel GJ, Prins MH, van der Meulen JH, Bossuyt PM. Empirical evidence of design-related bias in studies of diagnostic tests. *JAMA* 1999; **282**: 1061–1066.

Lumbreras-Lacarra B, Ramos-Rincon JM, Hernandez-Aguado I. Methodology in diagnostic laboratory test research in clinical chemistry and clinical chemistry and laboratory medicine. *Clinical Chemistry* 2004; **50**: 530–536.

Moher D, Jadad AR, Tugwell P. Assessing the quality of randomized controlled trials. Current issues and future directions. *International Journal of Technology Assessment in Health Care* 1996; **12**: 195–208.

Mulherin SA, Miller WC. Spectrum bias or spectrum effect? Subgroup variation in diagnostic test evaluation. *Annals of Internal Medicine* 2002; **137**: 598–602.

Naaktgeboren CA, Bertens LCM, Smeden Mv, Groot JAHd, Moons KGM, Reitsma JB. Value of composite reference standards in diagnostic research. *BMJ* 2013; **347**: f5605.

Naylor CD. Meta-analysis and the meta-epidemiology of clinical research. *BMJ* 1997; **315**: 617–619.

Pai M, Flores LL, Pai N, Hubbard A, Riley LW, Colford JM, Jr. Diagnostic accuracy of nucleic acid amplification tests for tuberculous meningitis: a systematic review and meta-analysis. *Lancet Infectious Diseases* 2003; **3**: 633–643.

Pepe MS, Feng Z, Janes H, Bossuyt PM, Potter JD. Pivotal evaluation of the accuracy of a biomarker used for classification or prediction: standards for study design. *Journal of the National Cancer Institute* 2008; **100**: 1432–1438.

Ransohoff DF, Feinstein AR. Problems of spectrum and bias in evaluating the efficacy of diagnostic tests. *New England Journal of Medicine* 1978; **299**: 926–930.

Reid MC, Lachs MS, Feinstein AR. Use of methodological standards in diagnostic test research. Getting better but still not good. *JAMA* 1995; **274**: 645–651.

Reitsma JB, Rutjes AW, Khan KS, Coomarasamy A, Bossuyt PM. A review of solutions for diagnostic accuracy studies with an imperfect or missing reference standard. *Journal of Clinical Epidemiology* 2009; **62**: 797–806.

Rutjes AW, Reitsma JB, Vandenbroucke JP, Glas AS, Bossuyt PM. Case-control and two-gate designs in diagnostic accuracy studies. *Clinical Chemistry* 2005; **51**: 1335–1341.

Rutjes AW, Reitsma JB, Di Nisio M, Smidt N, van Rijn JC, Bossuyt PM. Evidence of bias and variation in diagnostic accuracy studies. *Canadian Medical Association Journal* 2006; **174**: 469–476.

Slaar A, Fockens MM, Wang J, Maas M, Wilson DJ, Goslings JC, Schep NW, van Rijn RR. Triage tools for detecting cervical spine injury in pediatric trauma patients. *Cochrane Database of Systematic Reviews* 2017; **12**: CD011686.

Smidt N, Rutjes AW, van der Windt DA, Ostelo RW, Reitsma JB, Bossuyt PM, Bouter LM, de Vet HC. Quality of reporting of diagnostic accuracy studies. *Radiology* 2005; **235**: 347–353.

Stengel D, Bauwens K, Rademacher G, Mutze S, Ekkernkamp A. Association between compliance with methodological standards of diagnostic research and reported test accuracy: meta-analysis of focused assessment of US for trauma. *Radiology* 2005; **236**: 102–111.

Sterne JA, Jüni P, Schulz KF, Altman DG, Bartlett C, Egger M. Statistical methods for assessing the influence of study characteristics on treatment effects in 'meta-epidemiological' research. *Statistics in Medicine* 2002; **21**: 1513–1524.

Tullus K. Defining urinary tract infection by bacterial colony counts: a case for less than 100,000 colonies/mL as the threshold. *Pediatric Nephrology* 2019; **34**: 1651–1653.

van Rijkom HM, Verdonschot EH. Factors involved in validity measurements of diagnostic tests for approximal caries-a meta-analysis. *Caries Research* 1995; **29**: 364–370.

Verhagen AP, de Vet HC, de Bie RA, Boers M, van den Brandt PA. The art of quality assessment of RCTs included in systematic reviews. *Journal of Clinical Epidemiology* 2001; **54**: 651–654.

Whiting P, Rutjes AW, Reitsma JB, Bossuyt PM, Kleijnen J. The development of QUADAS: a tool for the quality assessment of studies of diagnostic accuracy included in systematic reviews. *BMC Medical Research Methodology* 2003; **3**: 25.

Whiting P, Rutjes AW, Dinnes J, Reitsma JB, Bossuyt PM, Kleijnen J. A systematic review finds that diagnostic reviews fail to incorporate quality despite available tools. *Journal of Clinical Epidemiology* 2005; **58**: 1–12.

Whiting P, Harbord R, Main C, Deeks JJ, Filippini G, Egger M, Sterne JA. Accuracy of magnetic resonance imaging for the diagnosis of multiple sclerosis: systematic review. *BMJ* 2006; **332**: 875–884.

Whiting PF, Rutjes AW, Westwood ME, Mallett S, Deeks JJ, Reitsma JB, Leeflang MM, Sterne JA, Bossuyt PM. QUADAS-2: a revised tool for the quality assessment of diagnostic accuracy studies. *Annals of Internal Medicine* 2011; **155**: 529–536.

Whiting PF, Rutjes AW, Westwood ME, Mallett S. A systematic review classifies sources of bias and variation in diagnostic test accuracy studies. *Journal of Clinical Epidemiology* 2013; **66**: 1093–1104.

Worster A, Carpenter C. Incorporation bias in studies of diagnostic tests: how to avoid being biased about bias. *Canadian Journal of Emergency Medicine* 2008; **10**: 174–175.

Yang B, Mallett S, Takwoingi Y, Davenport CF, Hyde CJ, Whiting PF, Deeks JJ, Leeflang MMG, Bossuyt PMM, Brazzelli MG, Dinnes J, Gurusamy KS, Jones HE, Lange S, Langendam MW, Macaskill P, McInnes MDF, Reitsma JB, Rutjes AWS, Sinclair A, de Vet HCW, Virgili G, Wade R, Westwood ME. QUADAS-C: a tool for assessing risk of bias in comparative diagnostic accuracy studies. *Annals of Internal Medicine* 2021a; **174**: 1592–1599.

Yang B, Olsen M, Vali Y, Langendam MW, Takwoingi Y, Hyde CJ, Bossuyt PMM, Leeflang MMG. Study designs for comparative diagnostic test accuracy: a methodological review and classification scheme. *Journal of Clinical Epidemiology* 2021b; **138**: 128–138.

Zhao S, Wang S, Pan P, Xia T, Chang X, Yang X, Guo L, Meng Q, Yang F, Qian W, Xu Z, Wang Y, Wang Z, Gu L, Wang R, Jia F, Yao J, Li Z, Bai Y. Magnitude, risk factors, and factors associated with adenoma miss rate of tandem colonoscopy: a systematic review and meta-analysis. *Gastroenterology* 2019; **156**: 1661–1674.

Zhou XH. Correcting for verification bias in studies of a diagnostic test's accuracy. *Statistical Methods in Medical Research* 1998; **7**: 337–353.

9

Understanding meta-analysis

Petra Macaskill, Yemisi Takwoingi, Jonathan J. Deeks and Constantine Gatsonis

KEY POINTS

- Statistical methods for systematic reviews of test accuracy combine estimates of the sensitivity and specificity of an index test from each study.
- Heterogeneity between the results of test accuracy studies is expected, thus requiring the use of random-effects models.
- Hierarchical random-effects models simultaneously combine estimates of sensitivity and specificity, allowing for correlation between them across studies.
- The bivariate model focuses on the estimation of a summary point, whereas the hierarchical summary receiver operating characteristic (HSROC) model focuses on the estimation of a summary ROC curve.
- When all studies included in an analysis apply the same threshold for test positivity, estimation of a summary point is appropriate.
- When studies included in an analysis apply different thresholds for test positivity, estimation of a summary curve is appropriate.
- Covariates can be included in the models to investigate heterogeneity and also to make comparisons between index tests.
- Analyses that include data from multiple thresholds per study require more complex extensions of the bivariate model.

9.1   Introduction

The statistical aspects of a systematic review of test accuracy are more challenging than those for reviews of interventions. It is therefore recommended that review teams include an individual with the statistical expertise needed to understand and implement the hierarchical models required for meta-analysis. This chapter has been written with this recommendation in mind. It aims first to provide guidance to the key

This chapter should be cited as: Macaskill P, Takwoingi Y, Deeks JJ, Gatsonis C. Chapter 9: Understanding meta-analysis. In: Deeks JJ, Bossuyt PM, Leeflang MM, Takwoingi Y, editors. *Cochrane Handbook for Systematic Reviews of Diagnostic Test Accuracy*. 1st edition. Chichester (UK): John Wiley & Sons, 2023: 203–248.

Cochrane Handbook for Systematic Reviews of Diagnostic Test Accuracy, First Edition. Edited by Jonathan J. Deeks, Patrick M. Bossuyt, Mariska M. Leeflang and Yemisi Takwoingi.
© 2023 The Cochrane Collaboration. Published 2023 by John Wiley & Sons Ltd.

researchers in the review team on the purpose, possibilities and interpretation of methods of meta-analysis, and second to provide the technical detail to assist a statistical expert in applying the methods recommended for Cochrane Reviews.

Sections 9.1, 9.2 and 9.3 outline the conceptual approach to meta-analysis, graphical presentations and the key meta-analysis methods that are recommended. Section 9.4 is the more technical guide to the routinely used meta-analytical models, while Section 9.5 introduces some more advanced methods. Both sections are intended to assist an informed statistician to apply the models using statistical software programs, and is necessarily written presuming a level of familiarity with statistical hierarchical modelling and so unlikely to be applicable to (or understood by) all readers. Section 9.4 includes examples with data sets, choice of model and interpretation of model estimates.

Chapter 10 is designed to complement this chapter by providing worked examples for a range of software packages used to implement the methods described in Section 9.4. Chapter 10 also provides technical explanations, examples and codes for some of the more advanced methods that are referred to in Section 9.5.

9.1.1 Aims of meta-analysis for systematic reviews of test accuracy

Reviews of diagnostic test accuracy provide information on how well tests distinguish patients with the target condition from those without. Hence, the statistical methods focus on two statistical measures of test accuracy, the sensitivity and the specificity of the test (see Chapter 4). Systematic reviews of diagnostic test accuracy aim to quantify and compare measures of test accuracy for one or more diagnostic tests to describe how accurately each test classifies individuals, and to estimate and compare the likely error rates (false positive and false negative diagnoses) that may be encountered.

Meta-analysis is a set of statistical techniques for combining results from two or more separate studies. Meta-analysis of test accuracy studies provides summaries of the results of relevant included studies, providing estimates of the average diagnostic accuracy of a test or tests, the uncertainty of these estimates and the variability between studies around the estimates.

Meta-analysis helps to make sense of heterogeneous and apparently inconsistent study results, as it identifies which differences are likely to be real, which are explicable by chance and which can be explained by known differences in study characteristics. As the precision of estimates typically increases with the quantity of data, meta-analysis may have more power to detect real differences in test accuracy between tests than single studies, and may yield more precise estimates of average sensitivity and specificity. Also, by quantifying the variability of test accuracy across many settings, meta-analysis may provide insights into the applicability of test results. Meta-analysis models also provide a framework for comparing the accuracy of tests (see Section 9.4.7).

9.1.2 When not to use a meta-analysis in a review

Meta-analysis is a powerful tool for summarizing study findings, provided that the estimates of test accuracy in the individual studies are both relevant and unlikely to be biased.

A common criticism of meta-analyses of studies of interventions is that 'they combine apples with oranges', implying that they may mix together estimates from studies that differ in important ways. This is one reason why Cochrane Reviews emphasize the importance of carefully defining eligibility criteria to identify studies that directly address the review question. In any analysis it is important to ensure that there are no major differences between the studies in terms of the participants they recruit and the tests they evaluate, which could lead to differences in the test performance that would make the results of the meta-analysis uninterpretable and potentially misleading. This is particularly important in reviews of test accuracy, as changes to patient selection criteria will alter the spectrum of those with and without the target condition in the population, which can strongly affect test accuracy, as discussed in Chapter 11.

In addition, it is important that the studies that are being combined in an analysis are methodologically rigorous. Meta-analysis of studies at risk of bias may be seriously misleading. If bias is present in individual studies, meta-analysis may compound the errors and produce an erroneous result that may be inappropriately interpreted as having credibility. Sensitivity analysis (Section 9.4.9) can be used to investigate how sensitive the results of the review are to the exclusion of poorer-quality studies.

9.1.3 How does meta-analysis of diagnostic test accuracy differ from meta-analysis of interventions?

The format of Cochrane Reviews of diagnostic test accuracy allows for greater flexibility for structuring and reporting meta-analysis than is available in Cochrane Reviews of interventions, and requires use of external statistical software. These differences arise for five main reasons.

- Systematic reviews of test accuracy can have diverse aims and address different types of question (as outlined in Section 9.1.4). Different comparisons and multiple aims may be addressed in a single review, often using data from the same studies in several analyses. Thus there is a need to develop both an appropriate data structure (see Chapter 4) and a clear analysis plan (see Section 9.1.5).
- Statistical methods for evaluating test accuracy require knowledge of two quantities: the test's sensitivity and its specificity. Meta-analysis methods for test accuracy thus have to deal with two statistics simultaneously rather than one (as is the case for reviews of interventions).
- A meta-analysis of test accuracy has to allow for the trade-off between sensitivity and specificity that occurs between studies that vary in the threshold value used to define test positives and test negatives. Meta-analysis methods have been devised to enable the combination of studies that have used a test(s) at different thresholds, a common occurrence in many systematic reviews of test accuracy (see Section 9.4.3 and Chapter 10, Section 10.7).
- Heterogeneity is to be expected in results of test accuracy studies, thus random-effects models are required to describe the variability in test accuracy across studies (see Section 9.3.2).
- Methods for undertaking analyses that account for both sensitivity and specificity, the relationship between them and the heterogeneity in test accuracy require fitting hierarchical random-effects models. Exploratory descriptive analyses can currently be undertaken in Cochrane's primary authoring tool, Review Manager (RevMan) (training.cochrane.org/online-learning/core-software-cochrane-reviews/revman),

whereas the definitive analyses need to be undertaken in statistical software packages and sophisticated statistical programming environments such as SAS, Stata, S-Plus, R, MLwiN or winBUGS/OpenBUGS/JAGS (see Chapter 10), for which collaboration with a statistical expert is highly recommended.

9.1.4 Questions that can be addressed in test accuracy analyses

Three main types of question can be addressed in a Cochrane Review of diagnostic test accuracy analysis concerning the accuracy of a test.

9.1.4.1 What is the accuracy of a test?

Such an analysis is restricted to characterizing the accuracy of a single test, and aims either to estimate an average summary value of sensitivity and specificity at a specified threshold, or to describe how sensitivity and specificity vary with changing threshold by estimating a summary ROC (SROC) curve. Which approach is used will depend on the nature of the test, and whether or not there is variability between studies in the criteria used to define a positive test (thresholds), which is discussed in more detail in Section 9.3.1.

9.1.4.2 How does the accuracy vary with clinical and methodological characteristics?

Planned investigations of heterogeneity investigate whether the observed test accuracy varies between studies according to characteristics associated with the setting in which the test is used, how the test is implemented, participants or methodology of the studies. For purposes of graphical presentation, it is best to group studies in categories to explore these factors. However, meta-regression models allow investigation of the relationship of accuracy to both categorical and continuous covariates, such as disease prevalence or test threshold. Differences in key parameters of SROC curves or summary points can be investigated depending on which is appropriate for a given analysis (Section 9.4.6).

9.1.4.3 How does the accuracy of two or more tests compare?

Comparison of the accuracy of tests is an important part of a Cochrane Review of diagnostic test accuracy, as it identifies which test (or tests) yields superior test accuracy. It is possible to compare multiple tests in a single analysis; there is no general restriction to comparing only pairs of tests, but it is often helpful to structure comparisons of multiple tests as a series of pairwise comparisons (bearing in mind problems caused by making an excessive number of multiple comparisons). Methodologically, comparing two tests can be considered as a form of subgroup analysis, with studies evaluating each test forming a subgroup, thereby allowing modelling techniques analogous to those used for investigating sources of heterogeneity to be applied. Review authors should consider which studies should be included in each pairwise test comparison. An 'indirect' comparison would use data from all studies that have evaluated one or both tests. A 'direct' comparison would generally be restricted to comparative studies that make direct (within-study) comparisons by testing all patients using both tests, or randomizing patients to undergo one of the tests. A within-study comparison of test performance between two independent but comparable groups of patients could also be considered for inclusion in such an analysis. Direct comparison has the advantage that each study acts as its own control, thereby dealing with potential confounding that may occur due to study characteristics. However, the number of comparative studies available may not be sufficient to allow such an analysis.

9.1.5   Planning the analysis

Undertaking meta-analyses for a Cochrane Review of diagnostic test accuracy involves first developing an analysis plan. Some of these decisions can be made at protocol stage (see Chapter 1), others only after the data have been extracted from the reports. The established and commonly used statistical methods for test accuracy meta-analysis use accuracy data for one threshold per study per index test. The following sections and examples used in Section 9.4 follow this approach. More advanced methods for dealing with data from multiple thresholds per study are discussed in Section 9.4.5 and dealt with in more detail in Chapter 10.

The planning stages can be organized as follows.

- Clearly stating the main questions that need answering, specifying which tests require estimates of test accuracy, and which tests should be compared with each other.
- Detailed planning of the way in which comparisons will be made, identifying the different tests or groups of tests that can be compared, the multiple and pairwise comparisons that will be made, and the studies and data that will be included in each analysis. Review authors need to decide whether comparative analyses should include all studies, or be restricted to studies that evaluate both tests. Covariates for any heterogeneity analyses similarly need to be specified and coded.
- From these decisions, a list of the planned main analyses, test comparisons and heterogeneity analyses will be produced. The quantity of data that are available for each analysis should be determined to guide the choice of analysis method, and to assess whether adequate data are available for planned heterogeneity analyses.
- Results can be plotted on forest plots and ROC plots to report study-specific estimates of sensitivity and specificity and the variability between these estimates across studies.
- A strategy needs to be developed to deal with the mixed reporting of thresholds that may occur across studies. A key issue is deciding whether an analysis should be restricted to studies that share a common threshold value (which allows estimation of the summary sensitivity and specificity of a test at that threshold) or to include all studies regardless of threshold value (which allows estimation of SROC curves but compromises the interpretation of summary points). This will depend on the thresholds at which tests were evaluated in the primary studies, and knowledge of how the tests are applied in clinical practice. Consideration should also be given to whether a more complex analysis is feasible that uses multiple thresholds per study (see Section 9.4.5 and Chapter 10, Section 10.7).
- If this analysis plan has been created using RevMan, the data should be exported from RevMan to the chosen statistics package, and appropriate models fitted. Results should be collated and tabulated as required, and parameter estimates copied back

into the RevMan graphics function to produce final graphical output showing summary points or SROC curves as appropriate.

9.2 Graphical and tabular presentation

A Cochrane Review of diagnostic test accuracy uses two main forms of graphical display: coupled forest plots and SROC plots. Review authors can create these figures within RevMan for each analysis that is specified.

9.2.1 Coupled forest plots

Forest plots for diagnostic test accuracy report the number of true positives and false negatives in participants with the target condition (diseased), and true negatives and false positives in participants who do not have the target condition (non-diseased) in each study, and the estimated sensitivity and specificity, together with confidence intervals (CIs). The plots are known as coupled forest plots as they contain two graphical sections: one depicting sensitivity and one specificity (Figure 9.2.a). The order of the studies can be sorted, for example by values of sensitivity, or grouped by test type or covariate values. While it is possible to observe heterogeneity in sensitivity and specificity individually on such plots, it is not easy to visualize whether there are threshold-like relationships. Summary statistics computed from meta-analyses are rarely added to coupled forest plots. In Cochrane Reviews of diagnostic test accuracy, an archive of coupled forest plots for all the tests for which data were entered into RevMan is published with the review to make the 2×2 tables of the index test result for those with the target condition (referred to as the diseased) and without the target condition (referred to as non-diseased) readily accessible.

9.2.2 Summary ROC plots

An SROC plot is a scatterplot of the results of individual studies in ROC space where each study is plotted as a single (specificity, sensitivity) point. The size of the symbol (e.g. rectangle, ellipse) used to mark each point can be controlled to depict the precision of the estimate (typically scaled according to their sample sizes). Using sample-size weights, the height of the symbol is proportional to the number of diseased (and hence the precision of the sensitivity estimate) and the width is proportional to the number of non-diseased (and hence the precision of the specificity estimate) (see Figure 9.2.b).

Both the within-study sampling variability and the heterogeneity between studies contribute to the total variability between studies. Even if the summary plots scale the symbols to indicate the precision of the estimates from individual studies, it is difficult to distinguish visually between these two sources of variability.

Two types of meta-analytical summary can be added to an SROC plot: SROC curves and summary points. Confidence regions for the summary points can be included, as can prediction regions that give an indication of between-study heterogeneity (see later Figure 9.4.a).

Studies can also be plotted using different symbols and/or colours to indicate different subgroups for investigations of heterogeneity or for test comparisons.

Study	TP	FP	FN	TN	Generation	Sensitivity	Specificity
Aotsuka 2005	115	17	16	73	CCP2	0.88 [0.81, 0.93]	0.81 [0.71, 0.89]
Bas 2003	110	24	86	215	CCP1	0.56 [0.49, 0.63]	0.90 [0.85, 0.93]
Bizzaro 2001	40	5	58	227	CCP1	0.41 [0.31, 0.51]	0.98 [0.95, 0.99]
Bombardieri 2004	23	0	7	39	CCP2	0.77 [0.58, 0.90]	1.00 [0.91, 1.00]
Choi 2005	236	20	88	231	CCP2	0.73 [0.68, 0.78]	0.92 [0.88, 0.95]
Correa 2004	74	11	8	130	CCP2	0.90 [0.82, 0.96]	0.92 [0.86, 0.96]
De Rycke 2004	89	4	29	142	CCP2	0.75 [0.67, 0.83]	0.97 [0.93, 0.99]
Dubucquoi 2004	90	2	50	129	CCP2	0.64 [0.56, 0.72]	0.98 [0.95, 1.00]
Fernandez-Suarez 2005	31	0	22	75	CCP2	0.58 [0.44, 0.72]	1.00 [0.95, 1.00]
Garcia-Berrocal 2005	69	8	18	38	CCP2	0.79 [0.69, 0.87]	0.83 [0.69, 0.92]
Girelli 2004	25	2	10	40	CCP2	0.71 [0.54, 0.85]	0.95 [0.84, 0.99]
Goldbach-Mansky 2000	43	1	63	120	CCP1	0.41 [0.31, 0.51]	0.99 [0.95, 1.00]
Greiner 2005	70	5	17	228	CCP2	0.80 [0.71, 0.88]	0.98 [0.95, 0.99]
Grootenboer-Mignot 2004	167	8	98	88	CCP2	0.63 [0.57, 0.69]	0.92 [0.84, 0.96]
Hitchon 2004	26	8	15	15	CCP1	0.63 [0.47, 0.78]	0.65 [0.43, 0.84]
Jansen 2003	110	3	148	118	CCP1	0.43 [0.37, 0.49]	0.98 [0.93, 0.99]
Kamali 2005	26	1	20	56	CCP2	0.57 [0.41, 0.71]	0.98 [0.91, 1.00]
Kumagai 2004	64	14	15	293	CCP2	0.81 [0.71, 0.89]	0.95 [0.92, 0.97]
Kwok 2005	71	2	58	66	CCP2	0.55 [0.46, 0.64]	0.97 [0.90, 1.00]
Lee 2003	68	14	35	132	CCP2	0.66 [0.56, 0.75]	0.90 [0.84, 0.95]
Lopez-Hoyos 2004	38	3	0	73	CCP2	1.00 [0.91, 1.00]	0.96 [0.89, 0.99]
Nell 2005	42	2	60	96	CCP2	0.41 [0.32, 0.51]	0.98 [0.93, 1.00]
Nielen 2005	149	7	109	114	CCP2	0.58 [0.51, 0.64]	0.94 [0.88, 0.98]
Quinn 2006	147	10	35	106	CCP2	0.81 [0.74, 0.86]	0.91 [0.85, 0.96]
Rantapaa-Dahlqvist 2003	47	7	20	375	CCP2	0.70 [0.58, 0.81]	0.98 [0.96, 0.99]
Raza 2005	24	3	18	79	CCP2	0.57 [0.41, 0.72]	0.96 [0.90, 0.99]
Saraux 2003	40	11	46	146	CCP1	0.47 [0.36, 0.58]	0.93 [0.88, 0.96]
Sauerland 2005	171	26	60	443	CCP2	0.74 [0.68, 0.80]	0.94 [0.92, 0.96]
Schellekens 2000	72	14	77	298	CCP1	0.48 [0.40, 0.57]	0.96 [0.93, 0.98]
Soderlin 2004	7	2	9	51	CCP2	0.44 [0.20, 0.70]	0.96 [0.87, 1.00]
Suzuki 2003	481	23	68	185	CCP2	0.88 [0.85, 0.90]	0.89 [0.84, 0.93]
Vallbracht 2004	190	12	105	408	CCP2	0.64 [0.59, 0.70]	0.97 [0.95, 0.99]
van Gaalen 2005	82	13	71	301	CCP2	0.54 [0.45, 0.62]	0.96 [0.93, 0.98]
van Venroooij 2004	865	79	252	2218	CCP2	0.77 [0.75, 0.80]	0.97 [0.96, 0.97]
Vincent 2002	139	7	101	464	CCP1	0.58 [0.51, 0.64]	0.99 [0.97, 0.99]
Vittecoq 2004	69	5	107	133	CCP2	0.39 [0.32, 0.47]	0.96 [0.92, 0.99]
Zeng 2003	90	7	101	313	CCP1	0.47 [0.40, 0.54]	0.98 [0.96, 0.99]

Figure 9.2.a Coupled forest plot of the sensitivity and specificity of Anti-CCP for the diagnosis of rheumatoid arthritis

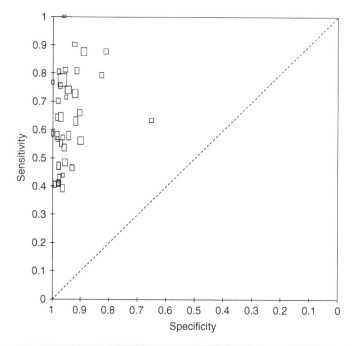

Figure 9.2.b SROC plot of Anti-CCP for the diagnosis of rheumatoid arthritis

9.2.3 Linked SROC plots

Linked SROC plots are used in analyses of paired test comparisons, where both tests have been evaluated within a study. The points are plotted as for a routine SROC plot, but the two estimates (one for each test) from each study are joined by a line. It is thus possible to get a sense of the difference in accuracy between tests within each study, and to assess visually the degree of consistency in this difference across studies. Summary estimates of sensitivity and specificity for each test, as well as SROC curves obtained from meta-analysis, can be added to these plots (see later Figure 9.4.g for an example plot).

9.2.3.1 Example 1: Anti-CCP for the diagnosis of rheumatoid arthritis – descriptive plots

These data are taken from a review (Nishimura 2007) of anti-cyclic citrullinated peptide antibody (anti-CCP). The reference standard was based on the 1987 revised American College of Rheumatology (ACR) criteria for clinical diagnosis. The meta-analysis included 37 studies and their sensitivities and specificities are shown on the forest plot (Figure 9.2.a); these study-specific estimates are also shown in a scatterplot in ROC space.

The forest plot shows the studies in alphabetical order. The figure gives the numbers for the 2×2 table (true positives (TP), false positives (FP), false negatives (FN), true negatives (TN)) for each study that will form the basis for statistical analyses. Study-specific estimates of sensitivity and specificity are shown, with their 95% confidence intervals. These estimates (and confidence intervals) are also represented graphically. The most striking features of this figure are the consistently high specificity and the greater uncertainty (indicated by the confidence interval width) and variability (indicated by the scatter of point estimates) in sensitivity than specificity. The studies can be ordered in different ways (e.g. in increasing order of sensitivity) to provide a visual representation of any association between sensitivity and specificity. Ordering studies by year of publication may also be useful to identify trends in test accuracy resulting from changes in methodology and/or selection criteria over time (Cohen 2016). The figure also includes information on a covariate, the CCP generation, which may be associated with heterogeneity in test accuracy. (This will be explored in Section 9.4.6.2.)

The SROC plot shown in Figure 9.2.b also illustrates the greater variability in estimated sensitivity than specificity across studies. Covariate information (e.g. generation of CCP) could be used to distinguish between studies in different subgroups (e.g. CCP1 vs CCP2). (See Section 9.4.6.3 for further exploration of these data.)

Formal statistical analyses are required to obtain a summary estimate of test accuracy and to explore heterogeneity. These will be covered in Section 9.4.6.3. Before proceeding to these statistical analyses, the review author should decide whether it is appropriate to focus on a summary point(s) or a summary curve(s) in the statistical analyses that follow. This will be influenced by the threshold(s) used by the included studies to define a positive test result (see Section 9.4).

9.2.4   Tables of results

Review authors need to construct additional tables to report results from their meta-analytical models. Review authors might consider creating tables to report the following.

- The numbers of studies and individuals available for each of the key analyses.
- Summary estimates of diagnostic accuracy for each test.
- Statistics for the comparative accuracy and tests of statistical significance for the pairwise comparisons between tests (a half-matrix display of all possible pairwise comparisons may be useful). Separate tables based on direct (within-study) comparisons and uncontrolled comparisons may be needed (see Section 9.4.7).
- Results of investigations of heterogeneity, including estimates of test accuracy in subgroups, summary statistics of comparative accuracy, and tests of statistical significance (see Section 9.4.6).
- Results of sensitivity analyses (see Section 9.4.9).

This list is not exhaustive, and review authors should explore and identify the best ways of communicating the results of their analyses.

Cochrane Reviews of diagnostic test accuracy also include 'Summary of findings' tables, which are described in Chapter 12.

9.3   Meta-analytical summaries

Test accuracy meta-analysis aims to compute the average accuracy of a test, compare estimates of accuracy between tests, and investigate the heterogeneity between studies. Review authors should choose which summary statistics to use. In Cochrane

Reviews that use one 2×2 table per study (per test), the choice is between estimating average values of sensitivity and specificity for a test at a common threshold (referred to as the average or summary operating point or summary point), or estimating the underlying ROC curve for a test across many thresholds (referred to as the summary ROC curve or SROC curve). In most scenarios estimation of a summary point is preferred, as it facilitates interpretation of the results in terms of the numbers of true positives, true negatives, false positives and false negatives (see Chapter 11 and Chapter 12). However, there are situations when estimation of an SROC curve is the only analysis possible, or there are benefits in terms of precision of estimates and comparisons.

9.3.1 Should I estimate an SROC curve or a summary point?

In a systematic review of test accuracy studies, it is likely that the collected data on test performance will have been measured at a mixture of different positivity thresholds. A threshold could, for instance, represent a cut-point on a quantitative scale or a judgement on an ordinal scale. A key principle underlying the choice of statistical summary in meta-analysis of test accuracy is that the sensitivity and specificity of a test will vary as the positivity thresholds vary, as graphically depicted using an ROC curve. It is important to note that both hierarchical models recommended for meta-analysis for Cochrane Reviews of diagnostic test accuracy account for correlation between sensitivity and specificity observed across studies that is due to the functional relationship between sensitivity and specificity as the criterion for test positivity (threshold) varies. This correlation is accounted for in the analysis regardless of whether an SROC curve or a summary point is the output of choice. Separate meta-analysis of sensitivity and specificity estimates fails to account for the trade-off between sensitivity and specificity, which may lead to under-estimates of test accuracy (Deeks 2001). Separate meta-analysis of likelihood ratios also ignores correlations between positive and negative likelihood ratios, and theoretically can produce estimates that are impossible (Zwinderman 2008).

While for some tests there is consensus about what value the positivity threshold should take, often tests are evaluated at different thresholds in different studies. Presentation of results at multiple thresholds within a single study is also possible, with some studies presenting estimates of ROC curves that depict the accuracy of the test at all possible thresholds. In addition, selective reporting of thresholds identified to optimize test accuracy can introduce bias, because sampling variability may influence which threshold is identified as 'optimal' when it is selected based on the observed data (Leeflang 2008).

Review authors need to decide whether they will use all the studies available and estimate an SROC curve, or select only studies that use a common threshold to estimate a summary point (an analysis that could be repeated across a set of different common thresholds). Estimating summary sensitivity and specificity by combining studies that mix thresholds will produce an estimate that relates to some notional unspecified average of the thresholds that occur in the included studies. This must be avoided, because it is clinically uninterpretable and not generalizable. More complex methods do allow use of all data to estimate both curves and summary points, but are not currently often used due to challenges in their implementation (see Section 9.4.5).

In some contexts, test positivity is based on an ordinal rating scale rather than an explicit numerical threshold requiring a judgement rather than measurement, which is likely to lead to variability between individual readers in how they interpret the thresholds on the rating scale. For a study-level meta-analysis of test accuracy, it is generally reasonable to assume a common threshold across studies if the same point on the rating scale was applied. At the study level, the estimated sensitivity and specificity represent average estimates of accuracy across readers in that study. Even when it is possible to define a common threshold on the basis of a numerical value or a point on a rating scale, it must be acknowledged that some variability will remain in the actual threshold between studies through calibration differences between equipment, differences between groups of raters or observers in terms of training and experience, as well as variation in the implementation of tests. The consequence of such variability will be additional heterogeneity in test results observed at the common threshold. The summary sensitivity and specificity point will reflect the average observed accuracy across studies, while the prediction region (see Section 9.3.2) will reflect the heterogeneity between studies, as illustrated in the example in Section 9.4.2.

Thus, the three main strategies used to handle mixed and variable thresholds in an analysis are as follows.

- Estimating summary sensitivity and specificity of the test for a common threshold, or at each of several different common thresholds if there are sufficient data. Each study can contribute to one or more analyses depending on what thresholds it reports. Studies that do not report at any of the selected thresholds are excluded.
- Estimating the underlying ROC curve that describes how sensitivity and specificity trade off with each other as thresholds vary. In this case, one threshold per study is selected to be included in the analysis. A range of thresholds across studies is needed to inform the shape of the SROC curve.
- Simultaneous analysis of multiple (one or more) estimates of sensitivity and specificity reported by each study. This approach allows estimation of an SROC curve and summary points on the curve for particular thresholds of interest.

For analyses that will include one threshold per study, the choice of analytical approach will be influenced by the variation of thresholds in the available studies. For example, if there is little consistency in the thresholds used, meta-analyses that are restricted to common thresholds will contain very few data, and estimating an SROC curve may be preferred. If there is little variation in threshold between studies, attempting to fit an SROC curve will be difficult, as the points are likely to be too tightly clustered in ROC space and there is little information in the data to estimate the shape of the underlying curve.

It can be reasonable to estimate both SROC curves and summary points in a review, as they may complement each other in providing clinically useful summaries and powerful ways of detecting effects. For example, separate analyses of test data at different thresholds may be used to provide clinically informative estimates of sensitivity and specificity based on the studies that provide data at each threshold. Including all studies to estimate how SROC curves depend on covariates or test type will be the most powerful way to test hypotheses and investigate heterogeneity when thresholds vary across studies.

When some studies provide data for multiple thresholds, more complex models that estimate an SROC curve and summary points on that curve may be applied (see Section 9.4.5 and Chapter 10, Section 10.7). However, the potential gain relative to the more straightforward approaches will be limited if only a small proportion of studies provide such data.

9.3.2 Heterogeneity

Heterogeneity is to be expected in meta-analyses of diagnostic test accuracy. A consequence of this is that meta-analyses of test accuracy studies tend to focus on computing *average* rather than *typical* effects. In systematic reviews of interventions it is sometimes noted that the estimates of the effect of the intervention in the different studies are very similar, the differences between them being small enough to be explicable by chance. In such situations it is appropriate to use a fixed-effect approach meta-analysis, which estimates the underlying common effect (and is interpreted as the actual effect of the intervention). In systematic reviews of test accuracy, large differences are commonly noted between studies, too big to be explained by chance, indicating that actual test accuracy varies between studies: there is heterogeneity in test accuracy. Random-effects meta-analysis methods are recommended when effects are heterogeneous. These methods focus on providing an estimate of the average accuracy of the test and describing the variability in accuracy between studies. In Cochrane Reviews of diagnostic test accuracy, heterogeneity is presumed to exist and random-effects models are fitted by default, only simplified to fixed-effect models where there are too few studies to estimate between-study variability, or analysis and forest or SROC plots demonstrate that fixed-effect models are appropriate (see Section 9.4.8).

Univariate tests for heterogeneity in sensitivity and specificity and estimates of the I^2 statistic (Higgins 2003) are not recommended for systematic reviews of test accuracy, as they do not account for heterogeneity explained by phenomena such as positivity threshold effects, whereby an increasing threshold for defining test positivity will decrease sensitivity and increase specificity. Problems with the I^2 statistic that could lead to misleading conclusions have also been highlighted in the literature (Rücker 2008, Wetterslev 2009, Zhou 2014); other measures such as the variance parameter of the random-effects model (Rücker 2008) and also multivariate and test accuracy-specific I^2 statistics (Zhou 2014) have been proposed but are not used routinely.

The numerical estimates of the random-effects terms in the hierarchical models do quantify the amount of heterogeneity observed, but they are not easily interpreted as they represent variation in parameters expressed on log odds scales. Graphical displays provide a more straightforward means of assessing the magnitude of the observed heterogeneity. For instance, if variation in threshold occurs in a meta-analysis, what matters is the degree to which the observed study results in an SROC plot lie close to the SROC curve, not how scattered they are in ROC space.

For a summary point estimate, the inclusion of a prediction region around the point provides a visual assessment of heterogeneity. The region takes account of the variance of the random effects for logit(sensitivity) and logit(specificity), as well as the correlation between them. The region provides a visual summary of the spread of the true underlying test accuracy across the studies included in the random-effects model (see the example in Section 9.4.2). Hence, a 95% prediction region represents the region within which one has 95% confidence that the true sensitivity and specificity of any future study should lie (Harbord 2007). Estimation of a prediction interval or region relies on the assumption of normal distributions for the effects across studies. This may be very problematic when the number of studies is small and can lead to spuriously large (or small) regions (Deeks 2019).

9.4 Fitting hierarchical models

In this section, the bivariate model (Reitsma 2005) and the hierarchical SROC (HSROC) model of Rutter and Gatsonis (Rutter 2001) are described and discussed for the meta-analysis of studies each of which contributes one threshold to the analysis. These hierarchical models include random study effects that account for the unexplained heterogeneity between studies that is typical in systematic reviews of test accuracy. They supersede the earlier, more limited fixed-effect SROC approach of Moses and Littenberg (Littenberg 1993, Moses 1993).

Both the bivariate and Rutter and Gatsonis HSROC models involve statistical distributions at two levels. At the lower level (level 1), they model the cell counts in the 2×2 tables extracted from each study using binomial distributions and logistic (log odds) transformations of proportions, thereby taking account of random sampling variability within studies. At the higher level (level 2), random study effects are assumed to account for heterogeneity in test accuracy between studies beyond that accounted for by sampling variability at the lower level.

The two models are mathematically equivalent when no covariates are fitted (Harbord 2007, Arends 2008), but differ in their parametrizations. The bivariate parametrization models sensitivity, specificity and the correlation between them directly, whereas the Rutter and Gatsonis HSROC parametrization models a function of sensitivity and specificity to define an SROC curve. Given their shared statistical properties, in the absence of covariates in the models SROC curves can be computed from bivariate models and summary points from HSROC models.

If review authors are using RevMan, the parameter estimates from either model can be input to produce an appropriate graphical display in ROC space of the summary estimates of test accuracy for a particular analysis, usually superimposed on the scatterplot of study specific estimates. The options are:

- the SROC curve; or
- the summary point (i.e. summary values for sensitivity and specificity);
- a confidence region around the summary point; and
- a prediction region around the summary point.

Although it is common to present 95% confidence and 95% prediction regions, RevMan offers options to use other values. The 95% prediction region around a summary point illustrates the extent of statistical heterogeneity by depicting a region within which, assuming the model is correct, we have 95% confidence that the true sensitivity and specificity of any future study should lie (Harbord 2007). There is also an option of plotting a 50% prediction region, in which the central half of the true values of future studies would lie (akin to an interquartile range).

Additional estimates can be derived from the models. Summary estimates for the positive and negative likelihood ratios and the diagnostic odds ratio, with corresponding confidence intervals, can be computed at the summary point or at any point on the SROC curve. From the SROC curve the average sensitivity at a given value of specificity (or the other way round) can also be computed (see Chapter 10). Not all of these possible summary measures will be relevant or appropriate for a given analysis.

The motivation for choosing one of these two alternative parameterizations becomes clear when covariates are added to explore heterogeneity in test accuracy or to compare tests. Ultimately, the choice of method will be determined by the focus one wishes to adopt, and which of the two models addresses the research question given the nature of the available data (see Section 9.3.1).

Both models require the use of external statistical software. The results given for the examples included in this chapter have been estimated using frequentist methods. Although this is the most commonly used approach, Bayesian estimation can also be used, as illustrated in Chapter 10. Publication-ready graphical output can be created in RevMan using the model parameter estimates to add model summaries to SROC plots.

Alternative specifications for summary curves based on functions of the bivariate model parameters have been proposed (Arends 2008, Chappell 2009). This chapter will focus on the Rutter and Gatsonis model, as it is the most established of the HSROC specifications.

9.4.1 Bivariate model

The bivariate method models sensitivity and specificity directly. The model can be regarded as having two levels corresponding to variation *within* and *between* studies. At the lower level, the within-study variability for both sensitivity and specificity is assumed to follow a binomial distribution. For sensitivity (denoted by A), the number testing positive $y_{Ai} \sim B(n_{Ai}, \pi_{Ai})$, where n_{Ai} and π_{Ai} respectively represent the total number of diseased individuals tested and the probability of a positive test result in that group in study i. Similarly, for specificity (denoted by B), the number testing negative $y_{Bi} \sim B(n_{Bi}, \pi_{Bi})$, where n_{Bi} and π_{Bi} respectively represent the total number of non-diseased individuals tested and the probability of a negative test result in that group in study i. The sensitivity–specificity pair for each study must be modelled jointly within the study at the lower level of the analysis, because they are linked by shared study characteristics including the positivity threshold. At the higher (between-study) level, the logit-transformed sensitivities are assumed to have a normal distribution with mean μ_A and variance σ^2_A, while the logit-transformed specificities have a normal distribution with mean μ_B and variance σ^2_B. Their correlation is included by modelling both at once by a single bivariate normal distribution

$$\begin{pmatrix} \mu_{Ai} \\ \mu_{Bi} \end{pmatrix} \sim N\left(\begin{pmatrix} \mu_A \\ \mu_B \end{pmatrix}, \Sigma \right) \text{ with } \Sigma = \begin{pmatrix} \sigma^2_A & \sigma_{AB} \\ \sigma_{AB} & \sigma^2_B \end{pmatrix}$$

where σ_{AB} is the covariance between logit(sensitivity) and logit(specificity). The model may also be parametrized using the correlation $\rho_{AB} = \sigma_{AB}/(\sigma_A \sigma_B)$, which may be more interpretable than the covariance. The bivariate model therefore has five parameters when no covariates are included: μ_A, μ_B, σ^2_A, σ^2_B and ρ_{AB}. (Note: we follow Harbord (2007) in using μ where Reitsma (Reitsma 2005) used θ in order to avoid confusion with the notation from that of the HSROC model that follows.)

The inclusion of a correlation parameter in the model allows for the expected trade-off in sensitivity and specificity. Where variation between studies arises through a trade-off resulting from variation in thresholds between studies, this correlation is expected to be negative. However, the correlation may be positive if there are other sources of heterogeneity.

Reitsma and colleagues originally proposed fitting these models by approximating the binomial within-study distributions by normal distributions (Reitsma 2005). Although this allows the model to be fitted in a slightly larger range of software (e.g. the MIXED procedure in SAS), Chu (2006) later demonstrated that the approximation can perform poorly and recommended that software be used that can explicitly model the binomial within-study distributions, as is done in the examples that follow and the sample programs provided in Chapter 10.

Meta-analysis of predictive values is possible using the bivariate method (Leeflang 2012), but this is not recommended as it is known that predictive values depend on the proportion of participants with the target condition, which is likely to vary between studies. Hence, the average predictive values will relate to use of the test at some average prevalence. Meta-analysis of predictive values may be appropriate when either sensitivity and specificity is not estimable due to partial verification (i.e. verification of only test positives or test negatives) or when there is differential verification.

9.4.2 Example 1 continued: anti-CCP for the diagnosis of rheumatoid arthritis

We now undertake the first stage of a formal statistical analysis of the data from a review of anti-cyclic citrullinated peptide antibody (anti-CCP) (Nishimura 2007). If it can be presumed that the anti-CCP test is deemed positive if any anti-CCP antibody is detected and that detection can be considered a common threshold, it is appropriate to focus on summary estimates for sensitivity and specificity.

As noted in the descriptive analyses of these data (Section 9.2.3), there appears to be variability across studies in estimates of test accuracy. This variability appears to be higher for sensitivity than specificity, which could arise either through heterogeneity or through estimates of sensitivity being based on smaller samples than estimates of specificity. Using the bivariate model to estimate a summary point based on the data for all studies, the parameter estimates from the bivariate model are shown in Table 9.4.a.

The parameter estimates can be input to RevMan to produce the summary point, 95% confidence region and 95% prediction region shown in Figure 9.4.a, superimposed on the individual study estimates. Computation of confidence and prediction regions also requires the standard error of the estimates for mean logit(sensitivity), mean logit(specificity) and the covariance between these estimates, which are 0.1275, 0.1459 and −0.00741, respectively. Note that the covariance shown in Table 9.4.a is the covariance between observed estimates of logit(sensitivity) and logit(specificity) across studies, not the covariance between the estimates for mean logit(sensitivity) and mean logit(specificity). The latter can be extracted as demonstrated in Chapter 10.

Table 9.4.a Bivariate model parameter estimates for accuracy of anti-CCP for the diagnosis of rheumatoid arthritis

Label	Parameter	Estimate	Standard error
Mean logit(sensitivity)	μ_A	0.6534	0.1275
Mean logit(specificity)	μ_B	3.1090	0.1459
Variance of random effects for logit(sensitivity)	σ^2_A	0.5426	0.1463
Variance of random effects for logit(specificity)	σ^2_B	0.5717	0.1873
Covariance of logit(sensitivity) and logit(specificity)	σ_{AB}	−0.2704	0.1199

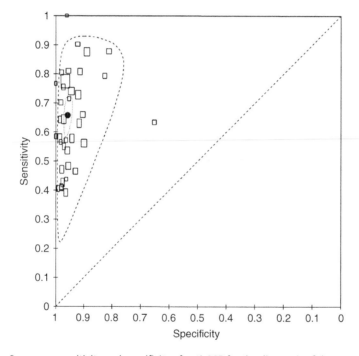

Figure 9.4.a Summary sensitivity and specificity of anti-CCP for the diagnosis of rheumatoid arthritis

The variance coefficients indicate similar heterogeneity in sensitivities and specificities on the logit scale. The magnitude of the heterogeneity in sensitivities and specificities (untransformed) is evident in the size of the prediction region on the SROC plot, with the variability in specificity being constrained on this scale because the underlying specificity is high. The summary estimates of sensitivity and specificity are shown by the solid black dot. The sensitivity and specificity at this point can be computed by inverse transformation of the logit estimates to give a sensitivity and specificity of 0.66 and 0.96, respectively. Confidence intervals can be computed by inverse transformation of the confidence intervals computed on the logit scale. (See Chapter 10 for further details.)

The plot shows a potential outlier, with a sensitivity of 0.63 and specificity of 0.65. A sensitivity analysis can be performed by omitting this study to assess its influence on the summary estimates (see Section 9.4.9).

9.4.3   The Rutter and Gatsonis HSROC model

The HSROC model proposed by Rutter and Gatsonis (Rutter 1995, Rutter 2001) is based on a latent scale logistic regression model (McCullagh 1980, Tosteson 1988). The HSROC model assumes that there is an underlying ROC curve in each study with parameters α and β that characterize the accuracy and asymmetry of the curve.

Accuracy, defined in terms of the lnDOR (natural logarithm of the diagnostic odds ratio), determines the position of the summary curve relative to the top left corner of the ROC axes. Each study contributes data at a single threshold to the analysis. The 2×2 table for each study then arises from dichotomizing at a positivity threshold denoted by θ. The parameters α and θ are assumed to vary between studies: both are assumed to have normal distributions, as in conventional random-effects meta-analysis.

The HSROC model can be regarded as having two levels corresponding to variation *within* and *between* studies. At the lower level, the number of diseased individuals who test positive is denoted by y_{i1} for the ith study, and the corresponding number of non-diseased who test positive is denoted by y_{i2}. For each study (i), the number testing positive in each disease group (j) is assumed to follow a binomial distribution such that $y_{ij} \sim B(n_{ij}, \pi_{ij})$, $j = 1, 2$, where n_{ij} and π_{ij}, respectively, represent the total number tested and the probability of a positive test result. The number testing positive in each diseased and non-diseased pair is analysed jointly within each study at the lower level in the analysis.

The model takes the form

$$logit(\pi_{ij}) = (\theta_i + \alpha_i dis_{ij}) \exp(-\beta dis_{ij})$$

where dis_{ij} represents the 'true' disease status (coded as −0.5 for the non-diseased and 0.5 for the diseased), thereby taking into account the within-study variability at the lower level. Using the terminology for this model, θ_i represents a proxy for positivity threshold calculated as the mean of the log odds of a positive test result for the diseased and the log odds of a positive test result for the non-diseased groups in study i. α_i (the lnDOR for study i) represents a measure of diagnostic accuracy in the ith study that incorporates both sensitivity and specificity for that study. The shape (scale) parameter (β) provides for asymmetry in the SROC curve by allowing accuracy to vary with threshold. Since each study contributes only one estimate of sensitivity and specificity at a single threshold, it is necessary to assume that the shape of the true underlying ROC curve in each study is the same, and hence β is fitted as a fixed effect.

The threshold and diagnostic accuracy for each study are specified as random effects and are assumed to be independent (uncorrelated) and normally distributed. The accuracy parameter has mean Λ (capital lambda) and variance σ_α^2, while the positivity (threshold) parameter has mean Θ (capital theta) and variance σ_θ^2. The shape parameter (β) is estimated using data from the studies considered jointly, assuming normally distributed random effects for test accuracy. When no covariates are included, the HSROC model has five parameters: Λ, Θ, β, σ_α^2 and σ_θ^2.

An SROC curve can be constructed from the HSROC model by choosing a range of values of 1–specificity and using the estimated average location parameter (Λ) and scale parameter (β) to compute the corresponding values for sensitivity. The average sensitivity at a chosen false positive fraction (1–specificity) is given by

$$\text{sensitivity} = 1 \Big/ \left[1 + \exp\left(-\left(\Lambda e^{-0.5\beta} + \text{logit}\left(1 - \text{specificity} \right) e^{-\beta} \right) \right) \right]$$

When β = 0, test accuracy can be summarized by Λ, which represents a common average accuracy (lnDOR) across all thresholds, and the resulting summary curve will be symmetrical.

9.4.4 Example 2: Rheumatoid factor as a marker for rheumatoid arthritis

In this example we will investigate the diagnostic performance of rheumatoid factor (RF) as a marker for rheumatoid arthritis (RA). The 50 studies included in the analysis are taken from the same review as Example 1 (Nishimura 2007). The reference standard was again based on the 1987 revised American College of Rheumatology (ACR) criteria or clinical diagnosis.

The threshold for test positivity for RF varied between studies and ranged from 3 to 100 U/mL. The variability in threshold used to define test positivity between studies is reflected in the variability in study-specific estimates of sensitivity and specificity in the SROC plot shown in Figure 9.4.b. Because of the variation in threshold across studies, a summary point does not have a useful interpretation. An SROC curve is appropriate to summarize these data and can be estimated by fitting an HSROC model. The

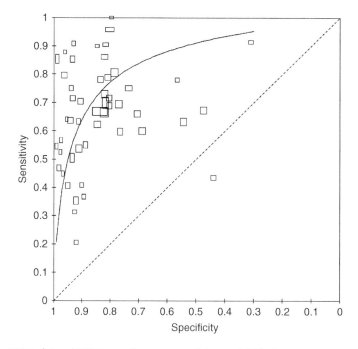

Figure 9.4.b SROC plot and SROC curve for accuracy of rheumatoid factor

Table 9.4.b HSROC parameter estimates for rheumatoid factor model

Label	Parameter	Estimate	Standard error
Mean accuracy	Λ	2.6016	0.1862
Mean threshold	Θ	−0.4370	0.1469
Shape of SROC curve	β	0.2267	0.1624
Variance of random effects for accuracy	σ_α^2	1.3014	0.3046
Variance of random effects for threshold	σ_β^2	0.5423	0.1237

parameter estimates shown in Table 9.4.b are extracted from the output of example programs for these data provided in Chapter 10.

The parameter estimates can be input to RevMan to draw the summary curve as shown in Figure 9.4.b; 2.6016 estimates the mean of the random effects for accuracy (Λ), −0.4370 estimates the mean of the random effects for threshold (Θ), 0.2267 estimates the shape parameter (β), 1.3014 estimates the variance of the random effects for accuracy, and 0.5423 estimates the variance of the random effects for threshold. All of these estimates are on the logit scale. The resulting curve shows the expected trade-off between sensitivity and specificity across thresholds. It is recommended that the fitted curve is displayed across the range of the observed study sensitivities and specificities, as shown here. The average sensitivity at a chosen specificity, or the other way round, can be computed from the fitted curve (see Chapter 10).

When interpreting the results of the analysis, it is important to note that RF constitutes part of the ACR criteria. Hence, there is risk of bias in the estimated curve since the index test is incorporated in the reference standard. This could result in an over-estimation of the diagnostic accuracy of RF, and consequently a distorted picture of the value of using RF as a first test for resolving uncertainty in a suspected case of rheumatoid arthritis.

9.4.5 Data reported at multiple thresholds per study

The key approaches that are described and illustrated in this chapter focus on methods of analysis that use data from one threshold per study. To estimate a summary point, we use data from a common threshold across studies. To estimate an SROC curve, data from a range of thresholds are required to inform the shape of the underlying curve across studies.

Some studies may report sensitivity and specificity at more than one threshold. Using data from all available thresholds has the potential to provide more accurate estimation of SROC curves and estimates of average sensitivity and specificity values at stated thresholds. The potential gain will increase as the number of studies that report multiple thresholds increases.

A range of methods has been proposed for the analysis of such data. An early approach by Dukic (2003) summarizes study-specific ROC curves to obtain an SROC curve within a Bayesian framework. However, single-threshold studies cannot be included and certain assumptions made in fitting the model can lead to sensitivities and specificities that are not monotonic (Hamza 2009). An alternative multivariate random-effects meta-analysis approach was proposed (Hamza 2009) that is applicable when there are specified thresholds of interest and all studies report sensitivity and specificity at these thresholds. This method can, in principle, be applied when studies do not provide data for all thresholds, but model convergence may be problematic in those circumstances. A subsequent approach based on survival analysis methods (Putter 2010) also requires that studies provide sensitivity and specificity at the specified thresholds of interest.

Recent approaches, including the methods of Steinhauser (2016) and Jones (2019), provide a more rigorous and robust approach for dealing with multiple thresholds per study. These methods can accommodate a variable number of thresholds and a range of different thresholds across studies. Studies that provide data for only one threshold can be included, thereby reducing possible bias resulting from the inclusion of an unrepresentative group of studies. Both methods allow for correlation between sensitivity and specificity across thresholds and also heterogeneity between studies through the inclusion of random study effects. An SROC curve is estimated and summary sensitivity and specificity can be computed at specified thresholds.

The Steinhauser method models the distribution of test results as a function of the continuous (or ordinal) thresholds for test positivity within both the diseased and non-diseased groups. Linear mixed-effects modelling is used to estimate the distribution parameters for a known underlying parametric distribution (usually assumed to be normal logistic) of the test results in the two groups. The more recent method of Jones (2019) fits multinomial distributions to tables of categorized test results in each of the diseased and non-diseased groups. The number of categories (equal to the number of thresholds + 1) is allowed to vary across studies. The Jones model assumes an underlying logistic distribution for some transformation (for example, the natural logarithm) of the underlying continuous results in each group. The approach is flexible in that the best-fitting transformation from the set of Box-Cox transformations can be estimated from the data. Covariates can also be included in the model to investigate sources of heterogeneity. The methods by Steinhauser and by Jones are described in more detail in Chapter 10, Section 10.4, and illustrated using an example.

9.4.6   Investigating heterogeneity

In systematic reviews of test accuracy it is usual to observe variability in test accuracy between studies that is considerably greater than would be expected from within-study sampling error alone. This is reflected in the model specifications for the bivariate and HSROC models, which both allow for random study effects. For the bivariate model, the summary estimates of sensitivity and specificity represent an *average* operating point across studies. Similarly, the estimated SROC curve represents an *underlying* ROC curve across studies.

Some of this heterogeneity in test accuracy between studies is likely to arise because of differences in patient characteristics, test methods, study design and other factors. Exploratory analyses can be conducted to investigate whether such study characteristics appear to be associated with test accuracy using symbols and colours in SROC plots to distinguish between studies belonging to different subgroups.

Statistically, it is generally more efficient to make use of all of the data available across studies when investigating heterogeneity by adding study-level covariates to a hierarchical model to identify factors associated with diagnostic test accuracy. This meta-regression approach also allows statistical inferences to be made. It is usually assumed that each covariate has a fixed effect when added to the model. This approach is also applicable to test comparisons, as discussed in Section 9.4.7.

The bivariate and HSROC models differ in how study-level covariates are included. The bivariate method focuses on the estimation of summary estimates of sensitivity and specificity, and estimating how these values vary with study-level covariates. The HSROC approach, by contrast, focuses on the estimation of the SROC curve as the basis for assessing test accuracy, and investigating how the position and shape of the curve may vary with study-level covariates.

Both models allow the use of categorical and continuous covariates. In practice, covariates relating to study characteristics are usually categorical and indicator variables are created as in standard regression modelling. For continuous covariates, particular care should be taken to check that the assumption of linear associations is valid. For the bivariate model, this refers to association with logit(sensitivity) and/or logit(specificity). For the HSROC model, this refers to association with the accuracy parameter (lnDOR) and/or the threshold parameter.

The uses and limitations of investigating heterogeneity using subgroup analysis and meta-regression in Chapter 10, Section 10.11.5 of the *Cochrane Handbook for Systematic Reviews of Interventions* (Deeks 2019) apply equally to diagnostic studies.

9.4.6.1 Criteria for model selection

Irrespective of which model is used, review authors should specify what modelling strategy will be used for adding or removing covariates and what criterion will be used to decide whether or not a covariate should be included in a model.

The decision as to whether a covariate should be retained in the model may be based in part on statistical tests. Commonly used software for fitting these models will provide P values for each estimate in the model based on Wald statistics. A P value based on the likelihood ratio Chi² statistic is generally more reliable than the Wald statistic, especially for small sample sizes (Agresti 2007). The likelihood ratio Chi² statistic is computed as the change in the −2Log likelihood when a covariate is added (or removed) from a model, with the degrees of freedom equal to the difference in the number of parameters fitted in these models. The effect of adding (or removing) covariates on measures of model fit such as Akaike's information criterion (AIC) or the Bayesian information criterion (BIC) can also be used. The deviance information criterion (DIC) is commonly used for models fitted by Markov chain Monte Carlo (MCMC) simulation. (See Chapter 10 for further details.)

Statistical tests can also be used to assess whether allowing for variance of the random effects to vary by test in a comparison of two or more index tests provides a better-fitting model (see Chapter 10).

9.4.6.2 Heterogeneity and regression analysis using the bivariate model

The bivariate model allows covariates to affect summary sensitivity or summary specificity, or both. Using the notation of Harbord (2007), and assuming that we have a single study-level covariate Z that may affect both sensitivity and specificity, then the model can be extended as follows:

$$\begin{pmatrix} \mu_{Ai} \\ \mu_{Bi} \end{pmatrix} \sim N\left(\begin{pmatrix} \mu_A + V_A Z_i \\ \mu_B + V_B Z_i \end{pmatrix}, \Sigma \right)$$

As before, Σ represents the covariance matrix for the random effects for logit(sensitivity) and logit(specificity). If the covariate does explain some of the heterogeneity in sensitivity and/or specificity, then we would expect the estimated variance for one or both random effects to be reduced. The estimated covariance (correlation) parameter may also change.

Assuming that we have a binary study-level covariate (Z) coded as 0 or 1 to represent the two groups of studies, then μ_A estimates the logit(sensitivity) at the summary point for the referent group (Z = 0), and $\mu_A + v_A$ estimates the logit(sensitivity) at the summary point for the other group (Z = 1). Hence, $exp(v_A)$ estimates the odds ratio for sensitivity in group 1 relative to the referent group. The average sensitivity is estimated as $exp(\mu_A)/(1 + exp(\mu_A))$ for the referent group of studies, and as $exp(\mu_A + v_A)/(1 + exp(\mu_A + v_A))$ for the other group. Comparisons of specificity between the two groups of studies follow the same approach as described earlier based on μ_B and v_B. The fit of the model, with and without the additional parameters v_A and v_B, can be used to assess whether the covariate is associated with sensitivity and/or specificity. This joint test will have 2 degrees of freedom if Z is binary. Separate tests of statistical significance of the covariate with sensitivity and specificity can also be conducted, first to assess whether v_A differs from 0 (a statistically significant result indicates that there is evidence that sensitivity differs between the two groups of studies) and secondly whether v_B differs from 0 (a statistically significant result indicates that there is evidence that specificity differs between the two groups of studies). See also Section 9.4.6.1 relating to criteria for model selection.

The standard error of a new estimate that is a function of the model parameter estimates can be obtained using the delta method, on the assumption that the error distribution of the new estimate is approximately normal (Oehlert 1992). The delta method is implemented in standard statistical software packages such as SAS and Stata (see Chapter 10).

The bivariate model is easily extended to allow for more than one covariate. However, this may not be feasible in practice unless the number of studies is large. Typically only one source of heterogeneity can be investigated at a time. Also, it is important to note that a covariate may only be associated with sensitivity and not specificity, or the other way round. It is not required that the same covariates are fitted for both sensitivity and specificity, although this may commonly be the case. Where a covariate (or covariates) is allowed to affect both the sensitivity and the specificity, the bivariate model is equivalent to an HSROC model in which the covariate (or covariates) is allowed to affect both the accuracy and the positivity threshold but not the shape parameter. However, using the estimates from the bivariate model to test for the effect of covariates on the shape and position of the SROC curve is not straightforward. Using the HSROC model parametrization allows this to be done in a more direct and straightforward manner.

It is usually assumed that the variance of the random effects (and their correlation in the case of the bivariate model) is not associated with the covariate. This is probably a reasonable assumption in most analyses investigating heterogeneity in test accuracy for a single index test. However, for analyses that compare different index tests, this assumption is less likely to hold (see Section 9.4.7).

9.4.6.3   Example 1 continued: Investigation of heterogeneity in diagnostic performance of anti-CCP

The studies included in the review to assess the diagnostic performance of anti-CCP used two different generations of the assay: first generation (CCP1, 8 studies) and second generation (CCP2, 29 studies). A binary covariate for test version (i.e. CCP1 or CCP2) with separate coefficients for sensitivity and specificity was added to the model. The covariate was coded as 0 for CCP1 (the referent group) and 1 for CCP2. Allowing both sensitivity and specificity to vary by test version in the model resulted in a –2Log likelihood of 533.4, a reduction of 12.2 compared with the model that contained no covariates. Hence, there is statistical evidence (Chi^2 = 12.2, 2 df, P = 0.002) that test accuracy is associated with the version of test used, but further investigation is required to ascertain whether this association is for sensitivity, specificity or both. The P values in Table 9.4.c are based on Wald statistics for each parameter estimate, adjusted for the other variables in the model. Based on these, there is strong evidence that sensitivity is associated with test version (P = 0.0005), but not specificity (P = 0.21).

The variances of the random effects for logit(sensitivity) and logit(specificity), and their covariance (σ_A^2, σ_B^2 and σ_{AB}, respectively), are assumed to be common for both generations of CCP. For the referent group (CCP1 in this case) the summary estimates for logit(sensitivity), logit(specificity) and the corresponding standard errors are denoted by μ_A and μ_B, respectively). The covariate parameter estimates (ν_A and ν_B) give the change in logit(sensitivity) and logit(specificity) for CCP2 relative to CCP1 – thus the logit(sensitivity) and logit(specificity) estimates for CCP2 are obtained by adding the covariate parameter estimates to those of the referent test ($\mu_A + \nu_A$ and $\mu_B + \nu_B$, respectively). The standard errors for the logit(sensitivity) and logit(specificity) for CCP2 are most easily computed by refitting the model and defining CCP2 to be the referent group (covariate coded as 0 for CCP2 and coded as 1 for CCP1). The model parameter estimates can be input to RevMan to display the summary points and corresponding confidence regions shown in Figure 9.4.c.

The summary point estimates and corresponding 95% confidence regions shown in the figure are consistent with the conclusion that the sensitivity varies by test type, but not specificity. Based on the model parameter estimates in Table 9.4.c, the summary estimates of specificity were 0.97 (95% CI 0.95 to 0.98) for CCP1 and 0.95 (95% CI 0.94 to 0.97) for CCP2. The summary estimates of sensitivity were 0.48 (95% CI 0.37 to 0.58) for CCP1 and 0.70 (95% CI 0.65 to 0.75) for CCP2. These results indicate an improvement in

Table 9.4.c Bivariate parameter estimates for comparison of the accuracy of CCP1 and CCP2 for the diagnosis of rheumatoid arthritis

Parameter	Estimate	Standard error	P value
μ_A	−0.09653	0.2203	0.66[*]
μ_B	3.4467	0.2982	< 0.0001[*]
σ_A^2	0.3598	0.1022	0.001
σ_B^2	0.5399	0.1802	0.005
σ_{AB}	−0.1969	0.09836	0.05
ν_A	0.9626	0.2513	0.0005
ν_B	−0.4302	0.3377	0.21

[*] These Wald statistics are ignored as they test whether μ_A = 0 and μ_B = 0, equivalent to testing hypotheses that sensitivity = 50% and specificity = 50%, respectively.

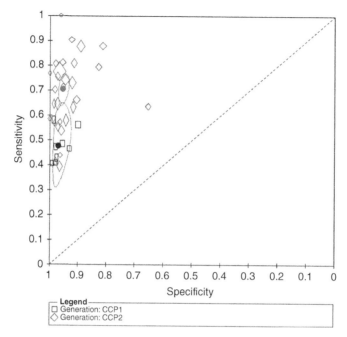

Figure 9.4.c Summary estimates of sensitivity and specificity for CCP1 and CCP2 with corresponding 95% confidence regions

sensitivity (P < 0.001), without loss of specificity (P = 0.21) for CCP2 compared with CCP1. (The model could be simplified by removing the covariate for specificity. The resulting estimate for specificity would then be assumed to be the same for CCP1 and CCP2.) For final presentation of the results we would wish to estimate the difference in sensitivity and specificity together with 95% confidence intervals. This is covered in Chapter 10.

Comparing the output from this model with that of the model with no covariates (see Section 9.4.2), it is clear that the variances of the random effects are smaller, particularly for sensitivity. Also, checks of the distributions of the random effects (not shown here) show that adjusting for the use of first- or second-generation anti-CCP tests results in distributions that more closely follow a normal distribution.

In these analyses, the variances of the random effects were assumed to be the same for logit(sensitivity) and logit(specificity) for both generations of the test. This assumption can be investigated by fitting additional models, as shown in Chapter 10. For the example here, allowing the variances to differ did not make a substantive change to the estimates or their interpretation. Chapter 10 also demonstrates how to compute the difference in sensitivity and also the difference in specificity, with corresponding confidence intervals, using the bivariate model from the example in Section 9.4.7.3 for illustration.

For analyses based on a small number of studies (unlike the example shown here), confidence intervals around the estimated difference in sensitivity and/or specificity may be large. Hence, it is important not to rely purely on tests of statistical significance to conclude that there is a lack of evidence of a difference, as the confidence interval for the estimated difference may cover a clinically important effect. In that situation, the results would be regarded as inconclusive.

9.4.6.4 Heterogeneity and regression analysis using the Rutter and Gatsonis HSROC model

The HSROC model allows covariates to be added to explore heterogeneity in test positivity (threshold), position of the curve (accuracy) and shape of the curve. A covariate may be associated with some but not all three model parameters.

Assuming that we have a binary study-level covariate (Z) coded as 0 or 1 to represent the two groups of studies, then the HSROC model can be extended to estimate the log odds of a positive test for study i and disease group j as follows

$$\text{logit}\left(\pi_{ij}\right)=\left(\left(\theta_i+\gamma Z_i\right)+\left(\alpha_i+\xi Z_i\right)dis_{ij}\right)\exp\left(-\left(\beta+\delta Z_i\right)dis_{ij}\right)$$

where each of γ, ξ and δ is assumed to be a fixed effect. Hence, the distributions of the random effects for threshold and accuracy are now given by $\theta_i \sim N(\Theta+\gamma Z_i,\sigma_\theta^2)$ and $\alpha_i \sim N(\Lambda+\xi Z_i,\sigma_\alpha^2)$, respectively. The shape parameter for the summary curves for the two groups is estimated as β for the referent group of studies (Z = 0) and $\beta + \delta$ for the other group (Z = 1). If the covariate does explain some of the heterogeneity in threshold and/or accuracy, then we would expect that the estimated variance for one or both random effects would be reduced.

The first step would be to investigate the shape of the summary curve. If $\delta \neq 0$, then the shape of the summary curve differs for the two groups of studies, which means that the relative accuracy of the test for the two groups of studies will vary with threshold (Figure 9.4.d (a)). This represents the most complex scenario, and the model would not generally be simplified any further. The power to detect differences in shape will be low

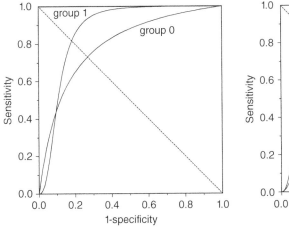

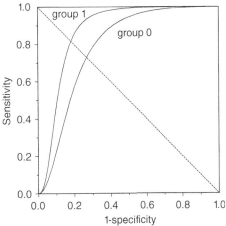

(a) Relative accuracy depends on particular specificity values, the curves crossing ($\delta \neq 0$)

(b) Group 1 dominates across all specificity values, the curves do not cross ($\delta = 0$)

Figure 9.4.d SROC curves with and without a difference in shape

when the number of studies in either group is limited. Also, it is important when investigating shape to consider the effect of outlying and potentially influential studies (see Section 9.4.9). When there is statistical evidence that the curves differ in shape, a plot of the estimated curves for the two groups will aid in interpretation. Focusing on the region of the plot that covers the observed data, it is then possible to compare the estimated curves. Where one curve consistently lies above another in the region of primary interest, there is evidence of superior accuracy even though the separation between the curves will vary across thresholds. If the curves cross, then the interpretation of which curve shows superior accuracy will depend on threshold.

If, based on statistical evidence, similarity of curve shapes and investigation of potentially influential studies, it can be assumed that $\delta = 0$, then the covariate can be removed for shape. The estimated SROC curves for the two groups will then have the same shape, even though they may not be symmetrical (Figure 9.4.d (b)), and the relative diagnostic accuracy of the two curves can be summarized using the relative diagnostic odds ratio (RDOR = exp (ξ)). The RDOR will be constant across all possible values of θ. If the model can be simplified further and both curves can be assumed to be symmetrical, i.e. $\beta = 0$, the RDOR again provides a measure of relative accuracy as already described, but in addition the DOR in each group will be constant across thresholds.

If the curves can be assumed to have the same shape (either both asymmetrical or both symmetrical), then the question is whether the covariate is associated with accuracy, i.e. the position of the curve. If there is evidence that $\xi \neq 0$, then the RDOR gives an estimate of the overall relative diagnostic accuracy. This would correspond to a clear separation between the SROC curves for the two groups. Alternatively, $\xi = 0$ implies that there is no separation between the curves and no association between the covariate and accuracy.

If ξ can be assumed to be 0, then the model can be further simplified by removing the covariate for accuracy, which will result in a single summary curve (assuming that the shape of the curve is the same for the two groups of studies). An association between the covariate and the threshold parameter (i.e. $\gamma \neq 0$) would indicate that the underlying test positivity rate for the two groups of studies differs. Such an association is often difficult to interpret unless the curves can be assumed to have the same shape and accuracy.

The RDOR is useful for the statistical comparison of two curves that have the same shape because the RDOR is constant across all values of the threshold parameter θ. However, it does not have a straightforward interpretation when the shapes of the curves differ. In that case, the estimated RDOR will represent the relative accuracy of the points on the curves where they intersect the diagonal line in ROC given by sensitivity = specificity. One approach that can be used to aid interpretation is to compute the estimated sensitivities at a chosen value of specificity (or the other way round) to compare the curves at selected points that are of clinical importance, as illustrated in Chapter 10.

9.4.6.5 Example 2 continued: Investigating heterogeneity in diagnostic accuracy of rheumatoid factor (RF)

We will now investigate whether the laboratory technique used to measure RF is associated with diagnostic performance. Of the 50 studies, 15 used nephelometry (N), 16 latex agglutination (LA), 16 ELISA, one study used RA hemagglutination and 2 did not report the method used. The analysis is restricted to studies that used N, LA or ELISA. The HSROC model was again used because of the variation in threshold used for test positivity across studies. In keeping with standard methods used in regression analysis, two covariates are defined to distinguish between the three techniques (indicator variables for N and ELISA to compare these groups of studies with LA, the referent group). These covariates were included in the model to assess whether accuracy, threshold or the shape of the SROC curve varied with technique. The variances of the random effects for threshold and accuracy are assumed to be common to all three techniques. (See Chapter 10 for example programs and output.)

The -2Log likelihood for the most complex model that included covariates for shape, accuracy and threshold parameters was 752.9. The increase in the -2Log likelihood was negligible (an increase to 753.1) when the covariates for shape were removed from the model (Chi^2 = 753.1 − 752.9 = 0.2, 2 df, P = 0.90). Parameter estimates for the model that assumes a common shape are given in Table 9.4.d, and the corresponding estimated HSROC curves shown in Figure 9.4.e. The estimates of alpha (Λ), theta (Θ) and beta (β) can be input to RevMan to obtain the summary curve for the referent group (LA).The threshold and accuracy parameter estimates for ELISA are given by $\Theta + \gamma_{ELISA}$ and $\Lambda + \xi_{ELISA}$, respectively, and for N are given by $\Theta + \gamma_N$ and $\Lambda + \xi_N$, respectively, on the logit scale. The standard errors of these estimates for ELISA and N are most easily obtained by refitting the model twice, first defining ELISA as the referent group and then defining N as the referent group.

From Figure 9.4.e, it appears that LA may be less accurate than the other two methods; however, removal of the covariate for accuracy (i.e. coefficients ξ_{ELISA} and ξ_N assumed to be 0) has a negligible effect on the fit of the model (Chi^2 = 753.7 − 753.1 = 0.6, 2 df, P = 0.74), indicating no statistical evidence of a difference in diagnostic accuracy of RF according to technique. This is consistent with the P values based on Wald statistics in Table 9.4.d. Hence, it is reasonable to fit a single SROC for RF, as there is no statistical evidence of a difference in test accuracy for the three techniques (see Chapter 10 for model estimates for the single common summary curve). These results indicate that it

Table 9.4.d HSROC parameter estimates to compare RF techniques

Parameter	Estimate	Standard error	P value
Λ	2.4552	0.3245	< 0.0001
Θ	−0.5490	0.2137	0.014[*]
β	0.1995	0.1702	0.25
σ_α^2	1.2865	0.3109	0.0002
σ_q^2	0.4786	0.1139	0.0001
ξ_{ELISA}	0.2483	0.4408	0.58
ξ_N	0.3328	0.4439	0.46
γ_{ELISA}	−0.1962	0.2614	0.46
γ_N	0.4960	0.2627	0.065

[*] This P value is ignored as it tests the uninformative hypothesis that the mean of the pseudo threshold parameter is zero.

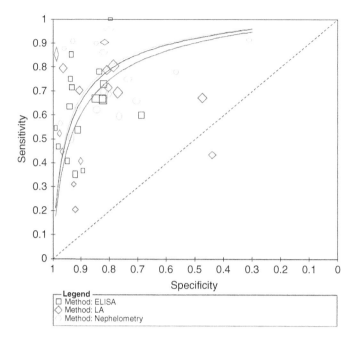

Figure 9.4.e SROC curves to compare accuracy of RF techniques

may be reasonable to treat the techniques as equivalent markers for RF (they have similar DOR, but the trade-off between sensitivity and specificity may still differ).

9.4.7   Comparing index tests

Many diagnostic reviews aim to compare the diagnostic accuracy of two alternative index tests that may be used to detect the same condition. In this section, the focus will be on the comparison of two index tests, but the approach can be extended to allow for more than two tests.

Two approaches are generally adopted for test comparisons. The first approach uses test accuracy data from all eligible studies that have evaluated one or both tests. The second approach restricts the analysis to studies that have either evaluated both tests in the same individuals, or have randomized individuals to undergo one or other of the two tests. The second approach has advantages because the comparison is less likely to be biased by confounding and hence these results should be relied upon where possible (Takwoingi 2013). However, the number of studies that report such direct comparisons is often very limited, which means that such an analysis may not be feasible or may only be considered as a sensitivity analysis (see Section 9.4.9).

9.4.7.1   Test comparisons based on all available studies
Often, many of the available studies evaluate only one of the tests of interest (Takwoingi 2013). By using all studies that have evaluated at least one of the tests, we maximize the number of studies in the analysis. However, the studies are likely to be heterogeneous

in terms of design and patient characteristics that are associated with test accuracy, and hence confounding may be an issue. In preliminary exploratory analyses this can be dealt with by comparing the tests within subgroups of studies that are homogeneous with respect to important potential confounders such as study design or spectrum of disease. The value and feasibility of such exploratory analyses will be affected by the number of available studies and missing or inconsistent reporting across studies of information on potential confounders.

The statistical methods described in this section follow directly from the description of hierarchical models in Section 9.4.6 and how they can be used to investigate heterogeneity in test accuracy. For the comparison of two index tests, the type of test is represented by a binary covariate, which is used to identify the test that gave rise to each 2×2 table included in the analysis. Confounders can potentially be adjusted for; however, this may be difficult to do in practice because the number of studies is often small and/or data on important confounders may be poorly recorded or incomplete.

Both the bivariate model and the Rutter and Gatsonis HSROC model can be used to investigate the relative accuracy of two index tests. However, as noted previously, the choice of approach will be influenced by the nature of the available data. The interpretation of the results will depend on which approach is used.

9.4.7.2 Test comparisons using the bivariate model

If, for each index test, the available studies have used a consistent threshold on a continuous or ordinal scale to define test positivity, then the bivariate model provides an appropriate framework for test comparisons. It may also be reasonable to assume a consistent threshold when a test comprises a 'test kit' that produces positive and negative results (such as a coloured line appearing on a device). By adopting the same strategy described earlier (Section 9.4.6.2), a binary covariate for test type can be included in the model to investigate whether sensitivity and/or specificity differs between two tests.

Care must be taken with the interpretation of the results of such a model, particularly if the common threshold for test positivity for either test is applied to a continuous or ordinal scale. Any inferences made about the relative diagnostic accuracy of the two tests is only valid at the chosen threshold for each of the two tests and cannot be extrapolated to other possible thresholds. Where other thresholds are reported, the analysis can be repeated using the available data to investigate the relative diagnostic accuracy of the tests at those alternative thresholds. However, such additional investigations should be restricted to thresholds reported by sufficient studies to allow a meaningful analysis.

Because we are analysing test accuracy data for two alternative index tests, it may not be reasonable to assume that the variances of the random effects for logit(sensitivity) and logit(specificity) are the same for the two tests. The bivariate model can be extended to allow the variance of the random effects for each test to depend on the covariate for test type (see Chapter 10). This will also affect the estimated correlation between them. Statistically, estimation of the variances of the random effects for logit(sensitivity) and logit(specificity) and correlation between them is subject to a higher level of uncertainty than for the main parameters of interest. However, when preliminary plots of the study-level estimates of sensitivity and specificity in ROC space show marked differences in heterogeneity between studies for the two tests, it is advisable to assess whether the assumption of equal variances of random effects for the two tests is reasonable. This can be done by comparing estimates for test accuracy between the alternative models to assess whether conclusions about the relative sensitivity and/or specificity of the tests are robust to assumptions about the variances of the random effects. Such an investigation may not be feasible if the number of studies is small.

It is usual for most of the studies in such an indirect analysis of test comparisons to have evaluated only one of the tests, but some studies may have evaluated both. If the proportion of studies that have evaluated both is very small, then treating the results of the two tests in a study as if they were obtained from different studies is unlikely to affect the results. Although this is often done in practice, such an approach is not recommended if the proportion of studies evaluating both tests is not small, because it is likely to result in inappropriate standard errors for the test comparison parameters for sensitivity and specificity. In that case the paired sensitivity/specificity data for both tests from each study should be at the lower level of the hierarchical analysis, and a binary covariate for test type included to identify which 2×2 table corresponds to each test.

9.4.7.3   Example 3: CT versus MRI for the diagnosis of coronary artery disease

Schuetz (2010) evaluated the diagnostic performance of multi-slice computed tomography (CT) and magnetic resonance imaging (MRI) for the diagnosis of coronary artery disease (CAD). The review included prospective studies that evaluated either CT or MRI (or both), used conventional coronary angiography (CAG) as the reference standard, and used the same index test threshold for clinically significant coronary artery stenosis (a diameter reduction of 50% or greater). A total of 103 studies provided a 2×2 table for one or both tests and were included in the meta-analysis: 84 studies evaluated only CT, 14 evaluated only MRI and 5 studies evaluated both CT and MRI. (See Chapter 10 for data and example programs.)

Because study selection was based on a common threshold for clinically significant coronary artery stenosis, the bivariate model was used for data synthesis and test comparison. In the first stage of the analysis, we base our test comparison on all studies that evaluated at least one test. The approach follows closely the method illustrated in Section 9.4.6.3 for exploring heterogeneity using the bivariate model and the same notation has been used.

A binary covariate is added to the model, which is coded as 0 if the 2×2 table is for MRI (the referent group) and coded as 1 if the 2×2 table is for CT. The 5 studies that evaluated both tests contribute a 2×2 table for each test, hence there are 19 studies included for MRI and 89 studies included for CT. Allowing both sensitivity and specificity to vary by type of test resulted in a –2Log likelihood of 953.0, a reduction of 42.5 compared with the model that contained no covariates. Hence, there is statistical evidence ($\text{Chi}^2 = 42.5$, 2 df, $P < 0.001$) that sensitivity and/or specificity are associated with test type. Removing the covariate for sensitivity from the model ($\text{Chi}^2 = 976.7 - 953.0 = 23.7$, 1 df, $P < 0.001$) shows strong statistical evidence of a difference in sensitivity between the two tests. Similarly, removing the covariate for specificity from the model ($\text{Chi}^2 = 976.2 - 953.0 = 23.2$, 1 df, $P < 0.001$) shows strong statistical evidence of a difference in specificity between the two tests. These results are consistent with the P values shown in Table 9.4.e that are based on Wald statistics.

Table 9.4.e gives the estimated mean logit(sensitivity) and mean logit(specificity) (μ_A and μ_B, respectively) for the referent category (MRI), the common variances of the

Table 9.4.e Bivariate model estimates for comparison of CT and MRI

Parameter	Estimate	Standard error	P value
μ_A	2.1771	0.2457	< 0.0001*
μ_B	0.8754	0.2111	< 0.0001*
σ_A^2	0.8749	0.2293	0.0002
σ_B^2	0.8447	0.1696	< 0.0001
σ_{AB}	0.1803	0.1384	0.20
ν_A	1.3033	0.2625	< 0.0001
ν_B	1.0415	0.2154	< 0.0001

* These Wald statistics are ignored as they test whether $\mu_A = 0$ and $\mu_B = 0$, equivalent to testing hypotheses that sensitivity = 50% and specificity = 50%, respectively.

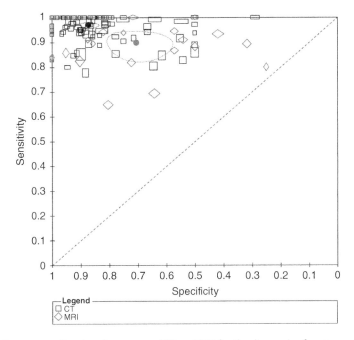

Figure 9.4.f Summary estimates of accuracy of CT and MRI for the diagnosis of coronary artery disease with corresponding 95% confidence regions

random effects (σ_A^2 and σ_B^2, respectively), their covariance (σ_{AB}) and the difference in mean logit(sensitivity) and mean logit(specificity) between CT and MRI (ν_A and ν_B, respectively). Estimates of the standard errors of mean logit(sensitivity) and mean logit(specificity) for CT are required for entry into RevMan and can be obtained easily from refitting the model with CT defined as the referent group.

Figure 9.4.f shows the SROC plot with summary points for MRI and CT and their 95% confidence regions superimposed as shown. The squares represent CT and the diamonds represent MRI. Because of the large number of studies for CT, the summary point and region are difficult to see. The figure could be redrawn without the individual study points to show just the summary points and regions, or the size of the study points can be reduced to improve visibility.

Inverse logit transformation of the model estimates and their confidence limits provide the relevant estimates in ROC space: summary estimates for sensitivity are 0.90 (95% CI 0.84 to 0.93) for MRI and 0.97 (95% CI 0.96 to 0.98) for CT. The summary estimates for specificity are 0.71 (95% CI 0.61 to 0.78) for MRI and 0.87 (95% CI 0.84 to 0.90) for CT. The P values for v_A and v_B show strong statistical evidence of an association between sensitivity and test type and also between specificity and test type.

Based on this analysis, there is strong evidence that CT has higher sensitivity and specificity than MRI for detecting clinically significant coronary artery stenosis, defined as a diameter reduction of 50% or more. Chapter 10 demonstrates how to compute the difference in sensitivity and difference in specificity, with corresponding confidence intervals, for the two tests.

Further descriptive analyses and modelling may be undertaken to assess whether the assumption of equal variances for the random effects for the two tests has a substantive effect on the results presented here (see Chapter 10).

9.4.7.4 Test comparisons using the Rutter and Gatsonis HSROC model

Comparisons of summary estimates of sensitivity (or specificity) of alternative tests can be misleading if the included studies have used different thresholds to define test positivity. In this situation, comparisons based on SROC curves provide a more informative approach.

The hierarchical modelling strategy used to investigate heterogeneity described earlier for the Rutter and Gatsonis HSROC model (Section 9.4.6.4) can be used for comparisons of test accuracy when there is variability in threshold between studies. The type of test is represented by a binary covariate that is used to identify the test that gave rise to each 2×2 table included in the analysis. This covariate then allows the review author to investigate whether test type is associated with the shape and position of the SROC curve. Interpretation of the results follows directly from the discussion of the interpretation of investigations of heterogeneity in Section 9.4.6.

Statistically, estimation of the variances of the random effects for threshold and accuracy is subject to a higher level of uncertainty than for the main model parameters of interest. If preliminary plots of the study-level estimates of sensitivity and specificity in ROC space show marked differences in heterogeneity between studies for the two tests, it is advisable to assess whether the assumption of equal variances of the random effects for the two tests is reasonable (see Chapter 10). This is usually done by comparing the fit of the alternative models (i.e. where variances do, or do not, depend on the covariate for test type). A comparison of the main estimates of interest between the alternative models is also useful to assess whether conclusions about the relative shape and accuracy of the summary curves for the two tests are robust to assumptions about the variances of the random effects. Again, such an investigation will not be feasible if the number of studies is small.

As noted for the bivariate model, it is usual for most of the included studies to have evaluated only one of the tests, but some studies will have evaluated both. If the proportion of studies that have evaluated both is very small, then treating the results of the two tests in a study as if they were obtained from different studies is unlikely to affect the results. However, more accurate standard errors will be obtained for the test comparison parameters if the data for both tests are modelled within the study at the lower level in the analysis.

9.4.7.5 Test comparison based on studies that directly compare tests
As noted in Section 9.1.3 and Section 9.3.2, heterogeneity in the estimated accuracy of a diagnostic test across studies is likely to occur. This could confound the comparison of two tests if different studies are used to estimate the diagnostic accuracy of each test. Ideally, the comparison should be based on studies that have made a direct comparison of the tests of interest, either by applying both tests to each study participant, or by randomizing each individual to receive one of the tests (Takwoingi 2013). A common reference standard should be applied to both tests. If there are sufficient studies of this type on which to base a test comparison, the results are less prone to bias than an analysis based on all available studies that have evaluated one or both tests.

A preliminary graphical analysis can be conducted by plotting the estimated sensitivity and specificity for both tests for each study in ROC space. The two points contributed by each study (one for each test) are joined by a line to highlight the relative test accuracy within each study to illustrate the pairing of test accuracy estimates at the study level (see Figure 9.4.g).

The rationale described earlier for choosing between the bivariate model and the HSROC model when making test comparisons is also applicable here, and the same

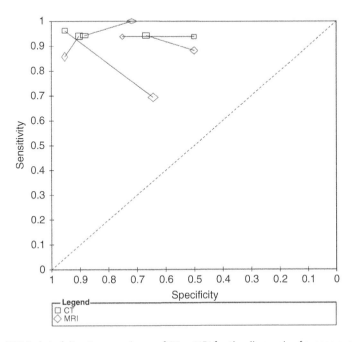

Figure 9.4.g SROC plot of direct comparisons of CT vs MRI for the diagnosis of coronary artery disease

issues relating to interpretation apply. The only major difference is that the analysis does not include any studies that have evaluated only one of the tests.

Because each study contributes a 2×2 table for each of the two tests to be compared, the data for the two tests should be analysed within the study at the lower level in the analysis. The random effect for that study is assumed to be common to both 2×2 tables for that study. A binary covariate for test type is included to identify which 2×2 table corresponds to each test. Entering a separate 2×2 table for each test (within each study) for analysis in a hierarchical model effectively assumes that the data arise from a randomized or independent groups design. This represents a conservative approach that is often necessitated by the lack of information on paired results at the individual level for truly 'paired' studies that have applied both tests to the same individual. At present, it is not common practice for researchers to publish a cross-classification of test results within both the diseased and non-diseased groups, or to provide individual patient data for analysis that would provide full information on the pairing of test results within an individual.

Meta-analytical models that account for pairing of test results within an individual within each study have been developed as an extension of the bivariate model. The method proposed by Trikalinos (2014) allows for comparisons of two tests based on studies that use a paired design and report fully cross-classified data. For studies that only report sensitivity and specificity for each test, counts for the cross-classification are imputed based on the associations observed in studies that report the full cross-classification. The approach of Dimou (2016) also allows for the inclusion of studies that report results for only one of the tests in the comparison. These methods require further evaluation before they are recommended for routine use. However, as suggested by Trikalinos (2014), they may be useful as a sensitivity analysis.

Network meta-analysis models have also been developed that use data from both direct and indirect comparisons of multiple tests, e.g. Ma (2018), Nyaga (2018), Lian (2019) and Owen (2018). Rücker (2018) provides a very useful overview of this topic. Veroniki (2022) also provides an overview and an empirical evaluation. However, further evaluation of these methods for dealing with complex correlational structures is required before they can be considered in Cochrane Reviews.

9.4.7.6 Example 3 continued: CT versus MRI for the diagnosis of coronary artery disease

The meta-analysis by Schuetz included five studies that made a direct comparison of CT and MRI. Basing the analysis on these five studies (10 2×2 tables) has the advantage that the results should be less prone to bias. However, the number of studies in the analysis is dramatically reduced, which reduces the precision of the summary estimates. As we will see in this example, simplifying assumptions may also be required to fit complex hierarchical models to these data. We will again apply the bivariate model for these data.

The SROC plot (Figure 9.4.g) shows the data for the five paired studies, with squares used to denote CT and diamonds used to denote MRI. A line is used to join the results for CT and MRI within each study. Examining this plot, we can see that sensitivity for CT is lower than for MRI in one study, equivalent in one study and higher in the other three studies. Specificity is higher for CT than for MRI in three studies and lower in the other two.

Fitting a model to these data is difficult, particularly for the bivariate model where convergence is more problematic than for the Rutter and Gatsonis model (see Section 9.4.8). Strategies need to be used to include only required terms in the model.

Based on the descriptive graphical display, a preliminary series of models were fitted to assess whether random effects should be included for both sensitivity and specificity (this model did not include the covariate for test type). The model that included random effects only for specificity gave a –2Log likelihood of 106.4, a better fit than the model that assumed a fixed effect for both sensitivity and specificity (–2Log likelihood 114.8). The model that assumed random effects only for sensitivity provided no improvement to the fit compared with the fixed-effect model. Hence, the covariate for test type was added to the model with random effects for specificity only and the parameter estimates for that model are given in Table 9.4.f.

The layout and interpretation of the output follow that for the indirect test comparison example discussed in Section 9.4.7.3. Note that the estimated common variance for logit(sensitivity) and the covariance are defined to be zero due to the simplification in the model, whereas there is an estimate of the variance of the random effects for logit(specificity). These estimates were input to RevMan to superimpose summary estimates and their 95% confidence regions on the SROC plot.

Inverse logit transformation of the estimates and their lower and upper 95% confidence limits gives estimated sensitivities of 0.86 (95% CI 0.76 to 0.92) for MRI and 0.94 (95% CI 0.87 to 0.98) for CT; and estimated specificities of 0.71 (95% CI 0.47 to 0.87) for MRI and 0.86 (95% CI 0.68 to 0.95) for CT. These estimates are consistent with the previous analysis, which showed that CT had higher sensitivity and specificity than MRI (Section 9.4.7.3).

The confidence regions shown on Figure 9.4.h are wider than would be indicated by the confidence regions shown in Figure 9.4.f because the number of studies is small.

Statistical evidence based on P values from changes in the –2Log likelihood show evidence of differences in sensitivity (P = 0.012) and specificity (P = 0.0011) between CT and MRI. (Note that the Wald tests in the output yield different P values (P = 0.07 and P = 0.04), which is expected given the small number of studies in this analysis and the

Table 9.4.f Bivariate model estimates for simplified model to compare CT and MRI

Parameter	Estimate	Standard error	P value
μ_A	1.8083	0.2412	0.0017[†]
μ_B	0.8910	0.3606	0.069[†]
σ_A^2	0[*]	–	–
σ_B^2	0.4239	0.3744	0.32
σ_{AB}	0[*]	–	–
ν_A	1.0051	0.4195	0.075
ν_B	0.9378	0.2955	0.034

[*] Variance for sensitivity and covariance term are assumed to be 0.
[†] These Wald statistics are ignored as they test whether $\mu_A = 0$ and $\mu_B = 0$, equivalent to testing hypotheses that sensitivity = 50% and specificity = 50%, respectively.

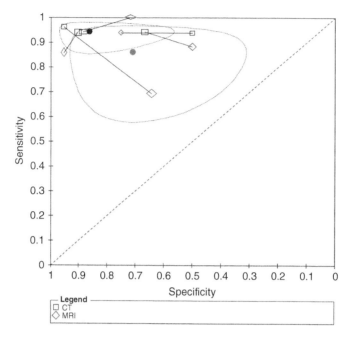

Figure 9.4.h Summary estimates of sensitivity and specificity for CT vs MRI for the diagnosis of coronary artery disease with corresponding 95% confidence regions

resulting difficulty in checking model assumptions.) The key message here is that the results of this analysis are consistent with the conclusions of the indirect comparison in Section 9.4.7.3, which was based on all available studies that evaluated at least one of the index tests.

9.4.8 Approaches to analysis with small numbers of studies

When the number of studies is small, it may be difficult to decide which terms should be included in a model and which is the 'best' model. For instance, when fitting an SROC curve, the uncertainty associated with the estimation of the shape parameter could be very high, and the estimate may also be strongly influenced by the inclusion/exclusion of individual studies. For both the bivariate and HSROC models, estimates of the variances of the random effects will be subject to a high level of uncertainty.

It is important to keep in mind that estimation of a single summary point using the bivariate model, or estimation of a single summary curve using the HSROC model, requires five parameters to be estimated in the full model specification. There is little information on which to base these estimates when the number of studies is small. In some situations the analyses based on frequentist methods may fail to converge. Model simplification may be appropriate in some circumstances to reduce the number of parameters to be estimated (Takwoingi 2017). Analysts should take into account such simplifying assumptions when interpreting the results and judgement should be exercised regarding whether a model is sufficiently reliable to report.

Failure of an analysis to converge may be symptomatic of several problems.

- In some cases, it may be due to poor choices of starting values for the parameter estimates. If so, it may help to fit the model first assuming a fixed effect for the model parameters, and then use these as the starting values for the random-effects model.
- For small data sets, convergence may also be affected by the inclusion/removal of individual studies. The effect of such influential studies should be investigated.
- Convergence problems can also arise when the observed heterogeneity is very small. This is a particular issue for the bivariate model parametrization, where an examination of the scatter plot may help to identify high heterogeneity in sensitivity but homogeneity in specificity, or the other way round. Restricting the model to have random effects for one parameter and a fixed effect for the other may then be warranted. This problem can also occur when the number of studies is relatively large.
- The standard error for the shape parameter in the HSROC model may be large. In this case, it is advisable to check how much the shape is influenced by the removal of individual studies. When the shape is uncertain and also very dependent on individual studies, then some analysts may choose to assume symmetry for the summary curve to acknowledge that the shape cannot be estimated reliably. Again, this needs to be reported and discussed in the report of the analyses.

Approaches to dealing with sparse data are discussed further and illustrated in Chapter 10, Section 10.6.

9.4.9 Sensitivity analysis

The process of undertaking a systematic review involves a sequence of decisions. While many of these decisions are clearly objective and non-contentious, some will be somewhat subjective. For instance, if eligibility criteria involve a numerical value, the choice of value is usually arbitrary: for example, defining groups of older people may reasonably have lower limits of 60, 65, 70 or 75 years, or any value in between. Other decisions may have to be based on assumptions because a study fails to include the required information. Further decisions involve judgement because there is no consensus on the best method to use for a particular problem, such as defining a reference standard or analysing missing data or inconclusive test results.

It is desirable to demonstrate that the findings from a systematic review are not dependent on potentially subjective decisions or assumptions. A sensitivity analysis is a repeat of the primary analysis or meta-analysis, substituting alternative decisions (or assumptions used to make decisions) for the original decisions. A sensitivity analysis asks the question 'Are the findings robust to the decisions made in the process of obtaining and analysing them?' For example, if the eligibility of some studies in the meta-analysis is questionable because they do not contain full details, sensitivity analysis may involve undertaking the meta-analysis twice: first including all studies, and second including only those that are definitely known to be eligible.

Many decision nodes within the systematic review process can generate a need for sensitivity analysis. Examples include the following.

Searching for studies
Should abstracts whose results cannot be confirmed in subsequent publications be included in the review?

Eligibility criteria
- Characteristics of participants: where a majority but not all people in a study meet the required presentation or demographic, should the study be included?
- Characteristics of tests: what versions of a test technology should be included? What threshold definition constitutes a common threshold?
- Characteristics of the reference standard: where there are variations in the information used in a clinical opinion-based reference standard, should they all be included? Where the reference standard involves follow-up, what lengths of follow-up are considered adequate?
- Study methods: should only studies that apply the same reference standard in all study participants be included? Should unblinded studies be included? Should case-control studies be included? Or should inclusion be restricted by any other methodological criteria?

What data should be analysed?
- Uninterpretable test results: how should they be handled in the analysis? Should they be classified as test negatives or excluded?
- Missing data: how should they be handled in the analysis?

Analysis methods
- Should a common or symmetrical shape for an SROC curve be presumed across subgroups or tests?
- Can equal variances be presumed for all tests in a comparison?

Reporting of sensitivity analyses in a systematic way may best be done by producing a summary table. Some sensitivity analyses can be pre-specified in the study protocol, but many issues requiring sensitivity analysis are only identified during the review process when the individual peculiarities of the studies under investigation are identified. If sensitivity analyses show that the overall result and conclusions are not affected by the different decisions or assumptions made during the review process, the results of the review can be regarded with a higher degree of certainty. If sensitivity analyses identify particular decisions or missing information that greatly influence the findings of the review, greater resources can be deployed to try to resolve uncertainties and obtain extra information, possibly through contacting study authors. If this cannot be achieved, the results must be interpreted with an appropriate degree of caution. Such findings may generate proposals for further investigations and future research.

Sensitivity analysis is sometimes confused with subgroup analysis. Although some sensitivity analysis may involve restricting the analysis to a subset of studies, the two methods differ in two ways. First, sensitivity analyses do not attempt to estimate the effect of the covariate in the group of studies removed from the analysis, whereas in subgroup analysis estimates are produced for all groups. Second, in sensitivity analysis informal comparisons are made between different ways of estimating the same thing to assess their impact on the magnitude of the estimate(s), whereas in subgroup analysis formal statistical comparisons are made across the subgroups.

The impact of individual study results on the summary estimates of test accuracy (including for example the shape of the SROC curve and the variance of the random effects) can be investigated by comparing analyses including and excluding individual influential studies. Where it is noted that the results of a single study have high influence, conclusions should be drawn with caution, particularly if the studies differ in some way or raise methodological concerns.

9.5 Special topics

9.5.1 Imperfect reference standard

The statistical models described so far in this chapter assume that there is a reference standard that it is accurate and that it has been applied to all study participants. However, for some conditions there may not be an accepted reference standard or the reference standard may be inaccurate. Misclassification of the true disease status of study participants in these situations leads to bias in study-level estimates of sensitivity, specificity and prevalence.

Latent class analysis (LCA) can be used to estimate test accuracy in these situations. LCA provides corrected estimates of sensitivity, specificity and disease prevalence under the assumption that true disease status cannot be observed directly and is represented by a latent (unobservable) variable. LCA models that have been proposed vary in complexity and in terms of the assumptions that are made to ensure that model parameters are identifiable (van Smeden 2014).

Walter (1999) proposed a latent class model for meta-analysis of test accuracy that assumed a fixed effect for both sensitivity and specificity, but random study effects for prevalence. Conditional independence, whereby test errors are not correlated in the underlying (true) diseased and non-diseased groups, is assumed. However, the resulting estimates of sensitivity and specificity may be biased given that conditional independence can be an inappropriate assumption in many settings where subgroups of patients share characteristics that make them more likely to be false positives (or false negatives) (Vacek 1985).

The application of Bayesian hierarchical modelling to latent class analyses has provided a more flexible framework whereby the constraints just outlined can be relaxed. Chu (2009) proposed an LCA extension of the bivariate model for the situation when there is no gold standard. The sensitivity and specificity of the index test and the reference test, as well as the prevalence, are treated as random study effects. Dendukuri (2012) developed an LCA extension of the HSROC model that includes random study effects for sensitivity and specificity. Both models can allow for conditional dependence between tests. Liu (2015) has demonstrated that the two models are mathematically equivalent in the absence of study-level covariates. Allowing for conditional dependence requires the addition of covariance parameters that make the model unidentifiable and necessitate the use of informative prior distributions to obtain a meaningful solution in some cases (Xie 2017). The LCA extension of the bivariate model is described further in Chapter 10 and illustrated using an example.

9.5.2 Investigating and handling verification bias

An examination of the potential for verification bias in a systematic review would ordinarily be part of the assessment of study quality. It may also be useful to investigate the presence of verification bias as a source of heterogeneity among studies. If verification bias is present, in some circumstances corrections for missing reference standard data can be implemented within individual studies before proceeding to the meta-analysis. The literature on methods for correcting verification bias in individual studies is extensive (Umemneku Chikere 2019), and commonly used methods for primary studies are covered in standard text books, e.g. Chapter 10 in Zhou (2011) and Chapter 7 in Pepe (2003). Issues arise in the extraction of study data when adjustments have been made for verification bias, as described in Chapter 7 of this handbook.

Bayesian hierarchical models that adjust for partial verification bias have been proposed, e.g. Ma (2016). These methods require further evaluation before any can be recommended for Cochrane Reviews of diagnostic test accuracy.

9.5.3 Investigating and handling publication bias

Systematic review authors should undertake comprehensive searches to attempt to locate all relevant studies. If the studies included in the review have results that differ systematically from relevant studies that are unavailable, estimates derived from the meta-analysis will be affected by publication bias (Begg 1994a).

Although there is a substantial literature relating to publication bias in systematic reviews of randomized trials of interventions, it is clear that the determinants of publication bias for reviews of randomized trials (Dickersin 1990, Ioannidis 1998) are unlikely to be generalizable to reviews of diagnostic accuracy studies. For instance, when considering the diagnostic accuracy of a single test, statistical significance is not particularly relevant, as few studies formulate and test hypotheses. The likely relationship between study size and methodological quality may also differ: whereas large randomized trials require large-scale funding and are generally conducted and analysed with greater methodological rigour than small randomized trials, large diagnostic studies may be no more than an analysis of a large laboratory database of routinely collected data.

Investigations of publication bias have identified possible factors that may influence the likelihood of publication of studies of diagnostic accuracy, but the findings vary. For diagnostic imaging studies, there is evidence that higher test accuracy is associated with faster publication (Dehmoobad Sharifabadi 2018) and conference abstracts with positive conclusions are more likely to be published (Treanor 2020). However, no association was found between ophthalmology conference abstracts reporting higher test accuracy and subsequent publication (Korevaar 2016).

Statistical tests to detect funnel plot asymmetry do not test for publication bias specifically (Page 2019), as there are several causes of relationships between study size and findings. Tests for funnel plot asymmetry designed primarily for use on reviews of randomized trials, including the Begg (1994b), Egger (1997), Harbord (2006) and Peters (2006) tests, should not be used with diagnostic studies. It is well established that the accuracy of such tests for funnel plot asymmetry is reasonable if the odds ratio is close to 1 (as occurs in many randomized trials), but deteriorates as the odds ratio moves away from 1 (Macaskill 2001, Schwarzer 2002, Deeks 2005). For diagnostic studies, the odds ratio is expected to be large. Applying such tests for funnel plot asymmetry in systematic reviews of test accuracy is likely to result in publication bias being incorrectly indicated by the test far too often (i.e. a Type I error rate that is too high) (Deeks 2005).

A more appropriate method for detecting funnel plot asymmetry in systematic reviews of test accuracy has been developed (Deeks 2005). It tests for association between the lnDOR and the 'effective sample size', a simple function of the number of diseased and non-diseased individuals. A simulation study has shown that the test has only modest power for detecting funnel plot asymmetry. Although it is the most appropriate of the commonly used methods (van Enst 2014), the Deeks test has particularly low power when there is heterogeneity in the DOR (Deeks 2005).

Since heterogeneity in test accuracy is to be expected in many systematic reviews of test accuracy, review authors are warned against interpreting statistical evidence of funnel plot asymmetry as necessarily implying publication bias, and absence of a relationship as excluding publication bias. Study size may be related to test accuracy for reasons other than publication bias. Heterogeneity in test accuracy should be explored, as patient and study characteristics may be associated with study size as well as test accuracy (Deeks 2005). Further research is required to improve our understanding of the determinants and extent of publication bias for test accuracy studies, for the evaluation of a single test and also for test comparisons.

9.5.4 Developments in meta-analysis for systematic reviews of test accuracy

This chapter reflects the currently established methods for meta-analysis of diagnostic test accuracy. Methodological developments continue to occur in this field, and the methods used in Cochrane Reviews of diagnostic test accuracy are certain to develop over time to extend the scope of the models and data structures that can be included. As new methods are shown to be robust and of importance, and software made available for their implementation, they will be included in updates of this chapter.

9.6 Chapter information

Authors: Petra Macaskill (*Sydney School of Public Health, University of Sydney, Australia*), Yemisi Takwoingi (*Institute of Applied Health Research, University of Birmingham, UK*), Jonathan J. Deeks (*Institute of Applied Health Research, University of Birmingham, UK*), Constantine Gatsonis (*School of Public Health, Brown University, USA*).

Sources of support: Yemisi Takwoingi is funded by a UK National Institute for Health Research (NIHR) Postdoctoral Fellowship. Jonathan J. Deeks is a UK National Institute for Health Research (NIHR) Senior Investigator Emeritus. Yemisi Takwoingi and Jonathan J. Deeks are supported by the NIHR Birmingham Biomedical Research Centre at the University Hospitals Birmingham NHS Foundation Trust and the University of Birmingham. The views expressed are those of the authors and not necessarily those of the NHS, the NIHR or the Department of Health and Social Care. No other authors declare sources of support for writing this chapter.

Declarations of interest: Petra Macaskill, Yemisi Takwoingi and Jonathan J. Deeks are members of Cochrane's Diagnostic Test Accuracy Editorial Team. Petra Macaskill and Yemisi Takwoingi are co-convenors of the Cochrane Screening and Diagnostic Tests

Methods Group. The authors declare no other potential conflicts of interest relevant to the topic of this chapter.

Acknowledgements: The authors thank Roger Harbord for contributions to a previous version of this chapter. The authors would like to thank Nandini Dendukuri, Kurinchi Gurusamy, Gerta Rücker, Alex Sutton and Bada Yang for helpful peer review comments.

9.7   References

Agresti A. *An introduction to categorical data analysis*. 2nd ed. Hoboken (NJ): John Wiley & Sons; 2007.

Arends LR, Hamza TH, van Houwelingen JC, Heijenbrok-Kal MH, Hunink MG, Stijnen T. Bivariate random effects meta-analysis of ROC curves. *Medical Decision Making* 2008; **28**: 621–638.

Begg CB. Publication bias. In: Cooper H, Hedges L, editors. *Handbook of Research Synthesis*. New York (NY): Sage Foundation; 1994a: 399–410.

Begg CB, Mazumdar M. Operating characteristics of a rank correlation test for publication bias. *Biometrics* 1994b; **50**: 1088–1101.

Chappell FM, Raab GM, Wardlaw JM. When are summary ROC curves appropriate for diagnostic meta-analyses? *Statistics in Medicine* 2009; **28**: 2653–2668.

Chu H, Cole SR. Bivariate meta-analysis of sensitivity and specificity with sparse data: a generalized linear mixed model approach. *Journal of Clinical Epidemiology* 2006; **59**: 1331–1332; author reply 1332-1333.

Chu H, Chen S, Louis TA. Random effects models in a meta-analysis of the accuracy of two diagnostic tests without a gold standard. *Journal of the American Statistical Association* 2009; **104**: 512–523.

Cohen JF, Korevaar DA, Wang J, Leeflang MM, Bossuyt PM. Meta-epidemiologic study showed frequent time trends in summary estimates from meta-analyses of diagnostic accuracy studies. *Journal of Clinical Epidemiology* 2016; **77**: 60–67.

Deeks JJ. Systematic reviews in health care: systematic reviews of evaluations of diagnostic and screening tests. *BMJ* 2001; **323**: 157–162.

Deeks JJ, Macaskill P, Irwig L. The performance of tests of publication bias and other sample size effects in systematic reviews of diagnostic test accuracy was assessed. *Journal of Clinical Epidemiology* 2005; **58**: 882–893.

Deeks JJ, Higgins JPT, Altman DG. Chapter 10: Analysing data and undertaking meta-analyses. In: Higgins JPT, Thomas J, Chandler J, Cumpston M, Li T, Page MJ, Welch VA, editors. *Cochrane Handbook for Systematic Reviews of Interventions* version 6.0. Cochrane, 2019.

Dehmoobad Sharifabadi A, Korevaar DA, McGrath TA, van Es N, Frank RA, Cherpak L, Dang W, Salameh JP, Nguyen F, Stanley C, McInnes MDF. Reporting bias in imaging: higher accuracy is linked to faster publication. *European Radiology* 2018; **28**: 3632–3639.

Dendukuri N, Schiller I, Joseph L, Pai M. Bayesian meta-analysis of the accuracy of a test for tuberculous pleuritis in the absence of a gold standard reference. *Biometrics* 2012; **68**: 1285–1293.

Dickersin K. The existence of publication bias and risk factors for its occurrence. *JAMA* 1990; **263**: 1385–1389.

Dimou NL, Adam M, Bagos PG. A multivariate method for meta-analysis and comparison of diagnostic tests. *Statistics in Medicine* 2016; **35**: 3509–3523.

Dukic V, Gatsonis C. Meta-analysis of diagnostic test accuracy assessment studies with varying number of thresholds. *Biometrics* 2003; **59**: 936–946.

Egger M, Davey Smith G, Schneider M, Minder C. Bias in meta-analysis detected by a simple, graphical test. *BMJ* 1997; **315**: 629–634.

Hamza TH, Arends LR, van Houwelingen HC, Stijnen T. Multivariate random effects meta-analysis of diagnostic tests with multiple thresholds. *BMC Medical Research Methodology* 2009; **9**: 73.

Harbord RM, Egger M, Sterne JA. A modified test for small-study effects in meta-analyses of controlled trials with binary endpoints. *Statistics in Medicine* 2006; **25**: 3443–3457.

Harbord RM, Deeks JJ, Egger M, Whiting PF, Sterne JA. A unification of models for meta-analysis of diagnostic accuracy studies. *Biostatistics* 2007; **8**: 239–251.

Higgins JP, Thompson SG, Deeks JJ, Altman DG. Measuring inconsistency in meta-analyses. *BMJ* 2003; **327**: 557–560.

Ioannidis JP. Effect of the statistical significance of results on the time to completion and publication of randomized efficacy trials. *JAMA* 1998; **279**: 281–286.

Jones HE, Gatsonis CA, Trikalinos TA, Welton NJ, Ades AE. Quantifying how diagnostic test accuracy depends on threshold in a meta-analysis. *Statistics in Medicine* 2019; **38**: 4789–4803.

Korevaar DA, Cohen JF, Spijker R, Saldanha IJ, Dickersin K, Virgili G, Hooft L, Bossuyt PM. Reported estimates of diagnostic accuracy in ophthalmology conference abstracts were not associated with full-text publication. *Journal of Clinical Epidemiology* 2016; **79**: 96–103.

Leeflang MM, Moons KG, Reitsma JB, Zwinderman AH. Bias in sensitivity and specificity caused by data-driven selection of optimal cutoff values: mechanisms, magnitude, and solutions. *Clinical Chemistry* 2008; **54**: 729–737.

Leeflang MM, Deeks JJ, Rutjes AW, Reitsma JB, Bossuyt PM. Bivariate meta-analysis of predictive values of diagnostic tests can be an alternative to bivariate meta-analysis of sensitivity and specificity. *Journal of Clinical Epidemiology* 2012; **65**: 1088–1097.

Lian Q, Hodges JS, Chu H. A Bayesian Hierarchical summary receiver operating characteristic model for network meta-analysis of diagnostic tests. *Journal of the American Statistical Association* 2019; **114**: 949–961.

Littenberg B, Moses LE. Estimating diagnostic accuracy from multiple conflicting reports: a new meta-analytic method. *Medical Decision Making* 1993; **13**: 313–321.

Liu Y, Chen Y, Chu H. A unification of models for meta-analysis of diagnostic accuracy studies without a gold standard. *Biometrics* 2015; **71**: 538–547.

Ma X, Chen Y, Cole SR, Chu H. A hybrid Bayesian hierarchical model combining cohort and case-control studies for meta-analysis of diagnostic tests: accounting for partial verification bias. *Statistical Methods in Medical Research* 2016; **25**: 3015–3037.

Ma X, Lian Q, Chu H, Ibrahim JG, Chen Y. A Bayesian hierarchical model for network meta-analysis of multiple diagnostic tests. *Biostatistics* 2018; **19**: 87–102.

Macaskill P, Walter SD, Irwig L. A comparison of methods to detect publication bias in meta-analysis. *Statistics in Medicine* 2001; **20**: 641–654.

McCullagh P. Regression models for ordinal data. *Journal of the Royal Statistical Society Series B (Methodological)* 1980; **42**: 109–142.

Moses LE, Shapiro D, Littenberg B. Combining independent studies of a diagnostic test into a summary ROC curve: data-analytic approaches and some additional considerations. *Statistics in Medicine* 1993; **12**: 1293–1316.

Nishimura K, Sugiyama D, Kogata Y, Tsuji G, Nakazawa T, Kawano S, Saigo K, Morinobu A, Koshiba M, Kuntz KM, Kamae I, Kumagai S. Meta-analysis: diagnostic accuracy of anti-cyclic citrullinated peptide antibody and rheumatoid factor for rheumatoid arthritis. *Annals of Internal Medicine* 2007; **146**: 797–808.

Nyaga VN, Aerts M, Arbyn M. ANOVA model for network meta-analysis of diagnostic test accuracy data. *Statistical Methods in Medical Research* 2018; **27**: 1766–1784.

Oehlert GW. A note on the Delta method. *American Statistician* 1992; **46**: 27–29.

Owen RK, Cooper NJ, Quinn TJ, Lees R, Sutton AJ. Network meta-analysis of diagnostic test accuracy studies identifies and ranks the optimal diagnostic tests and thresholds for health care policy and decision-making. *Journal of Clinical Epidemiology* 2018; **99**: 64–74.

Page MJ, Higgins JPT, Sterne JAC. Chapter 13: Assessing risk of bias due to missing results in a synthesis. In: Higgins JPT, Thomas J, Chandler J, Cumpston M, Li T, Page MJ, Welch VA, editors. *Cochrane Handbook for Systematic Reviews of Interventions* version 6.0. Cochrane, 2019.

Pepe M. *The statistical evaluation of medical tests for misclassification and prediction.* Oxford: Oxford University Press; 2003.

Peters JL, Sutton AJ, Jones DR, Abrams KR, Rushton L. Comparison of two methods to detect publication bias in meta-analysis. *JAMA* 2006; **295**: 676–680.

Putter H, Fiocco M, Stijnen T. Meta-analysis of diagnostic test accuracy studies with multiple thresholds using survival methods. *Biometrical Journal* 2010; **52**: 95–110.

Reitsma JB, Glas AS, Rutjes AW, Scholten RJ, Bossuyt PM, Zwinderman AH. Bivariate analysis of sensitivity and specificity produces informative summary measures in diagnostic reviews. *Journal of Clinical Epidemiology* 2005; **58**: 982–990.

Rücker G, Schwarzer G, Carpenter JR, Schumacher M. Undue reliance on I(2) in assessing heterogeneity may mislead. *BMC Medical Research Methodology* 2008; **8**: 79.

Rücker G. Network meta-analysis of diagnostic test accuracy studies. In: Biondi-Zoccai G, editor. *Diagnostic meta-analysis: A useful tool for clinical decision-making.* Springer; 2018: 183–197.

Rutter CM, Gatsonis CA. Regression methods for meta-analysis of diagnostic test data. *Academic Radiology* 1995; **2** Suppl 1: S48–S56; discussion S65-S67, S70-S71 pas.

Rutter CM, Gatsonis CA. A hierarchical regression approach to meta-analysis of diagnostic test accuracy evaluations. *Statistics in Medicine* 2001; **20**: 2865–2884.

Schuetz GM, Zacharopoulou NM, Schlattmann P, Dewey M. Meta-analysis: noninvasive coronary angiography using computed tomography versus magnetic resonance imaging. *Annals of Internal Medicine* 2010; **152**: 167–177.

Schwarzer G, Antes G, Schumacher M. Inflation of type I error rate in two statistical tests for the detection of publication bias in meta-analyses with binary outcomes. *Statistics in Medicine* 2002; **21**: 2465–2477.

Steinhauser S, Schumacher M, Rücker G. Modelling multiple thresholds in meta-analysis of diagnostic test accuracy studies. *BMC Medical Research Methodology* 2016; **16**: 97.

Takwoingi Y, Leeflang MM, Deeks JJ. Empirical evidence of the importance of comparative studies of diagnostic test accuracy. *Annals of Internal Medicine* 2013; **158**: 544–554.

Takwoingi Y, Guo B, Riley RD, Deeks JJ. Performance of methods for meta-analysis of diagnostic test accuracy with few studies or sparse data. *Statistical Methods in Medical Research* 2017; **26**: 1896–1911.

Tosteson AN, Begg CB. A general regression methodology for ROC curve estimation. *Medical Decision Making* 1988; **8**: 204–215.

Treanor L, Frank RA, Cherpak LA, Dehmoobad Sharifabadi A, Salameh JP, Hallgrimson Z, Fabiano N, McGrath TA, Kraaijpoel N, Yao J, Korevaar DA, Bossuyt PM, McInnes MDF. Publication bias in diagnostic imaging: conference abstracts with positive conclusions are more likely to be published. *European Radiology* 2020; **30**: 2964–2972.

Trikalinos TA, Hoaglin DC, Small KM, Terrin N, Schmid CH. Methods for the joint meta-analysis of multiple tests. *Research Synthesis Methods* 2014; **5**: 294–312.

Umemneku Chikere CM, Wilson K, Graziadio S, Vale L, Allen AJ. Diagnostic test evaluation methodology: a systematic review of methods employed to evaluate diagnostic tests in the absence of gold standard – an update. *PloS One* 2019; **14**: e0223832.

Vacek PM. The effect of conditional dependence on the evaluation of diagnostic tests. *Biometrics* 1985; **41**: 959–968.

van Enst WA, Ochodo E, Scholten RJ, Hooft L, Leeflang MM. Investigation of publication bias in meta-analyses of diagnostic test accuracy: a meta-epidemiological study. *BMC Medical Research Methodology* 2014; **14**: 70.

van Smeden M, Naaktgeboren CA, Reitsma JB, Moons KG, de Groot JA. Latent class models in diagnostic studies when there is no reference standard—a systematic review. *American Journal of Epidemiology* 2014; **179**: 423–431.

Veroniki AA, Tsokani S, Agarwal R, Pagkalidou E, Rücker G, Mavridis D, Takwoingi Y. Diagnostic test accuracy network meta-analysis methods: a scoping review and empirical assessment. *Journal of Clinical Epidemiology* 2022; **146**: 86–96.

Walter SD, Irwig L, Glasziou PP. Meta-analysis of diagnostic tests with imperfect reference standards. *Journal of Clinical Epidemiology* 1999; **52**: 943–951.

Wetterslev J, Thorlund K, Brok J, Gluud C. Estimating required information size by quantifying diversity in random-effects model meta-analyses. *BMC Medical Research Methodology* 2009; **9**: 86.

Xie X, Sinclair A, Dendukuri N. Evaluating the accuracy and economic value of a new test in the absence of a perfect reference test. *Research Synthesis Methods* 2017; **8**: 321–332.

Zhou XH, Obuchowski N, McClish D. *Statistical methods in diagnostic medicine*. 2nd ed. Chichester: John Wiley & Sons; 2011.

Zhou Y, Dendukuri N. Statistics for quantifying heterogeneity in univariate and bivariate meta-analyses of binary data: the case of meta-analyses of diagnostic accuracy. *Statistics in Medicine* 2014; **33**: 2701–2717.

Zwinderman AH, Bossuyt PM. We should not pool diagnostic likelihood ratios in systematic reviews. *Statistics in Medicine* 2008; **27**: 687–697.

10

Undertaking meta-analysis

Yemisi Takwoingi, Nandini Dendukuri, Ian Schiller, Gerta Rücker, Hayley E. Jones,
Christopher Partlett and Petra Macaskill

KEY POINTS

- Hierarchical models such as the bivariate and hierarchical summary receiver operating characteristic (HSROC) models are recommended for test accuracy meta-analysis. The models can be fitted in a frequentist or Bayesian statistics framework.
- To fit these hierarchical models, several statistical software packages and user-written programs are available for frequentist analyses, while Bayesian estimation within the R software environment facilitates analyses by applied health researchers.
- Convergence issues arising from analysis of sparse or atypical data are common, but there are potential solutions, including simplifying hierarchical models.
- For tests that produce a continuous numerical result, one of two promising approaches that extend the bivariate model to allow the inclusion of multiple thresholds per study can be used to obtain summary estimates of sensitivity and specificity at particular thresholds and a summary curve across thresholds.
- When the reference standard is imperfect, an extension of the bivariate model, assuming the target condition cannot be observed, can be implemented via latent class meta-analysis.

10.1   Introduction

Hierarchical models are recommended for meta-analysis of test accuracy studies, as explained in Chapter 9. Cochrane's primary authoring tool, Review Manager (RevMan; www. training.cochrane.org/online-learning/core-software/revman), which can be used to write systematic reviews of test accuracy, does not have the capability for fitting the bivariate and HSROC models described in Chapter 9. Therefore, external analysis using a statistical software package is required to fit such hierarchical models. If review authors are using RevMan,

This chapter should be cited as: Takwoingi Y, Dendukuri N, Schiller I, Rücker G, Jones HE, Partlett C, Macaskill P. Chapter 10: Undertaking meta-analysis. In: Deeks JJ, Bossuyt PM, Leeflang MM, Takwoingi Y, editors. *Cochrane Handbook for Systematic Reviews of Diagnostic Test Accuracy*. 1st edition. Chichester (UK): John Wiley & Sons, 2023: 249–326.

Cochrane Handbook for Systematic Reviews of Diagnostic Test Accuracy, First Edition. Edited by Jonathan J. Deeks, Patrick M. Bossuyt, Mariska M. Leeflang and Yemisi Takwoingi.
© 2023 The Cochrane Collaboration. Published 2023 by John Wiley & Sons Ltd.

parameter estimates can then be entered to generate summary receiver operating characteristic (SROC) plots showing summary points or summary curves as appropriate.

The bivariate model is a generalized linear mixed model (GLMM) and several statistical packages (e.g. SAS, Stata, R, BUGS and JAGS) are available for fitting the model using binomial likelihoods to model within-study variability rather than a normal approximation (see the model specification in Chapter 9, Section 9.4.1). The HSROC model is a non-linear generalized mixed model (GMM) and options for fitting this model are currently limited to packages that can fit nonlinear GMMs (e.g. SAS, BUGS and JAGS).

The meta-analysis methods introduced in Chapter 9 were presented using frequentist estimation methods. However, several of the more advanced analyses can also be undertaken using Bayesian estimation. Throughout this chapter we present analyses performed using both frequentist and Bayesian approaches wherever possible. The frequentist approach is typically preferred for simpler models and analyses; as there is substantial experience in the use of these methods, user-written programs are more widely available and easier to use. Frequentist methods also do not require the specification of prior distributions for the parameters that are estimated, which occasionally can have undesirable influence on the results.

This chapter complements Chapter 9. Depending on familiarity with the concepts underpinning test accuracy meta-analysis and the software packages, the reader may find some sections more challenging than others. The chapter gives an overview of how to fit the hierarchical models within a frequentist framework using three software packages (SAS, Stata and R) and within a Bayesian framework using rjags (an interface from R to the JAGS library for Bayesian data analysis).

A prerequisite to understanding the Bayesian estimation sections of this chapter is knowledge of basic methods for Bayesian inference (Spiegelhalter 2004, Gelman 2013, Kruschke 2015). Also, familiarity with using JAGS or BUGS languages (Lunn 2009, Plummer 2019) to fit simple models, such as models for estimating a single proportion or for logistic regression, will aid in understanding of the more complex models described in this chapter.

Bayesian model specification requires the user to provide (1) the likelihood function and (2) the prior distribution functions for all unknown parameters. The software takes care of implementing the necessary Monte Carlo Markov Chain (MCMC) algorithms in the background to provide the user with samples from the posterior distributions of the parameters of interest. Thus, the user needs only to be familiar with details of the syntax and does not have to carry out complex calculations. On the other hand, it is very important that the user is familiar with methods for verifying whether the MCMC algorithms have converged and for carrying out sensitivity analyses to assess the impact of different prior distribution functions.

Using examples introduced in Chapter 9, Sections 10.2, 10.3, 10.4 and 10.5 illustrate the estimation and comparison of summary points and curves when assuming a perfect reference standard. In addition to inbuilt software commands, user-written programs and macros that give outputs compatible with RevMan are highlighted. Section 10.6 provides suggestions on meta-analyses of problematic or atypical data sets, including simplifying hierarchical models, one of the approaches recommended in Chapter 9, Section 9.4.8, for meta-analysis of sparse data. Section 10.7 uses an example to elaborate on meta-analysis methods introduced in Chapter 9, Section 9.4.5, that allow multiple thresholds per study. Using a Cochrane Review of diagnostic test accuracy as an example, Section 10.8

illustrates latent class meta-analysis, an approach introduced in Chapter 9, Section 9.5.1, for meta-analysis with an imperfect reference standard. Section 10.9 concludes the chapter with a summary and information on additional resources.

The frequentist analyses were performed using SAS version 9.4 (SAS Institute, Cary, NC, USA), Stata version 16 (Stata-Corp, College Station, TX, USA) and R version 4.1.0. The corresponding SROC plots were produced using RevMan version 5.3.

10.2 Estimation of a summary point

The focus of the bivariate model is the estimation of a summary point. As described in Chapter 9, Section 9.4.1, the bivariate method models sensitivity and specificity directly and has five parameters when no covariates are included: μ_A, μ_B, σ^2_A, σ^2_B and σ_{AB}. The parameters μ_A and μ_B are the mean logit(sensitivity) and mean logit(specificity), respectively, σ^2_A and σ^2_B describe the between-study variability in logit(sensitivity) and logit(specificity), and σ_{AB} is the covariance between logit(sensitivity) and logit(specificity). The model may also be parametrized using the correlation $\rho_{AB} = \sigma_{AB}/(\sigma_A\sigma_B)$. Anti-CCP for diagnosis of rheumatoid arthritis is one of the two index tests in the review (Nishimura 2007) introduced in Chapter 9, Section 9.2.3.1. Meta-analysis of anti-CCP was illustrated using the bivariate model in Chapter 9, Section 9.4.2, and this example will be used throughout this section. The sensitivities and specificities of the 37 included studies are shown on the forest plot in Chapter 9, Figure 9.2.a.

10.2.1 Fitting the bivariate model using SAS

Hierarchical models can be fitted using the `NLMIXED` and `GLIMMIX` procedures in SAS. The `NLMIXED` procedure fits linear and nonlinear GMMs while `GLIMMIX` fits only GLMMs. This chapter focuses on the `NLMIXED` procedure because it can be used to fit both the bivariate and HSROC models. The `NLMIXED` procedure uses maximum likelihood to estimate the parameters of a model, and requires a regression equation and declaration of parameters with their starting values. These starting values are required for the iterative process, and it is essential to select good values in order to avoid excessively long computing time, and also to facilitate convergence of the optimization process for solving the maximum likelihood estimation problem. A single value can be chosen for each parameter or a set of values by using the TO and BY keywords to specify a number list for a grid search. For example, in the SAS code in the online supplementary material (10.S1 Code for undertaking meta-analysis, see Appendix 1), '`msens =1 to 2 by 0.5`' defines the grid of values to search for starting values for '`msens`', the logit(sensitivity) parameter.

The parameter estimates from the bivariate model fitted in SAS using the NLMIXED code in Appendix 1 of the online supplementary material (10.S1 Code for undertaking meta-analysis) are shown in Box 10.2.a. The parameter estimates in the red and blue boxes can be entered into the corresponding analysis in RevMan to generate the summary point, as can the 95% confidence and 95% prediction regions shown in Chapter 9, Figure 9.4.a. The bivariate output box in RevMan requires the estimate for mean logit(sensitivity), which is 0.6534; the estimate for mean logit(specificity), which is 3.1090; and the variances of the random effects for logit(sensitivity), logit(specificity)

Box 10.2.a SAS output of bivariate model parameters

Parameter Estimates

Parameter	Estimate	Standard Error	DF	t Value	Pr > |t|	95% Confidence Limits		Gradient
msens	0.6534	0.1275	35	5.13	<.0001	0.3946	0.9122	3.959E-6
mspec	3.1090	0.1459	35	21.31	<.0001	2.8128	3.4052	3.472E-8
s2usens	0.5426	0.1463	35	3.71	0.0007	0.2455	0.8397	-6.62E-6
s2uspec	0.5717	0.1873	35	3.05	0.0043	0.1914	0.9520	1.36E-6
covsesp	-0.2704	0.1199	35	2.26	0.0304	-0.5137	-0.02710	-1.59E-6

Covariance Matrix of Parameter Estimates

	msens	mspec	s2usens	s2uspec	covsesp
msens	0.01625	-0.00741	0.000890	-0.00004	-0.00004
mspec	-0.00741	0.02128	-0.00006	0.004287	-0.00116
s2usens	0.000890	-0.00006	0.02142	0.003997	-0.00874
s2uspec	-0.00004	0.004287	0.003997	0.03509	-0.01184
covsesp	-0.00004	-0.00116	-0.00874	-0.01184	0.01436

and their covariance, which are 0.5426, 0.5717, and –0.2704, respectively. Computation of confidence and prediction regions also requires the standard error of the estimates for mean logit(sensitivity), mean logit(specificity) and their covariance, which are 0.1275, 0.1459 and –0.00741, respectively (shown in the blue boxes).

The summary sensitivity and specificity can be obtained by inverse transformation of the estimates for mean logit(sensitivity) and logit(specificity) (0.6534 and 3.1090) to give a sensitivity and specificity of 0.66 and 0.96, respectively. This calculation can be done using the following equations.

$$Sensitivity = \frac{\exp(logit\ sensitivity)}{1+\exp(logit\ sensitivity)} = \frac{\exp(0.6534)}{1+\exp(0.6534)} = 0.66$$

$$Specificity = \frac{\exp(logit\ specificity)}{1+\exp(logit\ specificity)} = \frac{\exp(3.1090)}{1+\exp(3.1090)} = 0.96$$

The 95% confidence intervals (CI) for the summary estimates can be similarly obtained by inverse transformation of the 95% CI of the mean logit estimates.

The SAS macro MetaDAS is a wrapper for NLMIXED to automate fitting bivariate and HSROC models to produce parameter and summary estimates (Takwoingi 2010). The macro requires a minimum of two or three input parameters, depending on whether data import (e.g. from a spreadsheet) is required or a SAS data set already exists. The output from the analysis is saved in a rich text Word file and presented in tables, from which parameter estimates can be copied and pasted into RevMan to generate SROC plots. Example code is available in Appendix 1 of the online supplementary material (10.S1 Code for undertaking meta-analysis) and a user guide with a worked example can be found on the Cochrane Screening and Diagnostic Tests Methods Group website (www. methods.cochrane.org/sdt).

10.2.2 Fitting the bivariate model using Stata

The user-written programs `metandi` (Harbord 2008, Harbord 2009) and `midas` (Dwamena 2007) use the `xtmelogit` or `gllamm` commands to perform bivariate meta-analysis of sensitivity and specificity using a GLMM approach. However, `midas` does not give parameter estimates in the output and so cannot be used with RevMan. Therefore, only `metandi` will be illustrated in this section.

The GLMM estimation routine `xtmelogit` was introduced in Stata 10 and replaced with `meqrlogit` in Stata 13. In Stata 10 and above, `metandi` fits the model using the command `xtmelogit` by default. In Stata 8 or 9, `metandi` uses `gllamm`, which must also be installed. The `ssc` command allows users to download a user-written package from the Boston College Statistical Software Components (SSC) archive. For example, to download and install `metandi`, type the following in the command window in Stata:

```
ssc install metandi
```

The `metandi` command requires four input variables: the number of true positives (tp), false positives (fp), false negatives (fn) and true negatives (tn) within each study.

```
metandi tp fp fn tn
```

The results of the meta-analysis of anti-CCP using the metandi command are shown in Box 10.2.b.

Users of Stata 10 and above may choose to use option `gllamm` with `metandi`, which runs slower than `xtmelogit` but can sometimes solve convergence issues commonly encountered in meta-analysis of sparse data (see Section 10.6). Use the `help` command in Stata to learn more about `metandi` and its options, some of which are included in the code in Appendix 2 of the online supplementary material (10.S1 Code for undertaking meta-analysis). Although `metandi` only fits the bivariate model, it can output HSROC model parameters using functions of the parameter estimates from the bivariate model, since the two models are mathematically equivalent when no covariates are fitted (see Chapter 9, Section 9.4). Summary test accuracy measures are also reported as shown in the green box in Box 10.2.b. The parameter estimates in the red and blue boxes can be entered into RevMan as explained in Section 10.2.1. The metandi command is straightforward to use, but does not have an option for including a covariate in the bivariate model, i.e. one cannot perform meta-regression to investigate heterogeneity or compare test accuracy. Furthermore, there are limited options to try when convergence issues are encountered (see Section 10.6). Therefore it is useful to know how to fit the model using the `meqrlogit` command for greater flexibility.

The code provided in Appendix 3 of the online supplementary material (10.S1 Code for undertaking meta-analysis) uses `meqrlogit` but can be replaced with `xtmelogit`

Box 10.2.b Stata output of bivariate model parameters using metandi

Meta-analysis of diagnostic accuracy

Log likelihood   = -273.09555   Number of studies =   37

	Coef.	Std. Err.	z	P>|z|	[95% Conf. Interval]	
Bivariate						
E(logitSe)	.6534697	.1276188			.4033414	.9035981
E(logitSp)	3.108991	.1463993			2.822053	3.395928
Var(logitSe)	.5438584	.1467547			.3204777	.922941
Var(logitSp)	.5769244	.1896049			.3029517	1.098663
Corr(logits)	-.4820203	.1629024			-.7359252	-.1092559
HSROC						
Lambda	3.726636	.2679207			3.201521	4.251751
Theta	-1.206134	.2061505			-1.604182	-.796087
beta	.6295111	.1970895	0.15	0.881	-.3567771	.4157994
s2alpha	.58029	.2009854			.2943259	1.144094
s2theta	.415075	.1131522			.2432671	.7082225
Summary pt.						
Se	.6577919	.0287272			.5994902	.7116884
Sp	.9572621	.0059894			.943856	.967577
DOR	43.05422	6.517999			32.00015	57.9268
LR+	15.39129	1.988927			11.94756	19.82764
LR-	.3574863	.0291962			.3046079	.4195441
1/LR-	2.79731	.2284584			2.383539	3.282909

Covariance between estimates of E(logitSe) & E(logitSp) -.0074001

without changing the code syntax. The output in Box 10.2.c shows the meqrlogit command line that was executed along with the estimation log and two tables. The contents of the command line are explained alongside the code in Appendix 3 of the online supplementary material (10.S1 Code for undertaking meta-analysis). The estimation log includes a set of iterations used to refine starting values and a set of gradient-based iterations. By default, these are Newton-Raphson iterations, but other methods are available by specifying the appropriate maximize options. The first estimation table reports the fixed effects and the second table reports the variance components. The first section of the latter is labelled 'studyid: Unstructured', meaning these are random effects at the study level (the studyid variable identifies each study) with unstructured covariance, i.e. each variance and covariance are estimated uniquely from the data.

The five parameters (mean logits, variance and covariance estimates) of the bivariate model are shown in the red boxes. This covariance estimate is the covariance of the logits across studies. Unlike metandi, the output in Box 10.2.c shows the estimate for the covariance instead of the correlation parameter. This is because the variance option displays the random-effects parameter estimates as variances and covariances; to display them as standard deviations and correlations, use the option stddeviations to obtain the output in the red box in Box 10.2.d.

Box 10.2.c Stata output of bivariate model parameters using meqrlogit

```
. meqrlogit true sens spec, nocons|| studyid: sens spec, ///
> nocons cov(un) binomial(n) refineopts(iterate(3)) intpoints(5) variance

Refining starting values:

Iteration 0:   log likelihood = -279.47997
Iteration 1:   log likelihood = -273.46004
Iteration 2:   log likelihood = -273.13205
Iteration 3:   log likelihood = -273.21507

Performing gradient-based optimization:

Iteration 0:   log likelihood = -273.21507
Iteration 1:   log likelihood = -273.07355
Iteration 2:   log likelihood = -273.07286
Iteration 3:   log likelihood = -273.07286
```

Mixed-effects logistic regression			Number of obs	=	74

Binomial variable: n
Group variable: studyid   Number of groups = 37

Obs per group:
```
                                          min =         2
                                          avg =       2.0
                                          max =         2
```

Integration points =   5   Wald chi2(2)   =   668.10
Log likelihood = -273.07286   Prob > chi2   =   0.0000

true	Coef.	Std. Err.	z	P>|z|	[95% Conf. Interval]	
sens	.6534704	.1276192	5.12	0.000	.4033414	.9035994
spec	3.109004	.1464056	21.24	0.000	2.822054	3.395954

Random-effects Parameters	Estimate	Std. Err.	[95% Conf. Interval]	
studyid: Unstructured				
var(sens)	.5438606	.1467555	.3204787	.9229455
var(spec)	.5769862	.1896171	.3029926	1.09875
cov(sens,spec)	-.2699989	.1203215	-.5058247	-.0341731

The contents of the variance–covariance matrix need to be displayed using the `matrix list` command to obtain the covariance between mean logit(sensitivity) and logit(specificity), as shown in the blue box in Box 10.2.e. This covariance and the standard errors of the estimates for mean logit(sensitivity) and logit(specificity) are needed to draw confidence and prediction regions in RevMan.

There are negligible differences in results between `metandi` and `meqrlogit` due to the iterative nature of the maximum likelihood estimation and the choice of

---

Box 10.2.d Stata output of random-effects parameters of the bivariate model as standard deviations using meqrlogit

true	Coef.	Std. Err.	z	P>|z|	[95% Conf. Interval]	
sens	.6534704	.1276192	5.12	0.000	.4033414	.9035994
spec	3.109004	.1464056	21.24	0.000	2.822054	3.395954

Random-effects Parameters	Estimate	Std. Err.	[95% Conf. Interval]	
studyid: Unstructured				
sd(sens)	.7374691	.0994995	.5661083	.9607008
sd(spec)	.7595962	.1248144	.5504477	1.048213
corr(sens,spec)	-.4819871	.1629037	-.735899	-.109227

Box 10.2.e Stata output of variance–covariance matrix after estimation with meqrlogit

```
. matrix list e(V)

symmetric e(V)[5,5]
                       eql:        eql:     lns1_1_1:    lns1_1_2:   atr1_1_1_2:
                       sens        spec        _cons        _cons        _cons
   eql:sens         .01628658
   eql:spec        -.00740014    .02143278
lns1_1_1:_cons       .00082191   -.00005911    .01820336
lns1_1_2:_cons      -.00003298    .00376008    .00318077    .02700229
atr1_1_1_2:_cons     .00040708   -.00037087   -.00526803   -.00502673    .04503202
```

---

options – `intpoints()` and `refineopts()` – that control the process. The option `intpoints(5)` specifies the number of integration points for adaptive Gaussian quadrature, while option `refineopts(iterate(3))` controls the maximization process during the refinement of starting values. Two iterations is the default. Should the analysis fail to converge, one possible solution is to increase the number of integration points and/or iterations. An alternative is to use the `gllamm` command, which appears to be better at obtaining feasible starting values for the likelihood estimation than `xtmelogit` or `meqrlogit`. The code for fitting the bivariate model using `gllamm` and part of the output are available in Appendix 4 of the online supplementary material (10.S1 Code for undertaking meta-analysis). Other suggestions for dealing with convergence issues are considered in Section 10.6.

10.2.3   Fitting the bivariate model using R

Dewey (2018) provides an overview of a range of packages in R for meta-analysis, including meta-analysis of test accuracy studies. Table 10.2.a summarizes the functionality of R packages for meta-analysis of test accuracy that we were aware of in August 2021. It is important to note that not all of the packages in Table 10.2.a are compatible with RevMan,

Table 10.2.a Summary of packages for meta-analysis of test accuracy in R

Package (reference)	Model	Meta-regression	Compatible with RevMan	Other software requirements
lme4 (glmer function in lme4 for fitting GLMMs in R) (Bates 2016)	Bivariate binomial	Yes	Yes	None
mvmeta (Gasparrini 2015)[a]	Bivariate normal	Yes	Yes	None
mada (Doebler 2015)[a]	Bivariate normal[b]	Yes	Yes	None
CopulaDTA (Nyaga 2017)	Bivariate beta-binomial	Yes	No	None
meta4diag (Guo 2015)	Bivariate Bayesian	Yes	No	INLA
bamdit (Verde 2018)	Bivariate Bayesian	No	No	JAGS
diagmeta (Rücker 2020)	Bivariate	No	No	None
CopulaREMADA (Nikoloulopoulos 2015)	Trivariate[c]	No	No	None
NMADiagT (Lu 2020)	Network meta-analysis	No	No	JAGS

GLMM, generalized linear mixed model; INLA, Integrated Nested Laplace Approximation; JAGS, Just Another Gibbs Sampler.
[a] These packages implement the bivariate model with a normal within-study likelihood (i.e. a linear mixed model rather than a GLMM) and are not recommended for Cochrane Reviews of diagnostic test accuracy.
[b] If there are no covariates in the model, mada also generates parameters for the hierarchical summary receiver operating characteristic (HSROC) curve by exploiting the relationship between bivariate and HSROC models.
[c] The trivariate model jointly synthesizes the sensitivity, specificity and prevalence of the target condition.
Source: Adapted from Partlett 2021.

because RevMan is not set up for parameters from such analyses. Ideally, a binomial likelihood should be used to model within-study variability (Chu 2006). Therefore, packages such as mada and mvmeta that use a normal approximation (i.e. a linear mixed model rather than a GLMM), as described by Reitsma (2005), are not recommended for Cochrane Reviews of diagnostic test accuracy. The approximation may lead to biased results due to the unmet assumption of large sample sizes for the number of cases and non-cases, and the use of an ad hoc continuity correction when any of the cells of the 2×2 table is zero.

This section and Section 10.4.3 will focus on the glmer function in the R package lme4 because it fits a bivariate model using a GLMM approach, and also gives output that is compatible with RevMan for generating SROC plots with summary points. The diagmeta package performs meta-analysis using multiple thresholds from each study and will be illustrated in Section 10.7.1.

A free web-based interactive tool, MetaDTA, performs meta-analysis of test accuracy by using the glmer function (Freeman 2019, Patel 2021). MetaDTA is an app powered by RShiny and produces parameter estimates in a format compatible with RevMan. However, there is no option for meta-regression in the current version (version 2.0). MetaDTA supports the upload of different file formats; Figure 10.2.a shows the anti-CCP data uploaded from a .csv file.

The results of the meta-analysis can be viewed on the 'Meta-analysis' tab (Figure 10.2.b). The SROC plot is displayed and the parameter estimates needed for input into RevMan can be downloaded as a .csv file from the 'Parameters for RevMan' tab.

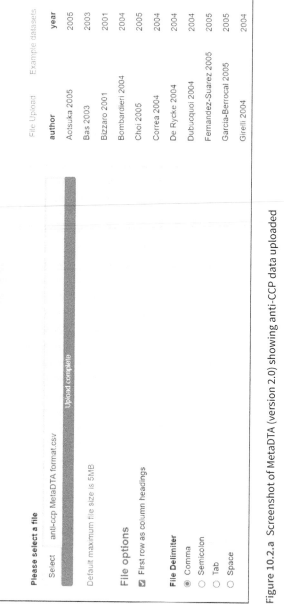

MetaDTA: Diagnostic Test Accuracy Meta-analysis   Home   **Load Data**   Meta-Analysis   Sensitivity Analysis   Prevalence   References   Privacy notice

Please select a file

Select   anti-ccp MetaDTA format.csv

Upload complete

Default maximum file size is 5MB

File options

☑ First row as column headings

File Delimiter

◉ Comma
○ Semicolon
○ Tab
○ Space

File Upload   Example datasets   Data for Analysis

author	year	TP	FN	FP	TN
Aotsuka 2005	2005	115	16	17	73
Bas 2003	2003	110	86	24	215
Bizzaro 2001	2001	40	58	5	227
Bombardieri 2004	2004	23	7	0	39
Choi 2005	2005	236	88	20	231
Correa 2004	2004	74	8	11	130
De Rycke 2004	2004	89	29	4	142
Dubucquoi 2004	2004	90	50	2	129
Fernandez-Suarez 2005	2005	31	22	0	75
Garcia-Berrocal 2005	2005	69	18	8	38
Girelli 2004	2004	25	10	2	40

Figure 10.2.a Screenshot of MetaDTA (version 2.0) showing anti-CCP data uploaded

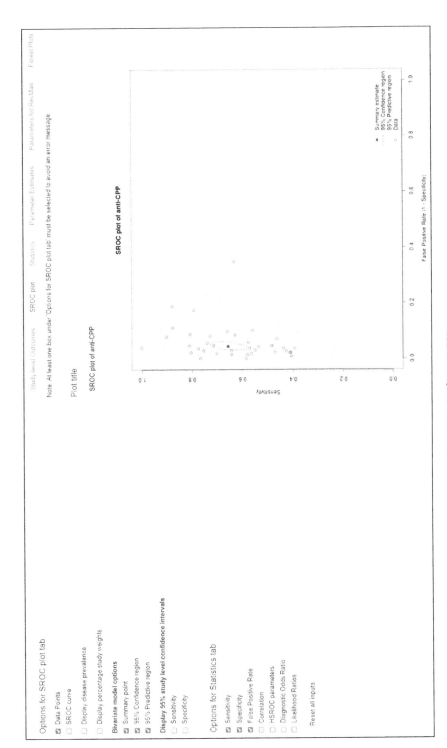

Figure 10.2.b Screenshot of MetaDTA (version 2.0) showing the SROC plot for anti-CCP

Box 10.2.f R output of bivariate model parameters using glmer

```
## Generalized linear mixed model fit by maximum likelihood (Laplace
##    Approximation) [glmerMod]
##  Family: binomial  (logit)
## Formula: cbind(true, n - true) ~ 0 + sens + spec + (0 + sens + spec |
##       Study.ID)
##    Data: Y
##
##      AIC      BIC   logLik deviance df.resid
##    555.6    567.1   -272.8    545.6       69
##
## Scaled residuals:
##     Min      1Q  Median      3Q     Max
## -1.9629 -0.2391  0.0097  0.2396  1.9864
##
## Random effects:
##  Groups    Name Variance Std.Dev.  Corr
##  Study.ID sens 0.5426   0.7366
##           spec 0.5712   0.7558   -0.49
## Number of obs: 74, groups:  Study.ID, 37
##
## Fixed effects:
##        Estimate Std. Error z value Pr(>|z|)
## sens    0.6534      0.1274   5.127 2.95e-07 ***
## spec    3.1084      0.1451  21.420  < 2e-16 ***
## ---
## Signif. codes:  0 '***' 0.001 '**' 0.01 '*' 0.05 '.' 0.1 ' ' 1
```

The code provided in Appendix 5 of the online supplementary material (10.S1 Code for undertaking meta-analysis) shows how to load the data, fit the bivariate model using `glmer`, and obtain the summary estimates. Box 10.2.f shows the output obtained after summarizing the `glmer` model output. The five parameters (mean logits, variances and correlation) of the bivariate model are shown in the red boxes. This correlation estimate is the correlation of the logits across studies. In the `glmer` function, the nAGQ argument controls the number of quadrature points. The default is nAGQ = 1, which equates to the Laplace approximation (see green box). Values greater than 1 produce greater accuracy in the evaluation of the log-likelihood. However, when there is more than one random-effects parameter in the model, the number of quadrature points used by `glmer` cannot be increased. This is a limitation of using `glmer` to fit the bivariate model, since the standard model without a covariate has two random-effects parameters.

The variance-covariance matrix can be displayed to obtain the covariance between the summary estimates of logit(sensitivity) and logit(specificity), as shown in the blue box in Box 10.2.g. This covariance and the parameter estimates are needed to generate the SROC plot in RevMan.

Box 10.2.g R output of variance–covariance matrix

```
(summary(MA_Y))$vcov
```

```
## 2 × 2 Matrix of class "dpoMatrix"
##              sens           spec
## sens   0.016241813  -0.007404185
## spec  -0.007404185   0.021058854
```

10.2.4   Bayesian estimation of the bivariate model

10.2.4.1   Specification of the bivariate model in rjags

Both levels of the bivariate model introduced in Chapter 9, Section 9.4.1, must be specified in rjags. This section covers the different components of this rjags model, which is the core of the code (see Box 10.2.h). The complete program is in Appendix 6 of the online supplementary material (10.S1 Code for undertaking meta-analysis), Section A6.1.

- Likelihood: The likelihood specifies that the observed data (TP and TN cells) in each study follow a binomial distribution, with the unknown parameters being the sensitivity (se) and specificity (sp) in each study.
- Prior distribution: To carry out Bayesian estimation, a prior distribution function must be specified for each unknown parameter in the likelihood. As this is a prior distribution for a meta-analysis model, it has a hierarchical structure. At the first level of the hierarchy, sensitivity and specificity parameters in the individual studies are assumed to have the same prior distribution. This is specified by assuming the logit sensitivities and logit specificities of the included studies follow a bivariate normal distribution whose mean is the vector (mean logit sensitivity (mu[1]), mean logit specificity (mu[2])) and whose variance–covariance matrix is parametrized by the between-study standard deviation in the logit sensitivities (tau[1]), the between-study standard deviation in the logit specificities (tau[2]) and the correlation between the logit sensitivities and the logit specificities (rho). Specifying the prior distribution for the logit(sensitivity) (l[,1]) and logit(specificity) (l[,2]) rather than for the sensitivity and specificity parameters directly makes it easier to expand the meta-analysis to a meta-regression model in Section 10.4.

At the second level of the hierarchy, prior distributions are provided for the parameters mu[1], mu[2], prec[1], prec[2] and rho, where prec[1] and prec[2] are the between-study precision in the logit sensitivities and logit specificities, respectively. The between-study precision is the inverse of the between-study variance, e.g. prec[1] = 1/tau.sq[1]. These prior distributions are typically defined to be vague, i.e. their parameter values are selected so they have a negligible influence on the results of the meta-analysis.

- Summary sensitivity and specificity: The mean logit(sensitivity) and mean logit(specificity) are transformed to the probability scale to obtain the summary sensitivity (Summary_Se) and summary specificity (Summary_Sp) across studies.

Box 10.2.h Specification of the bivariate model for Bayesian estimation in rjags

```
model {
#=== LIKELIHOOD ===#
for(i in 1:n) {
TP[i] ~ dbin(se[i],pos[i])
TN[i] ~ dbin(sp[i],neg[i])
# === PRIOR DISTRIBUTIONS FOR INDIVIDUAL LOGIT SENSITIVITY,
SPECIFICITY === #
logit(se[i]) <- l[i,1]
logit(sp[i]) <- l[i,2]
l[i,1:2] ~ dmnorm(mu[], T[,])
}
#=== HYPER PRIOR DISTRIBUTIONS MEAN LOGIT SENSITIVITY AND
SPECIFICITY === #
mu[1] ~ dnorm(0,0.25)
mu[2] ~ dnorm(0,0.25)
# Between-study variance-covariance matrix
T[1:2,1:2]<-inverse(TAU[1:2,1:2])
TAU[1,1] <- tau[1]*tau[1]
TAU[2,2] <- tau[2]*tau[2]
TAU[1,2] <- rho*tau[1]*tau[2]
TAU[2,1] <- rho*tau[1]*tau[2]
#=== HYPER PRIOR DISTRIBUTIONS FOR PRECISION OF LOGIT
SENSITIVITY ===#
#=== AND LOGIT SPECIFICITY, AND CORRELATION BETWEEN THEM === #
prec[1] ~ dgamma(2,0.5)
prec[2] ~ dgamma(2,0.5)
rho ~ dunif(-1,1)
# ===  PARAMETERS OF INTEREST === #
# BETWEEN-STUDY VARIANCE OF LOGIT SENSITIVITY AND SPECIFICITY
tau.sq[1]<-pow(prec[1],-1)
tau.sq[2]<-pow(prec[2],-1)
# BETWEEN-STUDY STANDARD DEVIATION OF LOGIT SENSITIVITY
AND SPECIFICITY
tau[1]<-pow(prec[1],-0.5)
tau[2]<-pow(prec[2],-0.5)
# SUMMARY SENSITIVITY AND SPECIFICITY
Summary_Se <- 1/(1+exp(-mu[1]))
Summary_Sp <- 1/(1+exp(-mu[2]))
# PREDICTED SENSITIVITY AND SPECIFICITY IN A NEW STUDY
l.predicted[1:2] ~ dmnorm(mu[],T[,])
Predicted_Se <- 1/(1+exp(-l.predicted[1]))
Predicted_Sp <- 1/(1+exp(-l.predicted[2]))
}
```

- Predicted sensitivity and specificity: Calculation of the predicted sensitivity and specificity parameters in a future study can be done by adding a line within the rjags model specifying the distribution of logit(sensitivity) and logit(specificity) (l.predicted) in a single, future study. This would be the same bivariate normal distribution as the observed studies in the meta-analysis. Transforming back to the probability scale gives posterior distributions for the predicted sensitivity (Predicted_Se) and predicted specificity (Predicted_Sp) in a future study.

10.2.4.2 Monitoring convergence

Convergence of the MCMC algorithm can be examined by running multiple MCMC chains with different starting values and examining the results using graphs such as those in Figure 10.2.c, created using the mcmcplots package in R (see Appendix 6 of the online supplementary material (10.S1 Code for undertaking meta-analysis) for the complete R script used to generate Figure 10.2.c). In Figure 10.2.c, results from three chains (identified by different colours) are superimposed. Panel (a) shows posterior density plots for Summary_Se; (b) the running posterior mean value; and (c) the history plots for Summary_Se. The very similar results from all three chains suggest that the algorithm converged to the same solution in each case.

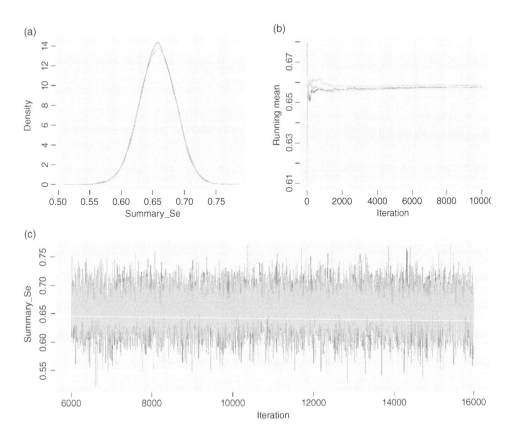

Figure 10.2.c MCMC diagnostics plots for a parameter (Summary_Se) from the bivariate model

Besides these graphs, many statistics for assessing convergence have been described. A well-known statistic for assessing convergence is the Gelman-Rubin statistic, which can be calculated separately for each parameter in the model. When this statistic diverges from 1 there is concern that the MCMC algorithm has not converged.

10.2.4.3 Summary statistics

Once convergence of the MCMC algorithm is achieved, summary statistics of the parameters of interest may be extracted from their posterior distributions. Output from the rjags program is given in Box 10.2.i. The focus here is on the mean and predicted values

---

Box 10.2.i Rjags output from Bayesian estimation of the bivariate model

```
Iterations = 26001:46000
Thinning interval = 1
Number of chains = 3
Sample size per chain = 20000
1. Empirical mean and standard deviation for each variable,
     plus standard error of the mean:
                   Mean       SD   Naive SE Time-series SE
Summary_Se     0.6575 0.028885 1.179e-04      1.924e-04
Summary_Sp     0.9568 0.005987 2.444e-05      5.896e-05
Predicted_Se   0.6427 0.155745 6.358e-04      6.469e-04
Predicted_Sp   0.9453 0.043130 1.761e-04      1.815e-04
mu[1]          0.6550 0.128844 5.260e-04      8.592e-04
mu[2]          3.1062 0.145372 5.935e-04      1.456e-03
rho           -0.4253 0.156699 6.397e-04      1.817e-03
tau.sq[1]      0.5546 0.151128 8.725e-04      2.040e-03
tau.sq[2]      0.5699 0.186720 1.078e-03      3.853e-03
2. Quantiles for each variable:
                  2.5%      25%      50%      75%     97.5%
Summary_Se     0.5996   0.6386   0.6578   0.6770   0.71300
Summary_Sp     0.9442   0.9530   0.9570   0.9609   0.96780
Predicted_Se   0.3045   0.5404   0.6590   0.7608   0.89549
Predicted_Sp   0.8303   0.9310   0.9569   0.9733   0.99033
mu[1]          0.4037   0.5692   0.6536   0.7401   0.90998
mu[2]          2.8282   3.0088   3.1028   3.2007   3.40312
rho           -0.6993  -0.5378  -0.4362  -0.3248  -0.09108
tau.sq[1]      0.3276   0.4482   0.5318   0.6367   0.91251
tau.sq[2]      0.2907   0.4373   0.5400   0.6714   1.01380
```

of sensitivity and specificity, but other parameters, such as the sensitivities and specificities in individual studies, may also be extracted. The logit-transformed mean sensitivity and specificity and the between-study variances and correlation are also reported (red box) in Box 10.2.i. Note that the posterior standard deviation (SD) estimated (blue box) is the standard error in frequentist terms. The results obtained using a Bayesian approach are similar to those obtained using a frequentist approach (see Box 10.2.b and Box 10.2.f).

It is common to report the posterior median values of the summary sensitivity and summary specificity, which would be 0.6578 and 0.9570, respectively, in this example, to cover the possibility that the posterior distribution is skewed. In the current example, it so happens that the posterior mean and posterior median values of the summary sensitivity and summary specificity are in fact quite similar. Obtaining a 95% credible interval is straightforward and does not require gathering values of the standard errors or the covariance parameters. To obtain a 95% equal-tailed credible interval for a parameter, use the 2.5% and 97.5% quantiles of its posterior distribution. These quantiles and the median are shown in the green boxes in Box 10.2.i. The 95% credible interval for the summary sensitivity is (0.5996, 0.7130), while the 95% credible interval for the summary specificity is (0.9442, 0.9678). Each of these intervals can be interpreted as having 95% probability of including the true value of the parameter given the observed data.

There is considerable between-study variability in both sensitivity and specificity. This is reflected in the much wider 95% prediction intervals (i.e. the 95% credible interval around the predicted values) compared to the 95% credible intervals for the mean values.

10.2.4.4 Generating an SROC plot
In this section we describe two ways of obtaining the SROC plot following Bayesian estimation with rjags.

- **SROC plot with the DTAplots package:** The package DTAplots within R was used to produce the plot in Figure 10.2.d with a 95% credible region (red line) and 95% prediction region (black dotted line) around the summary estimates of sensitivity and specificity (solid black circle). The posterior samples and the number of studies were provided as arguments to the SROC_rjags function (see Appendix 6 of the online supplementary material (10.S1 Code for undertaking meta-analysis), Section A6.1). The points on the plot represent sensitivity and specificity estimates in individual studies scaled according to sample size. The plot is very similar to Chapter 9, Figure 9.4.a, obtained with a frequentist approach. As already observed in Figure 9.4.a, the prediction region is much larger than the credible region due to considerable heterogeneity in the sensitivity and specificity estimates across studies. The DTAplots package uses the point estimates from the rjags output (Box 10.2.i) in the equations from Harbord (2007) to obtain the SROC plot.
- **SROC plot in RevMan:** In order to create a similar figure in RevMan, in addition to the point estimates of mu[1], mu[2], rho, tau.sq[1] and tau.sq[2] provided in the red and blue boxes in Box 10.2.i, the covariance between the posterior samples of the mean logit-transformed sensitivity and mean logit-transformed specificity must be provided. This term can be computed by adding an extra line to the R script (see Appendix 6 of the online supplementary material (10.S1 Code for undertaking meta-analysis), Section A6.1).

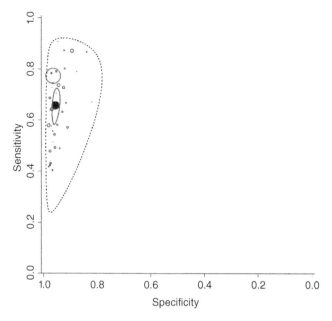

Figure 10.2.d SROC plot of anti-CCP for rheumatoid arthritis showing 95% credible and 95% prediction regions

10.2.4.5 Sensitivity analyses

As already noted, Bayesian estimation of the bivariate model typically relies on vague prior distribution functions. Since there is no unique way to specify a vague prior distribution, it is important to verify the impact of using an alternative vague prior distribution. It has been shown that when the number of studies is small (fewer than 10), results can be highly sensitive to the choice of prior distribution over the between-study variability parameters (Spiegelhalter 2004). In Box 10.2.h Gamma priors were used over the precision parameters. An alternative approach would be to use a uniform or half-normal prior distribution over the standard deviation parameters, tau[1] and tau[2].

10.3   Estimation of a summary curve

As described in Chapter 9, Section 9.4.3, the focus of the HSROC model is the estimation of a summary curve. When no covariates are included, the HSROC model has five parameters: the accuracy parameter with mean Λ (capital lambda) and variance σ_α^2; the positivity (threshold) parameter with mean Θ (capital theta) and variance σ_θ^2; and the shape parameter β. Rheumatoid factor (RF) for diagnosis of rheumatoid arthritis was used to illustrate the Rutter and Gatsonis HSROC model in Chapter 9, Section 9.4.4, and is the example used in this section. The sensitivities and specificities of the 50 included studies are shown on a forest plot (Figure 10.3.a) along with their thresholds for defining test positivity and RF measurement method.

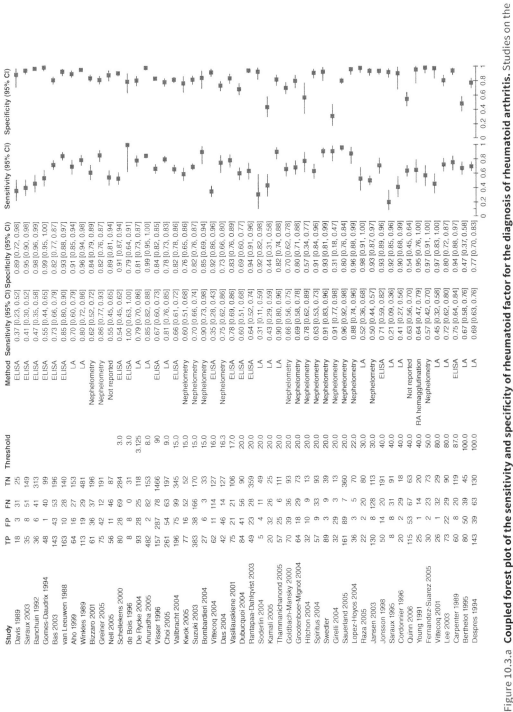

Study	TP	FP	FN	TN	Threshold	Method	Sensitivity (95% CI)	Specificity (95% CI)
Davis 1989	18	3	31	25		ELISA	0.37 [0.23, 0.52]	0.89 [0.72, 0.98]
Saraux 2003	35	8	51	149		ELISA	0.41 [0.30, 0.52]	0.95 [0.90, 0.98]
Banchuin 1992	36	6	41	313		ELISA	0.47 [0.35, 0.58]	0.98 [0.96, 0.99]
Gomes-Daudrix 1994	48	1	40	99		ELISA	0.55 [0.44, 0.65]	0.99 [0.95, 1.00]
Bas 2003	143	43	53	196		ELISA	0.73 [0.66, 0.79]	0.82 [0.77, 0.87]
van Leeuwen 1988	163	10	28	140		ELISA	0.85 [0.80, 0.90]	0.93 [0.88, 0.97]
Aho 1999	64	16	27	153		LA	0.70 [0.60, 0.79]	0.91 [0.85, 0.94]
Winkles 1989	113	19	29	481		LA	0.80 [0.72, 0.86]	0.96 [0.94, 0.98]
Bizzaro 2001	61	36	37	196		Nephelometry	0.62 [0.52, 0.72]	0.84 [0.79, 0.89]
Greiner 2005	75	42	12	191		Nephelometry	0.86 [0.77, 0.93]	0.82 [0.76, 0.87]
Nell 2005	56	11	46	87		Not reported	0.55 [0.45, 0.65]	0.89 [0.81, 0.94]
Schellekens 2000	80	28	69	284	3.0	ELISA	0.54 [0.45, 0.62]	0.91 [0.87, 0.94]
de Bois 1996	8	8	0	31	3.0	ELISA	1.00 [0.63, 1.00]	0.79 [0.64, 0.91]
De Rycke 2004	93	28	25	118	3.125	LA	0.79 [0.70, 0.86]	0.81 [0.73, 0.87]
Anuradha 2005	482	2	82	153	8.0	LA	0.85 [0.82, 0.88]	0.99 [0.95, 1.00]
Visser 1996	157	287	78	1466	90	ELISA	0.67 [0.60, 0.73]	0.84 [0.82, 0.85]
Choi 2005	261	54	63	197	9.0	LA	0.81 [0.76, 0.85]	0.78 [0.73, 0.83]
Vallbracht 2004	196	75	99	345	15.0	ELISA	0.66 [0.61, 0.72]	0.82 [0.78, 0.86]
Kwok 2005	77	16	52	52	15.0	Nephelometry	0.60 [0.51, 0.68]	0.76 [0.65, 0.86]
Suzuki 2003	383	38	166	170	15.0	Nephelometry	0.70 [0.66, 0.74]	0.82 [0.76, 0.87]
Bombardieri 2004	27	6	3	33	15.0	Nephelometry	0.90 [0.73, 0.98]	0.85 [0.69, 0.94]
Vittecoq 2004	62	11	114	127	16.0	ELISA	0.35 [0.28, 0.43]	0.92 [0.86, 0.96]
Das 2004	42	46	14	127	16.3	Nephelometry	0.75 [0.62, 0.86]	0.73 [0.66, 0.80]
Vasiliauskiene 2001	75	21	21	106	17.0	ELISA	0.78 [0.69, 0.86]	0.83 [0.76, 0.89]
Dubucquoi 2004	84	41	56	90	20.0	ELISA	0.60 [0.51, 0.68]	0.69 [0.60, 0.77]
Pantapaa-Dahlqvist 2003	49	23	28	359	20.0	ELISA	0.64 [0.52, 0.74]	0.94 [0.91, 0.96]
Soderlin 2004	5	4	11	49	20.0	LA	0.31 [0.11, 0.59]	0.92 [0.82, 0.98]
Kamali 2005	20	32	26	25	20.0	LA	0.43 [0.29, 0.59]	0.44 [0.31, 0.58]
Thammanichanond 2005	57	25	6	111	20.0	LA	0.90 [0.80, 0.96]	0.82 [0.74, 0.88]
Goldbach-Mansky 2000	70	39	36	93	20.0	Nephelometry	0.66 [0.56, 0.75]	0.70 [0.62, 0.78]
Grootenboer-Mignot 2004	64	18	29	73	20.0	Nephelometry	0.69 [0.58, 0.78]	0.80 [0.71, 0.88]
Hitchon 2004	32	10	9	13	20.0	Nephelometry	0.78 [0.62, 0.89]	0.57 [0.34, 0.77]
Spiritus 2004	57	9	33	93	20.0	Nephelometry	0.63 [0.53, 0.73]	0.91 [0.84, 0.96]
Swedler	89	3	9	39	20.0	Nephelometry	0.91 [0.83, 0.96]	0.93 [0.81, 0.99]
Girelli 2004	32	29	3	13	20.0	Nephelometry	0.91 [0.77, 0.98]	0.31 [0.18, 0.47]
Sauerland 2005	161	89	7	360	20.0	Nephelometry	0.96 [0.92, 0.98]	0.80 [0.76, 0.84]
Lopez-Hoyos 2004	36	3	5	70	22.0	Nephelometry	0.88 [0.74, 0.96]	0.96 [0.88, 0.99]
Raza 2005	22	2	20	80	30.0	LA	0.52 [0.36, 0.68]	0.98 [0.91, 1.00]
Jansen 2003	130	8	128	113	30.0	Nephelometry	0.50 [0.44, 0.57]	0.93 [0.87, 0.97]
Jonsson 1998	50	14	20	191	40.0	ELISA	0.71 [0.59, 0.82]	0.93 [0.89, 0.96]
Saraux 1995	8	8	31	91	40.0	LA	0.21 [0.09, 0.36]	0.92 [0.85, 0.96]
Cordonnier 1996	20	2	29	18	40.0	LA	0.41 [0.27, 0.56]	0.90 [0.68, 0.99]
Quinn 2006	115	53	67	63	40.0	Not reported	0.63 [0.56, 0.70]	0.54 [0.45, 0.64]
Young 1991	25	1	14	20	40.0	RA hemagglutination	0.64 [0.47, 0.79]	0.95 [0.76, 1.00]
Fernandez-Suarez 2005	30	3	23	73	50.0	Nephelometry	0.57 [0.42, 0.70]	0.97 [0.91, 1.00]
Vittecoq 2001	26	1	32	29	80.0	LA	0.45 [0.32, 0.58]	0.97 [0.83, 1.00]
Lee 2003	73	22	29	90	80.0	LA	0.72 [0.62, 0.80]	0.80 [0.72, 0.87]
Carpenter 1989	60	8	20	119	87.0	ELISA	0.75 [0.64, 0.84]	0.94 [0.88, 0.97]
Berthelot 1995	80	50	39	45	100.0	LA	0.67 [0.58, 0.76]	0.47 [0.37, 0.58]
Despres 1994	143	39	63	130	100.0	LA	0.69 [0.63, 0.76]	0.77 [0.70, 0.83]

Figure 10.3.a **Coupled forest plot of the sensitivity and specificity of rheumatoid factor for the diagnosis of rheumatoid arthritis.** Studies on the plot are sorted by threshold, method of measurement and sensitivity. ELISA, enzyme-linked immunosorbent assay; LA, latex agglutination; RA, rheumatoid arthritis. Source: Data taken from Nishimura 2007.

Box 10.3.a SAS output of HSROC model parameters

Parameter Estimates

Parameter	Estimate	Standard Error	DF	t Value	Pr > |t|	95% Confidence Limits		Gradient
alpha	2.6016	0.1862	48	13.97	<.0001	2.2273	2.9759	0.000069
theta	-0.4370	0.1469	48	-2.98	0.0046	-0.7323	-0.1417	0.000103
beta	0.2267	0.1624	48	1.40	0.1691	-0.09978	0.5532	0.000039
s2ua	1.3014	0.3046	48	4.27	<.0001	0.6890	1.9138	0.000020
s2ut	0.5423	0.1237	48	4.39	<.0001	0.2936	0.7909	-0.00012

10.3.1 Fitting the HSROC model using SAS

The HSROC model was used to estimate a summary curve using `Proc NLMIXED` in SAS (see code in Appendix 7 of the online supplementary material (10.S1 Code for undertaking meta-analysis)) to obtain the output shown in Box 10.3.a.

The parameter estimates in the red box can be entered into RevMan to draw the summary curve shown in Chapter 9, Figure 9.4.b; the estimate of the mean for accuracy (Λ, lambda) is 2.6016, −0.4370 for the mean for threshold (Θ, theta), 0.2267 for the shape parameter (β, beta), 1.3014 for the variance of the random effects for accuracy $\left(\sigma_\alpha^2\right)$, and 0.5423 for the variance of the random effects for threshold $\left(\sigma_\theta^2\right)$.

Estimation of a summary sensitivity and specificity are not clinically meaningful estimates for RF, since the 50 studies used different thresholds for RF. However, the expected sensitivity at a chosen specificity (or vice versa) can be computed from the fitted curve by using the equation given by

$$\text{logit}(\text{sensitivity}) = \Lambda e^{-0.5\beta} + \text{logit}(1 - \text{specificity})e^{-\beta}.$$

The equation can be included in an `ESTIMATE` statement in `NLMIXED` (see code in Appendix 7 of the online supplementary material (10.S1 Code for undertaking meta-analysis)). The `ESTIMATE` statement computes additional estimates as a function of parameter values and produces standard errors and confidence intervals using the delta method. For RF, the median (interquartile range) of specificities from the 50 studies was 0.87 (0.80 to 0.93). These three values of specificity were used in `ESTIMATE` statements to obtain the corresponding values of sensitivity and their 95% CIs. The estimates of logit(sensitivity) with their 95% CIs are presented in the additional estimates table in the SAS output, as shown in the red boxes in Box 10.3.b. Inverse transformations of the logit estimates (see equations in Section 10.2.1) give the estimates of sensitivity and their 95% CIs at the fixed values of specificity.

10.3.2 Bayesian estimation of the HSROC model

10.3.2.1 Specification of the HSROC model in rjags

The HSROC model equations introduced in Chapter 9, Section 9.4.3, are written out directly in rjags. This section covers the different components of this rjags model, which is the core of the program (comment lines separate the components in Box 10.3.c).

Box 10.3.b SAS output of additional estimates produced using HSROC model parameters

										Specificity	Sensitivity (95% CI)
		Additional Estimates									
Label	Estimate	Standard Error	DF	t Value	Pr > |t|	Alpha	Lower	Upper			
E(logitSe_sp80)	1.2177	0.1697	48	7.18	<.0001	0.05	0.8765	1.5589		0.80	0.77 (0.71 to 0.83)
E(logitSe_sp87)	0.8074	0.1553	48	5.20	<.0001	0.05	0.4952	1.1197		0.87	0.69 (0.62 to 0.75)
E(logitSe_sp93)	0.2608	0.1780	48	1.46	0.1494	0.05	-0.09713	0.6187		0.93	0.56 (0.48 to 0.65)

Box 10.3.c Specification of the HSROC model for Bayesian estimation in rjags

```
model {

# === LIKELIHOOD === #

for(i in 1:n) {

TP[i] ~ dbin(TPR[i],pos[i])
FP[i] ~ dbin(FPR[i],neg[i])

# === PRIOR DISTRIBUTIONS FOR TPR AND FPR === #

logit(TPR[i]) <- (theta[i] + 0.5*alpha[i])/exp(beta/2)
logit(FPR[i]) <- (theta[i] - 0.5*alpha[i])*exp(beta/2)
theta[i] ~ dnorm(THETA,prec[2])
alpha[i] ~ dnorm(LAMBDA,prec[1])

}

### === HYPER PRIOR DISTRIBUTIONS === ###

THETA ~ dunif(-10,10)
LAMBDA ~ dunif(-2,20)
beta ~ dunif(-5,5)
for(i in 1:2) {
prec[i] ~ dgamma(2.1,2)
tau.sq[i] <- 1/prec[i]
tau[i] <- pow(tau.sq[i],0.5)

}
}
```

- Likelihood: The likelihood specifies that the observed data in each study, the TP and FP cells, follow a binomial distribution with probability TPR (true positive rate) and FPR (false positive rate), respectively (Box 10.3.c).
- Prior distributions: The parameters logit TPR and logit FPR are expressed as functions of three additional parameters: the proxy for positivity threshold (theta) for each study, the lnDOR (alpha) for each study and the shape parameter (beta) (β in Chapter 9, Section 9.4.3), which is assumed to be common across studies. The parameters theta and alpha are assumed to follow hierarchical prior distributions, thus allowing for

both within-study and between-study variability. The theta parameters are assumed to have a normal prior distribution with mean THETA (Θ) and precision prec[2] ($=\frac{1}{\sigma_\theta^2}$, where σ_θ^2 is referred to as tau.sq[2] in Box 10.3.c and is the variance for the theta parameters). The alpha parameters are assumed to have a normal prior distribution with mean LAMBDA (Λ) and precision prec[1] ($=\frac{1}{\sigma_\alpha^2}$, where σ_α^2 is referred to as tau. sq[1] in Box 10.3.c and is the variance for the alpha parameters). The parameters THETA, prec[2], LAMBDA, prec[1] and beta are provided with vague prior distributions, with the intention that they have a negligible impact on the results.

10.3.2.2 Monitoring convergence

Detailed information on how to run the rjags program in Box 10.3.c is given in Appendix 6 of the online supplementary material (10.S1 Code for undertaking meta-analysis), Section A6.2. Here, the focus is on interpreting the results of the program when applied to the rheumatoid factor data of Nishimura (2007) introduced in Chapter 9. As in the case of the bivariate model (see Section 10.2.4.2), begin by examining whether the MCMC algorithm converged. Figure 10.3.b shows the diagnostics plots for LAMBDA, but similar plots can be obtained for all parameters. These plots, created using the mcmcplots

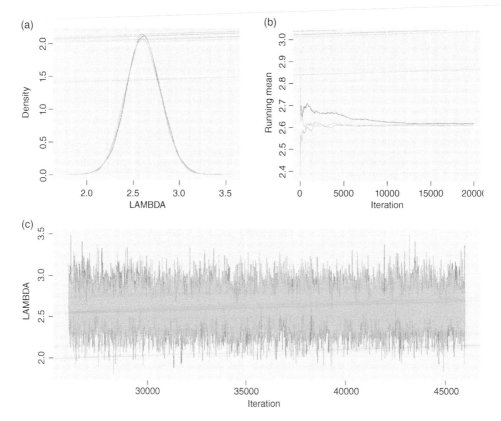

Figure 10.3.b MCMC diagnostics plots for a parameter (LAMBDA) from the HSROC model

---

Box 10.3.d Rjags output from Bayesian estimation of the HSROC model

```
Iterations = 6001:16000

Thinning interval = 1

Number of chains = 3

Sample size per chain = 10000

1. Empirical mean and standard deviation for each
variable,
    plus standard error of the mean:
              Mean        SD   Naive SE Time-series SE
LAMBDA      2.6187 0.191119 1.103e-03       3.787e-03
THETA      -0.4490 0.152213 8.788e-04       5.690e-03
beta        0.2155 0.163026 9.412e-04       8.912e-03
tau.sq[1]   1.3781 0.321925 1.859e-03       2.875e-03
tau.sq[2]   0.6241 0.139763 8.069e-04       1.133e-03

2. Quantiles for each variable:
             2.5%      25%      50%      75%     97.5%
LAMBDA     2.2434   2.4922   2.6167   2.7448   2.9985
THETA     -0.7518  -0.5516  -0.4476  -0.3460  -0.1534
beta      -0.1066   0.1069   0.2189   0.3256   0.5348
tau.sq[1]  0.8750   1.1481   1.3378   1.5589   2.1281
tau.sq[2]  0.4034   0.5243   0.6065   0.7036   0.9472
```

---

package in R, suggest that the MCMC algorithm has converged, as the results from the three independent MCMC chains (identified by different colours) with different initial values overlap nearly perfectly. The running mean plot in panel (b) shows some discordance between the chains when the number of iterations is small, but the values on the y-axis indicate that the apparent differences are in fact very small.

10.3.2.3 Summary statistics and SROC plot

Following successful convergence of the MCMC algorithm, the summary statistics of the parameters of interest can be calculated using a sample from the posterior distribution. Output from the rjags program (see red box in Box 10.3.d) gives the estimates for LAMBDA, THETA and beta, and the between-study variance of alpha (tau.sq[1]) and theta (tau.sq[2]). For comparison, see the results in Section 10.3.1 that were obtained using a frequentist approach in SAS.

The summary curve on the SROC plot (Figure 10.3.c) from the Bayesian estimation using the DTAplots package is very similar to the curve from the frequentist estimation (Chapter 9, Figure 9.4.b). Study points on the plot were scaled according to sample size. This plot can also be obtained in RevMan by providing the parameter estimates in the red box in Box 10.3.d.

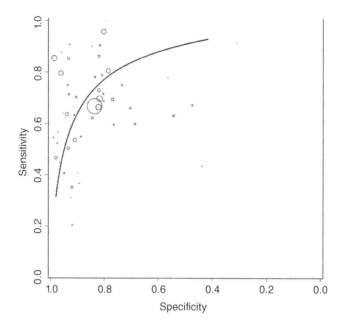

Figure 10.3.c SROC plot of rheumatoid factor for rheumatoid arthritis

10.3.2.4 Sensitivity analyses

As already noted, Bayesian estimation of the HSROC model typically relies on vague prior distribution functions. Since there is no unique way to specify a vague prior distribution, it is important to verify the impact of using an alternative vague prior distribution, as indicated in Section 10.2.4.5. In Box 10.3.c Gamma priors were used over the precision parameters. An alternative approach would be to use a uniform or half-normal prior distribution over the standard deviation parameters.

10.4 Comparison of summary points

The bivariate model is a regression model that can be extended to incorporate covariates (i.e. meta-regression) to compare summary points (see Chapter 9, Section 9.4.6.2 and Section 9.4.7.2). In Chapter 9, Section 9.4.6.3, a bivariate meta-regression was used to investigate heterogeneity by assessing differences in the sensitivity and specificity of two different generations of the anti-CCP test for diagnosis of rheumatoid arthritis. Similarly, a bivariate meta-regression was used in Chapter 9, Section 9.4.7.3, to compare the accuracy of two imaging modalities – multislice computed tomography (CT) and magnetic resonance imaging (MRI) – for diagnosis of coronary artery disease (CAD). For both analyses, the variances of the random effects were assumed to be equal for the logit sensitivities and the logit specificities.

The assumption of equal variances for the random effects of the logit sensitivities and the logit specificities of different subgroups may be reasonable in many situations when investigating heterogeneity in the accuracy of a single test, but less so when comparing the accuracy of different tests. For ease of reference, subgroups or tests will simply be referred to as 'group' in the model specifications. The model that allows for unequal vari-ances for each group can be written as

$$\begin{pmatrix} \mu_{Aik} \\ \mu_{Bik} \end{pmatrix} \sim N \left[\begin{pmatrix} \mu_A + v_A Z_k \\ \mu_B + v_B Z_k \end{pmatrix}, \begin{pmatrix} \sigma_{Ak}^2 & \sigma_{ABk} \\ \sigma_{ABk} & \sigma_{Bk}^2 \end{pmatrix} \right], \tag{10.1}$$

where μ_{Aik} and μ_{Bik} are the logit(sensitivity) and logit(specificity) for the kth group in the ith study; Z_k represents the study-level covariate; μ_A estimates the mean logit(sensitivity) for the referent group (note that for test comparisons this is not the reference standard but another index test); μ_B estimates the mean logit(specificity) for the referent group; $\mu_A + v_A Z_k$ estimates the mean logit(sensitivity) for the kth group; and $\mu_B + v_B Z_k$ estimates the mean logit(specificity) for the kth group. Hence, $exp(v_A)$ and $exp(v_B)$ estimate the odds ratio for sensitivity and specificity in the kth group relative to the referent group. The parameters σ_{Ak}^2 and σ_{Bk}^2 are the variances for the logit sensitivities and logit specifi-cities for the kth group; and σ_{ABk} is the covariance between the logits across studies evaluating the group (Takwoingi 2016). The variance–covariance structure in equa-tion 10.1 is typically modelled assuming independence between groups. For a binary covariate (e.g. two tests), this variance–covariance matrix can be expressed as

$$\begin{bmatrix} \mu_{Ai1} \\ \mu_{Ai2} \\ \mu_{Bi1} \\ \mu_{Bi2} \end{bmatrix} \sim N \left(\begin{pmatrix} \mu_A \\ \mu_B \end{pmatrix}, \Sigma \right) \text{with} \Sigma = \begin{bmatrix} \sigma_{A1}^2 & 0 & \sigma_{A1B1} & 0 \\ & \sigma_{A2}^2 & 0 & \sigma_{A2B2} \\ & & \sigma_{B1}^2 & 0 \\ & & & \sigma_{B2}^2 \end{bmatrix}. \tag{10.2}$$

The means $\mu_A = \begin{pmatrix} \mu_{A1} \\ \mu_{A2} \end{pmatrix}$ and $\mu_B = \begin{pmatrix} \mu_{B1} \\ \mu_{B2} \end{pmatrix}$ are column vectors of the means of logit sensi-tivities and logit specificities for the two groups. Since test comparisons may include only studies that used a paired design in which individuals received all index tests, the bivariate model can allow for correlation in test performance between tests by estimat-ing all between-study and between-test variability using the following unstructured variance-covariance matrix:

$$\begin{bmatrix} \mu_{Ai1} \\ \mu_{Ai2} \\ \mu_{Bi1} \\ \mu_{Bi2} \end{bmatrix} \sim N \left(\begin{pmatrix} \mu_A \\ \mu_B \end{pmatrix}, \Sigma \right) \text{with} \Sigma = \begin{bmatrix} \sigma_{A1}^2 & \sigma_{A1A2} & \sigma_{A1B1} & \sigma_{A1B2} \\ & \sigma_{A2}^2 & \sigma_{A2B1} & \sigma_{A2B2} \\ & & \sigma_{B1}^2 & \sigma_{B1B2} \\ & & & \sigma_{B2}^2 \end{bmatrix}. \tag{10.3}$$

Note that potential within-study correlation between tests is not taken into account in equation 10.3 – this would require individual participant data or aggregate data in the form of 2×4 tables of the results of two index tests cross-classified for individuals with and for those without the target condition. Such tables are seldom reported in primary studies. There may be biological/clinical justification for other variants of the variance–covariance matrix in equation 10.3, such as assuming independence between the sensitivity of one test and the specificity of another test (i.e. $\sigma_{A1B2} = 0$ and $\sigma_{A2B1} = 0$).

Sections 10.4.1, 10.4.2 and 10.4.3 revisit and extend the analyses presented in sections 9.4.6.3 and 9.4.7.3 to show how to fit models that allow for unequal variances using the variance–covariance matrix expressed in equation 10.2. Section 10.4.4 presents Bayesian estimation of the meta-regression analyses.

10.4.1   Fitting the bivariate model in SAS to compare summary points

The SAS code for the investigation of heterogeneity presented in Chapter 9, Section 9.4.6.3, is in Part I of Appendix 8 of the online supplementary material (10.S1 Code for undertaking meta-analysis). This appendix also contains code for meta-regression using MetaDAS. The parameter estimates required to draw the summary points and regions in RevMan can be extracted from the Proc NLMIXED output in Box 10.4.a. The variances of the random effects for logit(sensitivity) and logit(specificity), and their covariance, are common for both generations of CCP (see blue box in output). For the referent group (CCP1 in this example) the mean logit(sensitivity), mean logit(specificity), the corresponding standard errors and covariance are shown in the red boxes in the output. The covariate parameter estimates, se2 and sp2 (i.e. νA and νB), give the expected change in logit(sensitivity) and logit(specificity) for CCP2 relative to CCP1. The mean logit(sensitivity) for CCP2 is thus estimated by msens+se2, and the mean logit(specificity) is estimated by mspec+sp2. These additional estimates and their standard errors and covariance can be obtained as described in Chapter 9, Section 9.4.6.3, or using the ESTIMATE statement in Proc NLMIXED, as shown in the

---

Box 10.4.a SAS output of bivariate meta-regression of CCP generation: equal variances (model 1)

Fit Statistics	
-2 Log Likelihood	533.4
AIC (smaller is better)	547.4
AICC (smaller is better)	549.1
BIC (smaller is better)	558.6

Parameter Estimates

Parameter	Estimate	Standard Error	DF	t Value	Pr > |t|	95% Confidence Limits		Gradient
msens	-0.09653	0.2203	35	-0.44	0.6640	-0.5438	0.3507	0.000317
mspec	3.4467	0.2982	35	11.56	<.0001	2.8412	4.0522	-0.00005
s2usens	0.3598	0.1022	35	3.52	0.0012	0.1524	0.5673	8.325E-6
s2uspec	0.5399	0.1802	35	3.00	0.0050	0.1742	0.9057	0.000159
covsesp	-0.1969	0.09836	35	-2.00	0.0532	-0.3965	0.002825	-0.00004
se2	0.9626	0.2513	35	3.83	0.0005	0.4523	1.4728	0.000319
sp2	-0.4302	0.3377	35	-1.27	0.2111	-1.1158	0.2554	-0.00004

Covariance Matrix of Parameter Estimates							
	msens	mspec	s2usens	s2uspec	covsesp	se2	sp2
msens	0.04854	−0.02464	−0.00012	−0.00001	−0.00003	−0.04855	0.02465
mspec	−0.02464	0.08895	−0.00002	0.004772	−0.00065	0.02463	−0.08834
s2usens	−0.00012	−0.00002	0.01044	0.002118	−0.00440	0.000693	−0.00005
s2uspec	−0.00001	0.004772	0.002118	0.03246	−0.00860	−0.00006	−0.00039
covsesp	−0.00003	−0.00065	−0.00440	−0.00860	0.009674	0.000100	−0.00091
se2	−0.04855	0.02463	0.000693	−0.00006	0.000100	0.06317	−0.03160
sp2	0.02465	−0.08834	−0.00005	−0.00039	−0.00091	−0.03160	0.1141

Additional Estimates								
Label	Estimate	Standard Error	DF	t Value	Pr > |t|	Alpha	Lower	Upper
logitsens CCP2	0.8660	0.1209	35	7.16	<.0001	0.05	0.6207	1.1114
logitspec CCP2	3.0165	0.1622	35	18.59	<.0001	0.05	2.6871	3.3459
logLR+ CCP1	2.7355	0.2681	35	10.21	<.0001	0.05	2.1913	3.2797
logLR-CCP1	−0.6147	0.1018	35	−6.04	<.0001	0.05	−0.8213	−0.4081
logLR+ CCP2	2.7132	0.1458	35	18.60	<.0001	0.05	2.4171	3.0093
logLR-CCP2	−1.1693	0.08270	35	−14.14	<.0001	0.05	−1.3372	−1.0014

Covariance Matrix of Additional Estimates						
Label	Cov1	Cov2	Cov3	Cov4	Cov5	Cov6
logitsens CCP2	0.01461	−0.00697	−0.00001	5.023E-6	−0.00231	−0.00996
logitspec CCP2	−0.00697	0.02632	0.000598	−0.00002	0.02303	0.003674
logLR+ CCP1	−0.00001	0.000598	0.07185	−0.00301	0.000566	−0.00002
logLR-CCP1	5.023E-6	−0.00002	−0.00301	0.01035	−0.00002	−2.45E-6
logLR+ CCP2	−0.00231	0.02303	0.000566	−0.00002	0.02127	0.000554
logLR-CCP2	−0.00996	0.003674	−0.00002	−2.45E-6	0.000554	0.006840

program in Appendix 8 of the online supplementary material (10.S1 Code for undertaking meta-analysis). The additional estimates and their covariance matrix are shown in the green boxes in Box 10.4.a. The resulting SROC plot from entering parameter estimates, standard errors and covariances into RevMan is shown in Chapter 9, Figure 9.4.c, and panel (a) of Figure 10.4.a.

Part II of Appendix 8 of the online supplementary material (10.S1 Code for undertaking meta-analysis) fits the more complex model that allows for unequal variances for generations of anti-CCP (model 1). The regression equation specified in Proc NLMIXED is not in the same format as for model 1 because dummy variables have been created

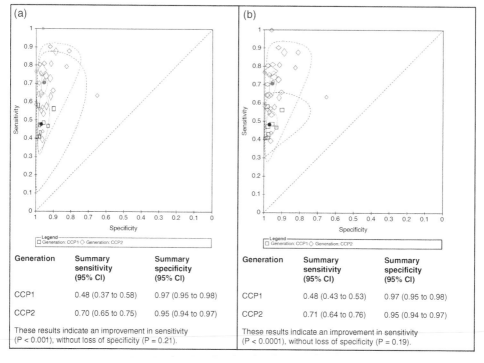

Generation	Summary sensitivity (95% CI)	Summary specificity (95% CI)
CCP1	0.48 (0.37 to 0.58)	0.97 (0.95 to 0.98)
CCP2	0.70 (0.65 to 0.75)	0.95 (0.94 to 0.97)

These results indicate an improvement in sensitivity (P < 0.001), without loss of specificity (P = 0.21).

Generation	Summary sensitivity (95% CI)	Summary specificity (95% CI)
CCP1	0.48 (0.43 to 0.53)	0.97 (0.95 to 0.98)
CCP2	0.71 (0.64 to 0.76)	0.95 (0.94 to 0.97)

These results indicate an improvement in sensitivity (P < 0.0001), without loss of specificity (P = 0.19).

Figure 10.4.a SROC plots produced using estimates from (a) model 1: equal variances and (b) model 2: unequal variances. The dotted region around each summary point (solid circle) is the 95% confidence region while the dashed region is the 95% prediction region

and included for both CCP1 and CCP2. This approach is more straightforward for directly obtaining all parameter estimates and for specifying the variance–covariance structure. The statistical significance of differences between the model that assumed equal variances (model 1) and the model that allowed for unequal variances (model 2) can be assessed using a likelihood ratio test (see Chapter 9, Section 9.4.6.1). The likelihood ratio Chi^2 statistic is the difference in the −2Log likelihood when covariate terms are added or removed from a model. The degrees of freedom used along with the Chi^2 statistic to obtain a P value are the difference in the number of parameters fitted in the two models being compared.

Prior to fitting model 1, it is useful to perform separate meta-analyses for CCP1 and CCP2 to explore whether or not the values of the variances are close or differ substantially between the two CCP generations. The output of these subgroup analyses are shown in Box 10.4.b. The variances of the random effects for the logit sensitivities (s2usens) are 0.04277 and 0.4830 for CCP1 and CCP2, respectively (see red boxes). This suggests much greater variation in sensitivity across CCP2 studies compared to CCP1 studies, which is also apparent from the scatter of the study points in Figure 10.4.a. The variances of the random effects for the logit specificities (s2uspec) also differ, but perhaps not to the extent that alone would justify fitting a model with unequal variances. It was evident from Box 10.4.a that the variances of the random effects have reduced, particularly for sensitivity, compared to the analysis without the covariate in Box 10.2.a. Nevertheless, it is worth investigating the assumption of equal variances, especially as

Box 10.4.b Subgroup analyses of CCP1 and CCP2 generations of anti-CCP test for rheumatoid arthritis

Meta-analysis of CCP1

Parameter	Estimate	Standard Error	DF	t Value	Pr > |t|	95% Confidence Limits		Gradient
msens	−0.07773	0.09375	6	−0.83	0.4387	−0.3071	0.1517	0.000033
mspec	3.4586	0.2910	6	11.89	<.0001	2.7466	4.1706	0.000043
s2usens	0.04277	0.03305	6	1.29	0.2432	−0.03811	0.1237	−0.00019
s2uspec	0.4793	0.3201	6	1.50	0.1850	−0.3040	1.2626	−0.00002
covsesp	−0.06258	0.07902	6	−0.79	0.4585	−0.2559	0.1308	−0.00008

Meta-analysis of CCP2

Parameter	Estimate	Standard Error	DF	t Value	Pr > |t|	95% Confidence Limits		Gradient
msens	0.8725	0.1377	27	6.33	<.0001	0.5899	1.1551	0.000025
mspec	3.0147	0.1655	27	18.21	<.0001	2.6750	3.3543	0.000489
s2usens	0.4830	0.1530	27	3.16	0.0039	0.1691	0.7968	−0.00004
s2uspec	0.5661	0.2185	27	2.59	0.0153	0.1177	1.0145	0.000055
covsesp	−0.2326	0.1303	27	−1.79	0.0854	−0.4999	0.03468	0.000114

there are many included studies and so model overfitting is not a concern. In addition to providing insight into whether or not an assumption of equal variances for the two generations is justifiable, the subgroup analyses can guide the choice of starting values. It is advisable not to use the exact values of the parameter estimates from the analyses, but rather values close to the estimates, e.g. in Box 10.4.b the estimate for 'msens' for CCP1 is −0.07773 and was used to inform a starting value of 0.1 for 'msens' in the meta-regression analysis (see Part II in Appendix 8 of the online supplementary material (10.S1 Code for undertaking meta-analysis)).

Box 10.4.c shows the parameter estimates obtained for CCP1 (red box) and for CCP2 (blue box) and their covariances (green boxes) from fitting model 2. The fit statistics table gives a −2Log likelihood of 524.6, a reduction of 8.8 (533.4−524.6) compared with model 1 that assumed equal variances. Hence, there is statistical evidence (Chi^2 = 8.8, 3 df, P = 0.032) that the variances are unequal for CCP1 and CCP2. The differences in mean logit sensitivity and mean logit specificity (i.e. v_A and v_B) are shown in Box 10.4.d (see red box). The P values based on Wald statistics indicate an improvement in sensitivity (P < 0.0001), without loss of specificity (P = 0.19); there is a similar conclusion based on the results of model 1 (Figure 10.4.a). Comparing the summary estimates

Box 10.4.c SAS output of parameter estimates and their covariance matrix from bivariate meta-regression of CCP generation: unequal variances (model 2)

Fit Statistics	
-2 Log Likelihood	524.6
AIC (smaller is better)	544.6
AICC (smaller is better)	548.1
BIC (smaller is better)	560.7

Parameter Estimates

Parameter	Estimate	Standard Error	DF	t Value	Pr > |t|	95% Confidence Limits		Gradient
msens1	-0.07780	0.09380	33	-0.83	0.4128	-0.2686	0.1130	1.38E-7
mspec1	3.4587	0.2918	33	11.85	<.0001	2.8650	4.0525	-2.5E-6
s2usens1	0.04285	0.03312	33	1.29	0.2046	-0.02452	0.1102	-1.13E-7
s2uspec1	0.4834	0.3238	33	1.49	0.1450	-0.1754	1.1422	-6.59E-6
covsesp1	-0.06258	0.07931	33	-0.79	0.4357	-0.2239	0.09878	8.354E-7
msens2	0.8725	0.1377	33	6.33	<.0001	0.5923	1.1527	-2.21E-7
mspec2	3.0146	0.1655	33	18.21	<.0001	2.6778	3.3514	-1.18E-6
s2usens2	0.4830	0.1530	33	3.16	0.0034	0.1717	0.7942	-5.45E-6
s2uspec2	0.5661	0.2185	33	2.59	0.0142	0.1215	1.0107	-0.00001
covsesp2	-0.2326	0.1303	33	-1.79	0.0834	-0.4976	0.03243	7.557E-6

Covariance Matrix of Parameter Estimates

	msens1	mspec1	s2usens1	s2uspec1	covsesp1	msens2	mspec2	s2usens2	s2uspec2	covsesp2
msens1	0.008798	-0.00772	-0.00028	0.000050	-0.00008	1.29E-14	0	3.57E-14	8.05E-14	0
mspec1	0.00772	0.08518	0.000068	0.01910	-0.00314	-603E-16	0	-709E-16	-238E-15	1.22E-13
s2usens1	0.00028	0.000068	0.001097	0.001066	-0.00119	-206E-16	0	-303E-16	-382E-16	0
s2uspec1	0.000050	0.01910	0.001066	0.1048	-0.01201	-88E-14	-183E-15	-835E-15	-178E-14	6.09E-13
covsesp1	0.00008	-0.00314	-0.00119	-0.01201	0.006290	-422E-16	-471E-16	-856E-16	-251E-15	0
msens2	1.29E-14	-603E-16	-206E-16	-88E-14	-422E-16	0.01897	-0.00819	0.001007	-0.00007	0.000119
mspec2	0	0	0	-183E-15	-471E-16	-0.00819	0.02740	-0.00012	0.006041	0.00198
s2usens2	3.57E-14	-709E-16	-303E-16	-835E-15	-856E-16	0.001007	-0.00012	0.02340	0.003848	0.00859
s2uspec2	8.05E-14	-238E-15	-382E-16	-178E-14	-251E-15	-0.00007	0.006041	0.003848	0.04776	0.01330
covsesp2	0	1.22E-13	0	6.09E-13	0	0.000119	-0.00198	-0.00859	-0.01330	0.01697

from model 1 and model 2, the results are also similar except for the narrower 95% CI for the sensitivity of CCP1 when variances were allowed to be unequal. This is also evident in the size of the 95% confidence region on the SROC plot in panel (b) compared to the region on the plot in panel (a) of Figure 10.4.a. Similarly, the 95% prediction region clearly indicates less heterogeneity in the sensitivity of CCP1 compared to CCP2, as would be expected since the variance of the random effects for logit(sensitivity) was 0.04285 for CCP1 and 0.4830 for CCP2. Note that MetaDAS version 1.3 does not have an

Box 10.4.d SAS output of additional estimates from bivariate meta-regression of CCP generation: unequal variances (model 2)

				Additional Estimates				
Label	Estimate	Standard Error	DF	t Value	Pr > |t|	Alpha	Lower	Upper
Diff logitsens CCP2-CCP1	0.9503	0.1666	33	5.70	<.0001	0.05	0.6113	1.2893
Diff logitspec CCP2-CCP1	-0.4441	0.3355	33	-1.32	0.1947	0.05	-1.1267	0.2385
logLR+ CCP1	2.7569	0.2732	33	10.09	<.0001	0.05	2.2010	3.3128
logLR-CCP1	-0.6240	0.04341	33	-14.37	<.0001	0.05	-0.7123	-0.5357
logLR+ CCP2	2.7134	0.1481	33	18.32	<.0001	0.05	2.4120	3.0148
logLR-CCP2	-1.1738	0.09464	33	-12.40	<.0001	0.05	-1.3663	-0.9813

option for fitting meta-regression models that allow for unequal variances, so model 2 will need to be fitted using Proc NLMIXED directly.

Meta-regression using categorical variables is not limited to binary covariates; when there are more than two subgroups or tests, create and include additional covariate terms in the model. For example if there was a third CCP generation, the data step for creating dummy variables given in Appendix 8 of the online supplementary material (10.S1 Code for undertaking meta-analysis) can be modified, as shown in the following:

```
data nishimura_accp;
      set nishimura_accp;
      ccpg2=0;
      ccpg2=0;
      ccpg3=0;
      if generation ="CCP1" then ccpg1=1;
      if generation ="CCP2" then ccpg2=1;
      if generation ="CCP3" then ccpg3=1;
  run;
```

For model 1, the Proc NLMIXED regression equation in Appendix 8 of the online supplementary material (10.S1 Code for undertaking meta-analysis) can then be modified as follows:

```
logitp=(msens+usens+se2*ccpg2+se3*ccpg3)*sens+(mspec+uspec+sp2*
ccpg2+sp3*ccpg3)*spec;
```

For model 2, the regression equation can be expressed as:

```
logitp=((msens1+usens1)*ccpg1+(msens2+usens2)*ccpg2+(msens3+
usens3)
*ccpg3)*sens+((mspec1+uspec1)*ccpg1+(mspec2+uspec2)*ccpg2+
(mspec3+
uspec3)*ccpg3)*spec;
```

Care is needed in specifying the RANDOM statement for this model to ensure the correct variance-covariance structure is specified as follows:

```
random usens1 uspec1 usens2 uspec2 usens3 uspec3 ~
normal ([0,0,0,0,0,0], [s2usens1,covsesp1,s2uspec1,0,0,s2usens2,0,0,
covsesp2,s2uspec2,0,0,0,0,s2usens3,0,0,0,0,covsesp3,s2uspec3])
```

First writing out the covariance matrix can be helpful, as in the following:

s2usens1					
covsesp1	s2spec1				
0	0	s2usens2			
0	0	covsesp2	s2uspec2		
0	0	0	0	s2usens3	
0	0	0	0	covsesp3	s2uspec3

Appendix 9 of the online supplementary material (10.S1 Code for undertaking meta-analysis) contains SAS code for the comparative meta-analysis of CT and MRI described in Chapter 9, Section 9.4.7.3 (based on all available studies), and Chapter 9, Section 9.4.7.5 (based on direct comparisons). Direct comparisons may require simplification of hierarchical models because there are often very few comparative studies; for the CT versus MRI example, there were only five comparative studies (see Section 10.6). To avoid repetition, further details will not be provided in this section because the same data will be used for the analyses in Stata described in Section 10.4.2.

10.4.2 Fitting the bivariate model in Stata to compare summary points

Meta-regression can also be performed using `meqrlogit` (or `xtmelogit`) in Stata by adding covariate terms to the regression equation. Since the focus of Section 10.4.1 was an investigation of heterogeneity, this section focuses on the comparative meta-analysis of CT and MRI for CAD (see Chapter 9, Section 9.4.7.3). However, for completeness the Stata code and output from fitting the models for investigation of CCP generation are provided in Appendix 10 of the online supplementary material (10.S1 Code for undertaking meta-analysis).

A tutorial that provides a detailed explanation of the comparative meta-analysis of CT versus MRI described here is available (Takwoingi 2023). As recommended in Section 10.4.1, preliminary assessment of the variances of the random effects for logit(sensitivity) and logit(specificity) for each test can be performed by examining the results from meta-analysis of each test (see the code for the analyses in Appendix 11 of the online supplementary material (10.S1 Code for undertaking meta-analysis)). The parameter estimates from the analyses of CT and MRI are shown in Box 10.4.e. The variance and covariance estimates in the red boxes indicate differences between the two tests, especially in the variance estimates for the random effects of the logit sensitivities (1.125 for CT and 0.112 for MRI).

Similar to the Stata code in Appendix 10 of the online supplementary material (10.S1 Code for undertaking meta-analysis), Part I of Appendix 11 of the online supplementary material (10.S1 Code for undertaking meta-analysis) fits the model that assumes equal variances (model 1), while Part II fits the model that allows for unequal variances (model 2). Using the `lrtest` command to perform a likelihood ratio test comparing the model with a covariate and equal variances (B) to the model without a covariate (A), provides strong statistical evidence (Chi^2 = 41.98, 2 df, P < 0.0001) of association of test type with sensitivity and/or specificity. However, further analyses are needed to assess whether the difference is in sensitivity, specificity or both.

```
. lrtest A B

Likelihood-ratio test                LR chi2(2)  =        41.98
(Assumption: A nested in B)          Prob > chi2 =       0.0000
```

Box 10.4.e Stata output of parameter estimates from separate meta-analysis of CT and MRI

Meta-analysis of CT

true	Coef.	Std. Err.	z	P>|z|	[95% Conf. Interval]	
sens	3.556827	.1742296	20.41	0.000	3.215343	3.898311
spec	1.932284	.1234624	15.65	0.000	1.690302	2.174266

Random-effects Parameters	Estimate	Std. Err.	[95% Conf. Interval]	
study_id: Unstructured				
var(sens)	1.125342	.3199718	.6445545	1.964758
var(spec)	.9009872	.1964317	.5876802	1.381326
cov(sens,spec)	.3205208	.178406	-.0291485	.6701901

Meta-analysis of MRI

true	Coef.	Std. Err.	z	P>|z|	[95% Conf. Interval]	
sens	1.966556	.162188	12.13	0.000	1.648673	2.284438
spec	.8405047	.2423615	3.47	0.001	.3654848	1.315525

Random-effects Parameters	Estimate	Std. Err.	[95% Conf. Interval]	
study_id: Unstructured				
var(sens)	.1116773	.1616462	.0065449	1.905583
var(spec)	.7268399	.3515484	.2816701	1.875585
cov(sens,spec)	-.1462588	.1381683	-.4170637	.1245461

To assess the difference in sensitivity, a model without the covariate for sensitivity (C) was fitted. Comparing this model with the model that included covariate terms for both sensitivity and specificity (B), the likelihood ratio test shows strong statistical evidence of a difference in sensitivity between the two tests (Chi^2 = 23.50, 1df, P < 0.0001).

```
.lrtest B C

Likelihood-ratio test                  LR chi2(1)  =         23.50
(Assumption: C nested in B)            Prob > chi2 =        0.0000
```

Similarly, to assess the difference in specificity, a model without the covariate for specificity (D) was fitted. There was strong statistical evidence of a difference in specificity between the two tests (Chi^2 = 23.01, 1 df, P < 0.0001).

```
.lrtest B D

Likelihood-ratio test                  LR chi2(1)  =         23.01
(Assumption: D nested in B)            Prob > chi2 =        0.0000
```

From these analyses, there is strong evidence that CT has higher sensitivity and specificity than MRI for detecting clinically significant coronary artery stenosis. The likelihood ratio test comparing the model with equal variances (B) to the model with unequal variances (E) provides statistical evidence (Chi^2 = 9.68, 2 df, P = 0.02) that the variances differ between the tests. The model with unequal variances (E) is chosen as the final model.

```
.lrtest B E

Likelihood-ratio test                  LR chi2(3)  =          9.68
(Assumption: B nested in E)            Prob > chi2 =        0.0215
```

To find the covariance between the estimated mean logit(sensitivity) and mean logit(specificity) for each test, display the contents of the variance–covariance matrix using the `matrix list` command in Appendix 11 of the online supplementary material (10.S1 Code for undertaking meta-analysis) to produce the output in Box 10.4.f (right half cropped). The estimate of the covariance of the logits is 0.003737 for CT and −0.00828709 for MRI.

These covariance estimates and the parameter estimates (see output in Appendix 11 of the online supplementary material (10.S1 Code for undertaking meta-analysis)) for CT and MRI from this model can be entered into the corresponding multiple tests analysis in RevMan to produce an SROC plot with summary points for CT and MRI, and their 95% confidence and 95% prediction regions. Figure 10.4.b shows the SROC plots produced using parameter estimates from the model with (panel a) and without (panel b) equal variances.

For the analysis with unequal variances, the summary estimates for sensitivity are 0.97 (95% CI 0.96 to 0.98) for CT and 0.88 (95% CI 0.84 to 0.91) for MRI. The summary estimates for specificity are 0.87 (95% CI 0.84 to 0.90) for CT and 0.70 (95% CI 0.59 to 0.79) for MRI (see Appendix 11 of the online supplementary material (10.S1 Code for

Box 10.4.f **Stata output of covariance estimates from comparative meta-analysis of CT and MRI**

```
. matrixliste(V)

symmetric e(V)[10,10]
                          eq1:          eq1:          eq1:
                         seCT          seMRI          spCT
     eq1:seCT        .03035595
    eq1:seMRI       4.662e-10      .02630489
     eq1:spCT         .003737      2.110e-10      .01524296
    eq1:spMRI      -9.127e-10     -.00828709     -1.165e-09
 lns1_1_1:_cons     .01115963      9.641e-10      .00002505
 lns1_1_2:_cons     .00016007      2.657e-10      .00280438
 atr1_1_1_2:_cons   .00265386      6.156e-10      .00027092
 lns1_2_1:_cons     1.001e-08      .02955113      8.255e-09
 lns1_2_2:_cons    -8.916e-10      .0001946      -1.505e-09
 atr1_2_1_2:_cons   5.250e-09      .01225547      3.470e-09
```

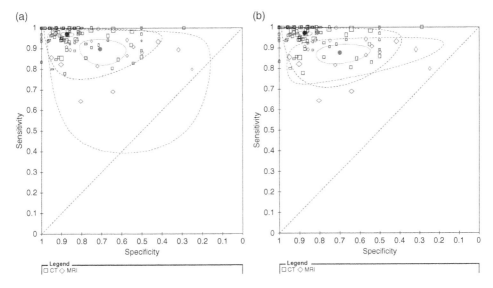

Figure 10.4.b **Summary estimates of accuracy of CT and MRI for the diagnosis of coronary artery disease with corresponding 95% confidence and 95% prediction regions.** (a) Model 1: equal variances; (b) model 2: unequal variances. The markers for each test on the SROC plots represent pairs of sensitivity and specificity from the included studies. The size of each marker was scaled according to the precision of sensitivity and specificity in the study. The solid circles (summary points) represent the summary estimates of sensitivity and specificity for each test. Each summary point is surrounded by a dotted line representing the 95% confidence region and a dashed line representing the 95% prediction region (the region within which one is 95% certain the results of a new study will lie). Source: Data taken from Schuetz 2010.

undertaking meta-analysis)). The estimates are similar to the results obtained for the model with equal variances (see Chapter 9, Section 9.4.7.3); the main difference as shown on Figure 10.4.b is the size of the prediction regions, leading to different conclusions about the extent of the observed heterogeneity, especially for MRI.

Box 10.4.g Estimates of absolute differences in sensitivity and specificity of CT and MRI

```
. nlcom diff_sensitivity: invlogit(_b[seCT])-invlogit(_b[seMRI])

diff_sensi~y:  invlogit(_b[seCT])-invlogit(_b[seMRI])
```

true	Coef.	Std. Err.	z	P>|z|	[95% Conf. Interval]	
diff_sensitivity	.0950214	.0180869	5.25	0.000	.0595718	.1304711

```
. nlcom diff_specificity: invlogit(_b[spCT])-invlogit(_b[spMRI])

diff_speci~y:  invlogit(_b[spCT])-invlogit(_b[spMRI])
```

true	Coef.	Std. Err.	z	P>|z|	[95% Conf. Interval]	
diff_specificity	.1749305	.0528258	3.31	0.001	.0713938	.2784673

Post estimation of the final model, absolute or relative differences in sensitivity and specificity can be computed using the `nlcom` command, which uses nonlinear combinations of the parameter estimates to compute point estimates. The standard errors of the estimates are computed by `nlcom` using the delta method. This is similar to using the ESTIMATE statement in SAS (see Section 10.3.1). Review authors need to choose between reporting absolute or relative differences (see Chapter 12). From the output in Box 10.4.g, the absolute differences in the sensitivity and the specificity of CT compared to MRI are 0.10 (95% CI 0.06 to 0.13) and 0.17 (95% CI 0.07 to 0.28), respectively. The point estimates are the same as the results obtained if the sensitivity (or specificity) of MRI is subtracted from that of CT using the output in Appendix 11 of the online supplementary material (10.S1 Code for undertaking meta-analysis). The P values in the output tables are from Wald tests.

In Appendix 11 of the online supplementary material (10.S1 Code for undertaking meta-analysis), the log of relative sensitivity and relative specificity were computed by taking the difference between the estimated summary sensitivities on the log scale, for example [log(sensitivity of CT) – log(sensitivity of MRI)], to ensure appropriate estimation of standard errors using the delta method. Exponents of the estimates in Box 10.4.h give a relative sensitivity and relative specificity of 1.11 (95% CI 1.06 to 1.15) and 1.25 (95% CI 1.08 to 1.45), respectively. The point estimates are the same as the results obtained if the sensitivity (or specificity) of CT is divided by that of MRI.

10.4.3   Fitting the bivariate model in R to compare summary points

Meta-regression can also be performed using `glmer` in R by adding covariate terms to the regression equation, allowing an investigation of sources of heterogeneity or test comparisons. The comparison of CT and MRI is illustrated in this section (see R code in Appendix 12 of the online supplementary material (10.S1 Code for undertaking meta-analysis)). Examining the variances of the two tests in the red boxes in Box 10.4.i, it is apparent that there is a difference between the variance of logit(sensitivity) of each test. Similarly, there is a difference between the correlation of the logits of the two tests.

Box 10.4.h Estimates of log relative sensitivity and specificity comparing CT and MRI

```
. nlcom log_relative_sensitivity: log(invlogit(_b[seCT]))-log(invlogit(_b[seMRI]))

log_relati~y:  log(invlogit(_b[seCT]))-log(invlogit(_b[seMRI]))
```

true	Coef.	Std. Err.	z	P>|z|	[95% Conf. Interval]	
log_relative_sensitivity	.1028441	.0204882	5.02	0.000	.0626879	.1430002

```
. nlcom log_relative_specificity: log(invlogit(_b[spCT]))-log(invlogit(_b[spMRI]))

log_relati~y:  log(invlogit(_b[spCT]))-log(invlogit(_b[spMRI]))
```

true	Coef.	Std. Err.	z	P>|z|	[95% Conf. Interval]	
log_relative_specificity	.2234729	.0747054	2.99	0.003	.077053	.3698929

Box 10.4.i R output for separate meta-analyses of CT and MRI

```
summary(ma_CT)
```

```
## Generalized linear mixed model fit by maximum likelihood (Laplace
##    Approximation) [glmerMod]
##  Family: binomial  ( logit )
## Formula: cbind(true, n -true)  ~ 0 + sens + spec + (0 + sens + spec |
##     Study_ID)
##    Data: Y.CT
##
##      AIC      BIC   logLik deviance df.resid
##    781.2    797.2   -385.6    771.2      173
##
## Scaled residuals:
##     Min      1Q   Median      3Q      Max
## -1.61587 -0.33545  0.04078  0.52705  1.25204
##
## Random effects:
##  Groups    Name Variance Std.Dev. Corr
##  Study_ID sens 1.107     1.0521
##           spec 0.880     0.9381   0.31
## Number of obs: 178, groups:  Study_ID, 89
##
## Fixed effects:
##      Estimate Std. Error z value Pr(>|z|)
## sens   3.5594    0.1739   20.46   <2e-16 ***
## spec   1.9316    0.1225   15.77   <2e-16 ***
```

```
summary(ma_MRI)
```

```
## Generalized linear mixed model fit by maximum likelihood (Laplace
##   Approximation) [glmerMod]
##  Family: binomial  ( logit )
## Formula: cbind(true, n - true) ~ 0 + sens + spec + (0 + sens + spec |
##      Study_ID)
##     Data: Y.MRI
##
##       AIC      BIC   logLik deviance df.resid
##     182.1    190.3    -86.0    172.1       33
##
## Scaled residuals:
##       Min       1Q   Median       3Q      Max
## -2.09808 -0.32879  0.01733  0.55890  1.43670
##
## Random effects:
##  Groups    Name Variance Std.Dev. Corr
##  Study_ID sens 0.1126   0.3355
##           spec 0.7118   0.8437   -0.52
## Number of obs: 38, groups:  Study_ID, 19
##
## Fixed effects:
##       Estimate Std. Error z value Pr(>|z|)
## sens    1.9670     0.1622  12.127  < 2e-16 ***
## spec    0.8408     0.2401   3.502 0.000461 ***
```

The R package lmtest contains a function lrtest for performing likelihood ratio tests to compare nested models. Comparing the model with a covariate and equal variances (B) to the model without a covariate (A), there is statistical evidence (Chi^2 = 42.45, 2 df, P < 0.0001) that sensitivity and/or specificity differs between CT and MRI (Box 10.4.j).

Box 10.4.j R output of likelihood ratio test comparing model with and without covariate

```
lrtest(A,B)
```

```
## Likelihood ratio test
##
## Model 1: cbind(true, n - true) ~ 0 + sens + spec + (0 + sens + spec |
##      Study_ID)
## Model 2: cbind(true, n - true) ~ 0 + seCT + seMRI + spCT + spMRI + (0 +
##      sens + spec | Study_ID)
##   #Df  LogLik Df  Chisq Pr(>Chisq)
## 1   5 -497.73
## 2   7 -476.50  2 42.452  6.049e-10 ***
## ---
## Signif. codes:  0 '***' 0.001 '**' 0.01 '*' 0.05 '.' 0.1 ' ' 1
```

Table 10.4.a Summary sensitivity and specificity (and 95% confidence intervals) of CT and MRI from different models

Model	CT		MRI	
	Sensitivity(95% CI)	Specificity(95% CI)	Sensitivity(95% CI)	Specificity(95% CI)
Separate meta-analysis for each test	97.2 (96.2 to 98.0)	87.3 (84.4 to 89.8)	87.7 (83.9 to 90.8)	69.9 (59.2 to 78.8)
Test comparison assuming equal variances (model B)	97.0 (95.8 to 97.8)	87.2 (84.2 to 89.5)	89.8 (86.5 to 93.5)	70.6 (60.0 to 78.4)
Test comparison allowing for unequal variances (model E)	97.2 (96.2 to 98.0)	87.3 (84.4 to 89.8)	87.7 (83.9 to 90.8)	69.9 (59.1 to 78.8)

Summary sensitivities and specificities are presented as percentages.

However, further analysis is required to determine if the difference is in sensitivity, specificity or both (see Section 10.4.2). Table 10.4.a summarizes the results from some of the models that were fitted and the summary sensitivity and specificity obtained for each test (see code in Appendix 12 of the online supplementary material (10.S1 Code for undertaking meta-analysis)). The parameter estimates (red boxes) for CT and MRI from the model with unequal variances (E), and the covariance between the estimated mean logit sensitivity and mean logit specificity for each test (blue boxes), are shown in Box 10.4.k.

10.4.4 Bayesian inference for comparing summary points

See Appendix 6 of the online supplementary material (10.S1 Code for undertaking meta-analysis), Section A6.3, for the complete Bayesian program. The rjags model involves specification of the following components.

- Likelihood: The observed data (TP and TN cells) follow a binomial distribution, with the unknown probability being the sensitivity (se) and specificity (sp) in each study.
- Prior distribution: Assuming one observation per study here, we define a dichotomous observed variable Z_i that takes the value 1 if the ith study evaluated CCP2 and 0 if CCP1. At the first level of the prior distribution, the logit(sensitivity) and logit(specificity) in the ith study follow a bivariate normal distribution, with mean values mu[1] + nu[1]*Z[i] and mu[2] + nu[2]*Z[i], respectively. The variance–covariance matrix is parameterized similarly to the one described in Section 10.2.4, i.e. by the between-study standard deviation in the logit sensitivities (tau[1]), the between-study standard deviation in the logit specificities (tau[2]) and the correlation between the logit sensitivities and the logit specificities (rho). At the second level, prior distributions need to be provided for mu[1], mu[2], prec[1], prec[2] and rho, like before, as well as for nu[1] and nu[2], which correspond to the logit mean difference between CCP2 and CCP1 in sensitivity and specificity, respectively. These prior distributions are typically vague, as stated in Section 10.2.4.1.

287

Box 10.4.k R output of parameter and covariance estimates for unequal variance model

i. Parameter estimates

```
summary(E)
```

```
## Generalized linear mixed model fit by maximum likelihood (Laplace
##    Approximation) [glmerMod]
##  Family: binomial  ( logit )
## Formula: cbind(true, n - true) ~ 0 + seCT + seMRI + spCT + spMRI + (0 +
##     seMRI + spMRI | Study_ID) + (0 + seCT + spCT | Study_ID)
##    Data: Y
##
##      AIC      BIC   logLik deviance df.resid
##    963.3    997.1   -471.7    943.3      206
##
## Scaled residuals:
##       Min       1Q   Median       3Q      Max
## -2.09753 -0.33455  0.04077  0.53006  1.43650
##
## Random effects:
##  Groups      Name   Variance Std.Dev. Corr
##  Study_ID    seMRI  0.1127   0.3357
##              spMRI  0.7122   0.8439   -0.52
##  Study_ID.1  seCT   1.1070   1.0521
##              spCT   0.8801   0.9381   0.31
## Number of obs: 216, groups:  Study_ID, 103
##
## Fixed effects:
##         Estimate Std. Error z value Pr(>|z|)
## seCT    3.5594     0.1739   20.464  < 2e-16 ***
## seMRI   1.9671     0.1624   12.109  < 2e-16 ***
## spCT    1.9317     0.1225   15.773  < 2e-16 ***
## spMRI   0.8410     0.2406    3.495 0.000474 ***
```

ii. Covariance between the mean logits

```
(vcovE = (summary(E))$vcov)
```

```
## 4 x 4 Matrix of class "dpoMatrix"
##                 seCT          seMRI           spCT          spMRI
## seCT    3.025237e-02   2.055647e-09   3.550535e-03  -2.960073e-09
## seMRI   2.055647e-09   2.638712e-02   8.912427e-10  -8.289464e-03
## spCT    3.550535e-03   8.912427e-10   1.499821e-02  -3.943513e-09
## spMRI  -2.960073e-09  -8.289464e-03  -3.943513e-09   5.791074e-02
```

- Comparing summary points: To compare summary points, we add a few lines to the rjags model to calculate the difference between the summary sensitivity of CCP2 and summary sensitivity of CCP1 (Difference_Se) and difference between the summary specificity of CCP2 and summary specificity of CCP1 (Difference_Sp). Using the step()

function in rjags, we can calculate the probability that the summary sensitivity of CCP2 is greater than the summary sensitivity of CCP1 (prob_Se), and similarly for specificity (prob_Sp).

10.4.4.1 Summary statistics

After ensuring that the MCMC algorithm successfully converged, the summary statistics for the parameters of interest can be calculated based on a sample from the posterior distribution. In the output from the rjags program in Box 10.4.l, the logit transformed summary sensitivity and specificity for CCP1 (mu[1] and mu[2]) and the between-study standard deviations and correlation are reported as well as the difference in logit mean sensitivities and specificities between CCP2 and CCP1 (nu[1] and nu[2]). These results are similar to the ones reported in Section 10.4.1. The difference in mean sensitivities and specificities between CCP2 and CCP1 is also reported on

---

Box 10.4.l Rjags output from Bayesian bivariate meta-regression of CCP generation

```
Iterations = 26001:46000
Thinning interval = 1
Number of chains = 3
Sample size per chain = 20000
1. Empirical mean and standard deviation for each
variable,
     plus standard error of the mean:
```

	Mean	SD	Naive SE	Time-series SE
Summary_Sp_CCP1	0.96791	0.009514	3.884e-05	1.586e-04
Summary_Sp_CCP2	0.95258	0.007405	3.023e-05	7.236e-05
Summary_Se_CCP1	0.47494	0.056278	2.298e-04	8.337e-04
Summary_Se_CCP2	0.70383	0.025918	1.058e-04	1.860e-04
mu[1]	-0.10161	0.228722	9.338e-04	3.388e-03
mu[2]	3.44889	0.301046	1.229e-03	5.130e-03
nu[1]	0.97037	0.260469	1.063e-03	3.936e-03
nu[2]	-0.43651	0.341737	1.395e-03	5.917e-03
tau.sq[1]	0.39251	0.112203	4.581e-04	1.170e-03
tau.sq[2]	0.56943	0.194723	7.950e-04	2.933e-03
rho	-0.38057	0.174221	7.113e-04	2.391e-0
Difference_Se	0.22888	0.061937	2.529e-04	9.445e-04
Difference_Sp	-0.01533	0.012038	4.914e-05	1.971e-04
prob_Se	0.99980	0.014141	5.773e-05	1.900e-04
prob_Sp	0.09882	0.298418	1.218e-03	3.755e-03

	2.5%	25%	50%	75%	97.5%
Summary_Sp_CCP1	0.94600	0.96264	0.96914	0.974560	0.98292
Summary_Sp_CCP2	0.93696	0.94789	0.95299	0.957715	0.96596
Summary_Se_CCP1	0.36477	0.43696	0.47499	0.512617	0.58609
Summary_Se_CCP2	0.65157	0.68684	0.70431	0.721308	0.75340
mu[1]	-0.55471	-0.25350	-0.10013	0.050479	0.34781
mu[2]	2.86329	3.24917	3.44701	3.645675	4.05251
nu[1]	0.46336	0.79715	0.96846	1.142235	1.49064
nu[2]	-1.10806	-0.66086	-0.43822	-0.214684	0.24391
tau.sq[1]	0.22526	0.31331	0.37531	0.452647	0.659967
tau.sq[2]	0.28326	0.43244	0.53753	0.671007	1.037957
rho	-0.68655	-0.50609	-0.39200	-0.267176	-0.01105
prob_Se	1.00000	1.00000	1.00000	1.000000	1.00000
prob_Sp	0.00000	0.00000	0.00000	0.000000	1.00000
Difference_Se	0.10751	0.18769	0.22887	0.270338	0.35087
Difference_Sp	-0.03735	-0.02328	-0.01598	-0.008228	0.01051

the probability scale. The median of the difference in summary sensitivities of CCP2 versus CCP1 is about 22.9 percentage points (95% credible interval ranging from 10.8 to 35.1 percentage points, see red boxes). The median of the difference in summary specificities (see green boxes) is −1.6 percentage points (with a 95% credible interval of −3.7 to 1.1 percentage points). The blue box highlights that there is a 0.999 probability that the summary sensitivity of CCP2 will be greater than the summary sensitivity of CCP1. However, there is only a 0.099 probability that the summary specificity of CCP2 will be higher than that of CCP1. Figure 10.4.c shows the diagnostics plots of the

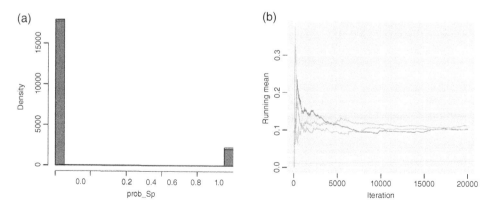

Figure 10.4.c MCMC diagnostics plots for a parameter (prob_Sp) from the Bayesian bivariate meta-regression model

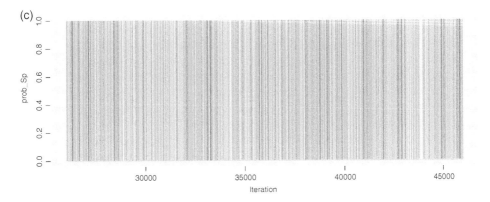

Figure 10.4.c (Continued)

probability that the summary specificity of CCP2 will be higher than that of CCP1. We can see that at any given iteration this probability is either 0 or 1. Its posterior mean is the desired summary statistic.

10.5 Comparison of summary curves

The Rutter and Gatsonis HSROC model, like the bivariate model, can be extended to a meta-regression model for investigating heterogeneity (Chapter 9, Section 9.4.6.4) or comparing test accuracy (Chapter 9, Section 9.4.7.4). HSROC meta-regression models were illustrated in Chapter 9, Section 9.4.6.4, using the RF data to investigate whether the laboratory technique (nephelometry, latex agglutination (LA) and ELISA) used to measure RF is associated with diagnostic performance. Covariate terms were included in the HSROC model to assess whether accuracy, threshold or the shape of the SROC curve varied with technique. The variances of the random effects for threshold (θ) and accuracy (α) were assumed to be equal for all three techniques (see Part I of Appendix 13 of the online supplementary material (10.S1 Code for undertaking meta-analysis) for SAS code) and modelled as follows:

$$\theta_i \sim N\left(\Theta, \sigma_\theta^2\right) \text{ and } \alpha_i \sim N\left(\Lambda, \sigma_\alpha^2\right). \tag{10.4}$$

Similar to the bivariate model, the variance parameters of the HSROC model can be allowed to differ between subgroups or tests. For example, if Z_i represents a vector of study-level covariates ($i = 1, \ldots, I$) from I studies included in a meta-analysis, allowing the difference in threshold and accuracy between tests to vary gives

$$\text{logit}\left(\pi_{ij}\right) = \left(\left(\theta_i + \gamma_i Z_i\right) + \left(\alpha_i + \xi_i Z_i\right)dis_{ij}\right)\exp\left(-\left(\alpha + \beta Z_i\right)dis_{ij}\right) \tag{10.5}$$

$$\begin{pmatrix} \theta_i \\ \gamma_i \end{pmatrix} \sim N\left(\begin{pmatrix} \Theta \\ \Gamma \end{pmatrix}, \begin{pmatrix} \sigma_\theta^2 & \sigma_\theta\sigma_\gamma \\ \sigma_\theta\sigma_\gamma & \sigma_\gamma^2 \end{pmatrix}\right) \text{ and } \begin{pmatrix} \alpha_i \\ \xi_i \end{pmatrix} \sim N\left(\begin{pmatrix} \Lambda \\ \Xi \end{pmatrix}, \begin{pmatrix} \sigma_\alpha^2 & \sigma_\alpha\sigma_\xi \\ \sigma_\alpha\sigma_\xi & \sigma_\xi^2 \end{pmatrix}\right). \tag{10.6}$$

Covariance terms are needed between the random effects for accuracy (i.e. α_i and ξ_i) and between the random effects for threshold (i.e. θ_i and γ_i), otherwise the variances for the referent test will be larger than those of the comparator test(s) (Macaskill 2003). Therefore, $\sigma_\alpha \sigma_\xi$ is the covariance between the random effects for accuracy and $\sigma_\theta \sigma_\gamma$ is the covariance between the random effects for threshold. The variances of the random effects for the comparator can be obtained using the expression for the variance of a sum that is $\sigma_\alpha^2 + \sigma_\xi^2 + 2\sigma_\alpha \sigma_\xi$ for accuracy and $\sigma_\theta^2 + \sigma_\gamma^2 + 2\sigma_\theta \sigma_\gamma$ for threshold. The computation of these variances will be illustrated in Section 10.5.1.

To investigate the effect of laboratory technique on the diagnostic performance of RF, HSROC meta-regression models will be fitted using SAS in Section 10.5.1 and Bayesian estimation will be illustrated in Section 10.5.2. Following the notation of equation 10.5, since laboratory technique has three categories, we define two dichotomous vectors of data Z_{1i} and Z_{2i}, where Z_{1i} takes the value 1 if the laboratory technique is nephelometry and 0 otherwise, while Z_{2i} takes the value 1 if the laboratory technique is ELISA and 0 otherwise. The laboratory technique LA is arbitrarily chosen to be the reference group that corresponds to the situation where Z_{1i} and Z_{2i} are simultaneously equal to 0.

10.5.1 Fitting the HSROC model in SAS to compare summary curves

The SAS code for this analysis is in Appendix 13 of the online supplementary material (10.S1 Code for undertaking meta-analysis). The output of the model that included covariate terms for the shape, accuracy and threshold parameters but assumed equal variances is shown in Box 10.5.a. The parameter estimates for LA, the reference group, are shown in the red box in the parameter estimates table, while the estimates for the accuracy, threshold and shape parameters for ELISA and nephelometry are shown in the blue box in the additional estimates table. Since the variances were assumed to be equal for the three techniques, the variance estimates in the red box (s2ua = 1.2817 and s2ut = 0.4780) are also the estimates for ELISA and nephelometry.

Further modelling was undertaken by removing the covariate terms for shape from the model, i.e. assuming a common shape for the three curves. The increase in the −2Log likelihood was negligible (Chi² = 753.1−752.9 = 0.2, 2 df, P = 0.90). Parameter estimates for the model that assumes a common shape are given in Chapter 9, Table 9.4.d, with the corresponding HSROC curves shown in Chapter 9, Figure 9.4.e. Since there appeared to be no difference in shape, covariate terms for accuracy were removed from the common shape model to assess the effect on the accuracy parameter. The output from fitting this model is shown in Box 10.5.b. The removal of the covariate terms for accuracy has a negligible effect on the fit of the model (Chi² = 753.7−753.1 = 0.6 on 2 df, P = 0.74), indicating no statistical evidence of a difference in diagnostic accuracy of RF according to technique (see Chapter 9, Section 9.4.6.4).

Fitting HSROC meta-regression models with a more complex variance–covariance structure (equation 10.6) is computationally intensive and prone to convergence issues. Such models may require simplification, e.g. assumption of same or no shape parameter (see Section 10.6.2). For an example of an HSROC meta-regression with unequal variances and the accompanying code, see Takwoingi (2016).

Box 10.5.a SAS output of HSROC meta-regression of RF technique: differences in shape, accuracy and threshold parameters, equal variances

Fit Statistics	
-2 Log Likelihood	752.9
AIC (smaller is better)	774.9
AICC (smaller is better)	778.1
BIC (smaller is better)	795.2

Parameter Estimates								
Parameter	Estimate	Standard Error	DF	t Value	Pr > |t|	95% Confidence Limits		Gradient
alpha	2.4233	0.3314	45	7.31	<.0001	1.7559	3.0907	-0.00026
theta	-0.5019	0.2449	45	-2.05	0.0463	-0.9952	-0.00853	-0.00033
beta	0.2796	0.2670	45	1.05	0.3006	-0.2582	0.8174	-0.00028
s2ua	1.2817	0.3104	45	4.13	0.0002	0.6565	1.9069	-0.00083
s2ut	0.4780	0.1139	45	4.20	0.0001	0.2486	0.7074	-0.00062
a1	0.2962	0.5141	45	0.58	0.5674	-0.7393	1.3316	-0.00028
a2	0.3730	0.4521	45	0.83	0.4137	-0.5375	1.2836	0.000267
t1	-0.2569	0.3708	45	-0.69	0.4919	-1.0038	0.4899	-0.00037
t2	0.3965	0.3601	45	1.10	0.2766	-0.3287	1.1217	-0.00027
b1	-0.1016	0.4274	45	-0.24	0.8132	-0.9625	0.7593	2.043E-6
b2	-0.1614	0.3983	45	-0.41	0.6872	-0.9637	0.6408	0.000412

Additional Estimates								
Label	Estimate	Standard Error	DF	t Value	Pr > |t|	Alpha	Lower	Upper
alpha ELISA	2.7194	0.3935	45	6.91	<.0001	0.05	1.9269	3.5120
theta ELISA	-0.7588	0.2785	45	-2.72	0.0091	0.05	-1.3198	-0.1978
beta ELISA	0.1780	0.3338	45	0.53	0.5964	0.05	-0.4943	0.8503
alpha Nephelometry	2.7963	0.3079	45	9.08	<.0001	0.05	2.1761	3.4165
theta Nephelometry	-0.1054	0.2637	45	-0.40	0.6914	0.05	-0.6364	0.4257
beta Nephelometry	0.1182	0.2955	45	0.40	0.6912	0.05	-0.4771	0.7134

Box 10.5.b SAS output of HSROC meta-regression of RF technique: differences in threshold parameter, equal variances

Fit Statistics	
-2 Log Likelihood	753.7
AIC (smaller is better)	767.7
AICC (smaller is better)	769.0
BIC (smaller is better)	780.6

Parameter Estimates

Parameter	Estimate	Standard Error	DF	t Value	Pr > |t|	95% Confidence Limits		Gradient
alpha	2.6574	0.1923	45	13.82	<.0001	2.2702	3.0447	0.000052
theta	−0.5565	0.2133	45	−2.61	0.0123	−0.9860	−0.1269	0.000080
beta	0.1912	0.1651	45	1.16	0.2529	−0.1413	0.5236	−0.00005
s2ua	1.2994	0.3148	45	4.13	0.0002	0.6653	1.9335	0.000011
s2ut	0.4784	0.1139	45	4.20	0.0001	0.2490	0.7079	−0.00009
t1	−0.1939	0.2614	45	−0.74	0.4621	−0.7203	0.3325	0.000174
t2	0.4971	0.2626	45	1.89	0.0648	−0.03171	1.0259	−0.00005

10.5.2 Bayesian estimation of the HSROC model for comparing summary curves

See Appendix 6 of the online supplementary material (10.S1 Code for undertaking meta-analysis), Section A6.4, for the complete Bayesian program. The rjags model involves specification of the following components.

- Likelihood: The likelihood of the observed data (TP and FP cells) follows a binomial distribution, with the unknown parameters being the TPR and FPR in each study.
- Prior distributions: The logit TPR and the logit FPR are expressed as functions of the positivity threshold (theta) for each study (i), the lnDOR (alpha) for each study and a regression equation of the shape parameter (beta, which is assumed to be common across studies) and the covariates Z_{1i} and Z_{2i} (delta[1] and delta[2]). At the first level of the prior distribution, theta and alpha parameters in the included studies are assumed to follow normal distributions with precision (i.e. 1/variance) prec[2] and prec[1], respectively, assumed to be equal for all three techniques. The mean of the prior distribution is expressed as a function of the covariates Z_{1i} and Z_{2i} via a regression equation. The mean of theta is expressed as a function of THETA, gamma[1] and gamma[2], where THETA, THETA+gamma[1] and THETA+gamma[2] are the mean positivity threshold parameters of the laboratory techniques LA, nephelometry and ELISA, respectively. Similarly, the mean of alpha is a function of LAMBDA, epsilon[1] and epsilon[2], where LAMBDA, LAMBDA+epsilon[1] and LAMBDA+epsilon[2] are the mean lnDOR parameters of LA, nephelometry and ELISA, respectively.

- At the second level of the prior distribution, vague prior distributions are provided for THETA, gamma[1], gamma[2], prec[2], LAMBDA, epsilon[1], epsilon[2], prec[1], beta, delta[1] and delta[2].

10.5.2.1 Monitoring convergence

The rjags program and the detailed script on how to run it are provided in Appendix 6 of the online supplementary material (10.S1 Code for undertaking meta-analysis). Before interpreting the results, the MCMC algorithm should be checked for convergence. As an illustrative example, Figure 10.5.a represents the convergence behaviour of LAMBDA, the mean lnDOR parameter of nephelometry. The overlapping results from three independent MCMC chains in each of the panels indicate that convergence was achieved.

10.5.2.2 Summary statistics

With convergence successfully achieved, we display the rjags output of the summary statistics of the parameters of interest based on their posterior distributions in Box 10.5.c. For comparison with the results obtained with the frequentist analysis in Section 10.5.1, the output returns posterior estimates of the variances of the random effects for threshold (tau.sq[1]) and accuracy (tau.sq[2]), THETA, LAMBDA and beta parameters for LA; THETA_nephelometry (THETA+gamma[1]), LAMBDA_ nephelometry (LAMBDA+epsilon[1]) and beta_ nephelometry (beta+delta[1]) parameters for nephelometry; and THETA_ELISA (THETA+gamma[2]), LAMBDA_ELISA (LAMBDA+epsilon[2]) and beta_ELISA (beta+delta[2]) parameters for ELISA.

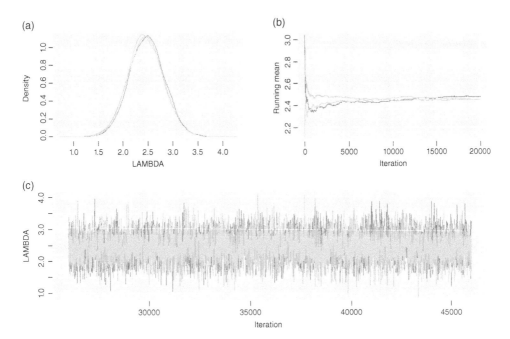

Figure 10.5.a MCMC diagnostics plots for a parameter (LAMBDA) from the HSROC meta-regression model

---

Box 10.5.c Rjags output from Bayesian HSROC meta-regression of RF laboratory techniques

---

```
Iterations = 26001:46000

Thinning interval = 1

Number of chains = 3

Sample size per chain = 20000

1. Empirical mean and standard deviation for each variable,
     plus standard error of the mean:
```

	Mean	SD	Naive SE	Time-series SE
LAMBDA	2.46056	0.35761	1.460e-03	0.0053571
LAMBDA_ELISA	2.77382	0.42765	1.746e-03	0.0153399
LAMBDA_Nephelometry	2.83999	0.32917	1.344e-03	0.0023498
THETA	-0.52722	0.26313	1.074e-03	0.0084638
THETA_ELISA	-0.77078	0.30704	1.253e-03	0.0128415
THETA_Nephelometry	-0.12863	0.28407	1.160e-03	0.0081274
beta	0.25933	0.27488	1.122e-03	0.0168935
beta_ELISA	0.17310	0.35237	1.439e-03	0.0195180
beta_Nephelometry	0.08596	0.30435	1.243e-03	0.0116891
tau.sq[1]	0.59907	0.14225	5.807e-04	0.0008611
tau.sq[2]	1.45742	0.36373	1.485e-03	0.0026122

```
2. Quantiles for each variable:
```

	2.5%	25%	50%	75%	97.5%
LAMBDA	1.759833	2.22213	2.45811	2.695339	3.169631
LAMBDA_ELISA	1.984570	2.48382	2.75725	3.041644	3.661214
LAMBDA_Nephelometry	2.198794	2.62092	2.83738	3.058208	3.497508
THETA	-1.047216	-0.70485	-0.52802	-0.351234	-0.007843
THETA_ELISA	-1.392830	-0.97026	-0.76279	-0.563522	-0.193243
THETA_Nephelometry	-0.688319	-0.31738	-0.12788	0.061554	0.425279
beta	-0.266138	0.07160	0.25477	0.442268	0.813086
beta_ELISA	-0.497171	-0.06738	0.17259	0.414194	0.855344
beta_Nephelometry	-0.517020	-0.11818	0.08346	0.291679	0.684564
tau.sq[1]	0.378056	0.49776	0.57973	0.679221	0.929534
tau.sq[2]	0.896167	1.19925	1.40845	1.658469	2.306908

10.6 Meta-analysis of sparse data and a typical data sets

When fitting hierarchical meta-analytical models within a frequentist framework using a maximum likelihood approach, estimation problems such as unreliable parameter estimates or lack of convergence often occur due to small number of studies or sparse data. Bayesian analyses of such data can also be challenging and checking convergence

Study	TP	FP	FN	TN	Sensitivity (95% CI)	Specificity (95% CI)	Sensitivity (95% CI)	Specificity (95% CI)
Li 2009	21	1	7	74	0.75 [0.55, 0.89]	0.99 [0.93, 1.00]		
Fenton 1989	19	6	0	131	1.00 [0.82, 1.00]	0.96 [0.91, 0.98]		
Montariol 1998	41	3	0	171	1.00 [0.91, 1.00]	0.98 [0.95, 1.00]		
Silverstein 1998	14	0	0	76	1.00 [0.77, 1.00]	1.00 [0.95, 1.00]		
Wu 2005	23	0	0	67	1.00 [0.85, 1.00]	1.00 [0.95, 1.00]		

0 0.2 0.4 0.6 0.8 1 0 0.2 0.4 0.6 0.8 1

Figure 10.6.a **Forest plot of intraoperative cholangiography for diagnosis of common bile duct stones.** Studies are ordered by sensitivity and study identifier. Source: Adapted from Gurusamy 2015

of the MCMC algorithm is critical. In addition, priors for variance parameters can have more influence than intended when the number of studies is small (Lambert 2005).

Sparse data are a common occurrence in meta-analysis of very accurate tests where most of the studies have 100% sensitivity and/or specificity. For example, in a Cochrane Review of intraoperative cholangiography (IOC) for diagnosis of common bile duct stones, four of the five IOC studies had a sensitivity of 100% (Figure 10.6.a) (Gurusamy 2015)).

There are also atypical situations where data are only available in a 2×1 (e.g. only sensitivity or only specificity estimated) rather than a 2×2 table format, or where false positives are impossible and thus are structural zeros. An example of the latter is a Cochrane Review of the accuracy of laparoscopy following CT scanning for assessing resectability with curative intent in pancreatic and periampullary cancer (Allen 2016). Since laparotomy (the reference standard) will be performed only if histopathology of the biopsy of the suspicious lesion on diagnostic laparoscopy shows no evidence of cancer, false positives are not possible, i.e. specificity is always 1. In the Cochrane Review of serum screening tests used in the first trimester of pregnancy, although studies reported results at different thresholds, it is common in this clinical field for studies to report sensitivity (detection rate) at a fixed specificity (usually a 5% FPR). The chosen FPR level is determined as the FPR deemed acceptable in a particular screening programme and so all studies report the same specificity. In both of these examples there is no need to account for correlation between sensitivity and specificity across studies in a hierarchical meta-analytical model.

Approaches for dealing with sparse data were introduced in Chapter 9, Section 9.4.8, and will be explained further and illustrated in this section with a focus on frequentist analyses.

10.6.1 Facilitating convergence

Irrespective of the model fitted or the software program used for frequentist estimation, adaptive Gaussian quadrature is commonly used for the maximum likelihood estimation. In sparse data situations, the variance–covariance parameters are often on the boundary of the parameter space (Riley 2007, Chung 2013); the maximum likelihood estimate on the boundary will have at least one of the variances in an HSROC model equal to 0 or the correlation parameter in a bivariate model equal to +1 or –1.

The direct comparison of CT versus MRI for CAD included five comparative accuracy studies (see Chapter 9, Section 9.4.7.5). The forest plot of CT and MRI shows that except for one study, the studies reported the same sensitivity for CT (Figure 10.6.b). This lack of heterogeneity in the sensitivity of CT, in addition to the small number of studies, may lead to estimation problems when a bivariate model is fitted to the data.

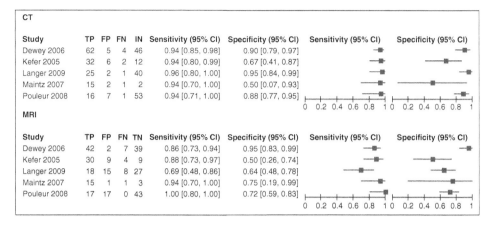

Figure 10.6.b **Forest plot of comparative studies of CT versus MRI for coronary artery disease.**
Source: Data taken from Schuetz 2010

Box 10.6.a Large gradient values in SAS for bivariate model parameters for CT and MRI comparative studies (model without test type covariate)

			Parameter Estimates					
Parameter	Estimate	Standard Error	DF	t Value	Pr > |t|	95% Confidence Limits		Gradient
msens	2.0000	0.4686	3	4.27	0.0236	0.5086	3.4914	−6.88008
mspec	1.0000	0.2041	3	4.90	0.0163	0.3504	1.6496	−25.4401
s2usens	−111E-14	0.4240	3	−0.00	1.0000	−1.3493	1.3493	−0.31355
s2uspec	2.21E-11	0.01977	3	0.00	1.0000	−0.06291	0.06291	−188.328
covsesp	−108E-15	-	3	-	-	-	-	−44.9080

To assess the effect of test type on sensitivity and specificity, models with and without the covariate were fitted. The output of fitting a bivariate model without the test type covariate to the data using Proc NLMIXED in SAS showed that the convergence criterion was satisfied. However, all the parameter estimates have large gradient values, indicating poor estimation (Box 10.6.a). A model may satisfy a convergence criterion but may be unstable (e.g. changing the starting values results in a change in parameter estimates), or have missing standard errors for one or more parameter estimates. Therefore, in addition to meeting a convergence criterion, meta-analysts should check for missing standard errors and if the program output permits, also check that gradient values for all model parameters are very close to zero before concluding that the analysis has successfully converged.

Several attempts were made to improve estimation of the parameters by specifying different options for fitting the model (see code in Appendix 9 of the online supplementary material (10.S1 Code for undertaking meta-analysis)). The options included

Box 10.6.b Improved estimation in SAS of bivariate model parameters for CT and MRI comparative studies by changing model fitting options

						Parameter Estimates		
Parameter	Estimate	Standard Error	DF	t Value	Pr > |t|	95% Confidence Limits		Gradient
msens	2.2554	0.3569	3	6.32	0.0080	1.1194	3.3913	0.000057
mspec	1.3083	0.3375	3	3.88	0.0304	0.2342	2.3823	0.000543
s2usens	0.006812	0.5582	3	0.01	0.9910	−1.7695	1.7831	1.70698
s2uspec	0.4138	0.3633	3	1.14	0.3374	−0.7424	1.5701	−0.02091
covsesp	−0.03331	0.1724	3	−0.19	0.8592	−0.5821	0.5155	−0.21665

increasing the number of quadrature points; changing the optimization technique from the default quasi-Newton technique to the Newton-Raphson technique; trying different starting values, e.g. using a grid search; and setting boundary constraints for the variance parameters (i.e. variance ≥ 0). Imposing boundary constraints can reduce the risk of convergence problems. If boundary constraints are triggered for variance parameters, then estimation of these parameters is truncated at zero. The same options explored here for fitting the bivariate model can be applied when fitting the HSROC model in SAS. For the CT versus MRI example, trying each of the options separately failed to improve estimation of the bivariate model parameters and there were error and/or warning messages. Finally, setting boundary constraints for the variance parameters and using a different set of starting values resulted in more reliable parameter estimates (Box 10.6.b).

The gradient for the variance of the random effects for logit(sensitivity) is large (1.70698), and there is concern about the analysis. Since the estimate of the variance of logit(sensitivity) is close to zero (s2usens = 0.006812) and given the previous observation about limited heterogeneity in the sensitivity estimates for CT, simplifying the model by removing either a variance or covariance parameter may be a reasonable strategy. Such an analysis will be explored in Section 10.6.2.

When the bivariate model was fitted to this data set in Stata using meqrlogit (see Appendix 11 of the online supplementary material (10.S1 Code for undertaking meta-analysis)), the results were similar to those obtained using SAS and all the gradient values were close to zero (Box 10.6.c). In Stata, the default optimization technique for meqrlogit and xtmelogit is a Newton-Raphson technique. Starting values are determined by the commands and are not specified by the user.

As stated in Section 10.2.3, it is not possible to increase the number of quadrature points used by glmer to fit a bivariate model in R. Different optimization options can be explored simultaneously using the allFit function (see code in Appendix 14 of the online supplementary material (10.S1 Code for undertaking meta-analysis)). The options are (1) bound optimization by quadratic approximation (BOBYQA); (2) an algorithm derived from BOBYQA named NLOPT_LN_BOBYQA in Box 10.6.d; (3) limited memory Broyden–Fletcher–Goldfarb–Shanno bound-constrained (L-BFGS-B) optimization; (4) Nelder-Mead

---

Box 10.6.c Estimation in Stata of bivariate model parameters for CT and MRI comparative studies (model without test type covariate)

```
Iteration 3:
                                              log likelihood = -53.173887
Gradient vector (length =   .000245):
              eq1:            eq1:      lns1_1_1:     lns1_1_2:   atr1_1_1_2:
              sens            spec       _cons          _cons        _cons
r1       .0000374        .0000781     .0000129       .0002278     -.0000219
```

Mixed-effects logistic regression	Number of obs	=	20
Binomial variable: n			
Group variable: study_id	Number of groups	=	5

	Obs per group:		
	min =		4
	avg =		4.0
	max =		4

Integration points = 5	Wald chi2(2)	=	145.10
Log likelihood = -53.173887	Prob > chi2	=	0.0000

---

true	Coef.	Std. Err.	z	P>|z|	[95% Conf. Interval]	
sens	2.249856	.204119	11.02	0.000	1.84979	2.649922
spec	1.308397	.3386634	3.86	0.000	.6446286	1.972165

Random-effects Parameters	Estimate	Std. Err.	[95% Conf. Interval]	
study_id: Unstructured				
var(sens)	.001594	.0147132	2.22e-11	114638.5
var(spec)	.4178528	.366883	.074757	2.335581
cov(sens,spec)	-.0258082	.1205167	-.2620166	.2104002

Using option `stddev` to output standard deviations and correlation instead of the variances and covariance above gives the following output.

Random-effects Parameters	Estimate	Std. Err.	[95% Conf. Interval]	
study_id: Unstructured				
sd(sens)	.0399259	.1842611	4.71e-06	338.5475
sd(spec)	.6464237	.2837953	.2734133	1.528322
corr(sens,spec)	-1	.0011101	-1	1

Box 10.6.d Estimation in R of bivariate model parameters for CT and MRI comparative studies (model without test type covariate)

```
ss$fixef                ## table of fixed effects
```

```
##                                    sens      spec
## bobyqa                           2.249866 1.308946
## Nelder_Mead                      2.249865 1.308946
## nlminbwrap                       2.249866 1.308946
## nmkbw                            2.249880 1.309040
## optimx.L-BFGS-B                  2.249866 1.308946
## nloptwrap.NLOPT_LN_NELDERMEAD    2.249860 1.308935
## nloptwrap.NLOPT_LN_BOBYQA        2.249818 1.308969
```

```
ss$sdcor                ## table of random effect SDs and correlations
```

##	Study_ID.sens	Study_ID.spec.sens	Study_ID.spec
## bobyqa	0.03989542	0.6429813	-1.0000000
## Nelder_Mead	0.03989567	0.6429822	-1.0000000
## nlminbwrap	0.03989607	0.6429808	-1.0000000
## nmkbw	0.03977192	0.6429379	-0.9999521
## optimx.L-BFGS-B	0.03989560	0.6429822	-1.0000000
## nloptwrap.NLOPT_LN_NELDERMEAD	0.03990032	0.6429883	-0.9999998
## nloptwrap.NLOPT_LN_BOBYQA	0.03977226	0.6429241	-0.9999665

---

method; (5) Nelder-Mead simplex algorithm (NLOPT_LN_NELDERMEAD in Box 10.6.d); (6) nonlinear minimization with box constraints (nlminb); and (7) Nelder-Mead algorithm for derivative-free optimization (nmkb). In this example, the seven optimization options in the red box produced similar results (Box 10.6.d). The help files of the functions and commands in different software packages are a useful source of information on the quadrature and optimization options available for model estimation.

10.6.2 Simplifying hierarchical models

Hierarchical models can be simplified by removing parameters from the regression equation and editing the covariance structure. Prior to simplifying the models, plot the data on forest and SROC plots to assess heterogeneity visually and to gain a better understanding of the data (e.g. all or most studies report 100% sensitivity and/or specificity with no indication of a threshold effect). If the bivariate model described in Chapter 9, Section 9.4.1, is simplified by assuming that the covariance or correlation is zero (i.e. an independent variance–covariance structure), the model reduces to two univariate random-effects logistic regression models for sensitivity and specificity as follows:

$$\begin{pmatrix} \mu_{Ai} \\ \mu_{Bi} \end{pmatrix} \sim N\left(\begin{pmatrix} \mu_A \\ \mu_B \end{pmatrix}, \Sigma \right) \text{ with } \Sigma = \begin{pmatrix} \sigma_A^2 & 0 \\ 0 & \sigma_B^2 \end{pmatrix}. \tag{10.7}$$

Study	TP	FP	FN	TN	Sensitivity (95% CI)	Specificity (95% CI)	Sensitivity (95% CI)	Specificity (95% CI)
Zar 2019	31	0	108	51	0.22 [0.16, 0.30]	1.00 [0.93, 1.00]		
Nicol 2018	64	0	206	97	0.24 [0.19, 0.29]	1.00 [0.96, 1.00]		
Sabi 2018	22	2	67	105	0.25 [0.16, 0.35]	0.98 [0.93, 1.00]		

0   0.2 0.4 0.6 0.8   1 0   0.2 0.4 0.6 0.8   1

Figure 10.6.c **Forest plot of Xpert Ultra against a composite reference standard.** Studies on the plot are sorted by sensitivity and then by specificity. Source: Adapted from Kay 2020

If there is little or no observed variation in sensitivity and/or specificity, these univariate models can be further simplified by dropping one or both variance parameters. Without the variance parameters, the models reduce to fixed-effect logistic regression models. For example, a Cochrane Review included three studies that assessed Xpert Ultra against a composite reference standard using sputum specimens from children (Kay 2020). The estimates of sensitivity and specificity were similar in the three studies (Figure 10.6.c). Given the small number of studies and lack of heterogeneity, a fixed-effect meta-analysis was considered appropriate. In Stata the `meqrlogit` or `xtmelogit` command cannot be used for fitting fixed-effect logistic regression models; instead use the `blogit` command (see code in Appendix 15 of the online supplementary material (10.S1 Code for undertaking meta-analysis)).

For the IOC example introduced in Section 10.6, when the covariance matrix for the random effects for logit(sensitivity) and logit(specificity) was unstructured (model A) – i.e. no constraints imposed so that the variances and covariance were uniquely estimated – the variances were poorly estimated, especially the variance parameter for the logit(sensitivity) of IOC. It is unsurprising that the variances were poorly estimated given the small number of studies and sparse data. Alternative models were investigated, as shown in Table 10.6.a. In model B, the exchangeable covariance structure estimated a common variance and a covariance for the random effects of the logit(sensitivity) and logit(specificity). The independent covariance structure used in model C estimated distinct variances for the random effects, but the covariance was assumed to be zero (i.e. two separate univariate random-effects logistic regression models). In model D the variance parameter for logit(sensitivity) was dropped and so there was no covariance. Stata code for the four models is in Appendix 16 of the online supplementary material (10.S1 Code for undertaking meta-analysis).

To check the robustness of the assumptions about the variances of the random effects, the estimates of sensitivity and specificity were also compared between models (Table 10.6.a). The analytical approach adopted was based on the reasoning that it is inappropriate to overfit models by estimating too many parameters from few studies, and to simplify models when parameter estimates cannot be reliably estimated. The validity of this approach has been investigated in a simulation study that concluded that simpler hierarchical models are valid in situations with few studies or sparse data (Takwoingi 2017). For estimating summary sensitivity and specificity, simplifying the bivariate model to univariate random-effects logistic regression models is appropriate. For estimating a summary curve, an HSROC model without the shape parameter (i.e. a symmetrical curve) can be used. If there is very little or no observed heterogeneity, fixed-effect equivalents of the models can be applied.

The output of the bivariate model fitted to the CT and MRI comparative studies in Stata (Box 10.6.c) and R (Box 10.6.d) show that the correlation of the logits was

Table 10.6.a Parameter and summary estimates for IOC from models with different variance–covariance structure

Parameter	Models			
	A: Unstructured variance–covariance structure	B: Exchangeable variance–covariance structure	C: Independent variance–covariance structure	D: Fixed effects for sensitivity of IOC
Mean logit sensitivity (SE)	7.06 (4.53)	4.43 (1.45)	6.12 (3.2)	2.82 (0.39)
Mean logit specificity (SE)	4.15 (0.52)	4.80 (1.00)	4.19 (0.57)	4.19 (0.57)
Variance of random effects for logit sensitivity (SE)	16.7 (26.9)	2.85 (2.71)	9.74 (12.7)	0
Variance of random effects for logit specificity (SE)	0.25 (0.54)	2.85 (2.71)	0.34 (0.67)	0.34 (0.67)
Correlation of the logits (SE)	−0.73 (0.98)	0.03 (0.76)	0	0
Sensitivity (95% CI)	99.9 (14.1, to 100)	98.8 (83.1 to 99.9)	99.8 (42.3 to 100)	94.4 (88.7 to 97.3)
Specificity (95% CI)	98.5 (95.8 to 99.4)	99.2 (94.5 to 99.9)	98.5 (95.6 to 99.5)	98.5 (95.6 to 99.5)

estimated on the boundary of the parameter space as –1 (see Section 10.6.1). Therefore, simplifying the model to two univariate random-effects logistic regression models for sensitivity and specificity, by removing the correlation or covariance parameter, seems a reasonable first step (see SAS code in Appendix 9 of the online supplementary material (10.S1 Code for undertaking meta-analysis)). The output of fitting this model in SAS shows that the boundary constraint for the variance of logit(sensitivity) was triggered (see Active BC column in (i) in Box 10.6.e). Thus the next step is to simplify further by also removing this variance parameter, i.e. assume a fixed effect for sensitivity. Covariate terms can now be added to this model to compare the sensitivity and specificity of CT and MRI (see SAS code in Appendix 9 of the online supplementary material (10.S1 Code for undertaking meta-analysis)). The difficulty encountered in the analysis of CT and MRI when using `Proc NLMIXED` in SAS was not experienced when using Stata (see code in Appendix 11 of the online supplementary material (10.S1 Code for undertaking meta-analysis)) and R (Appendix 14 of the online supplementary material (10.S1 Code for undertaking meta-analysis)). It is possible for the analysis of sparse data to be problematic in one program and not as problematic in another program due to differences in the implementation of the programs.

Univariate models can also be used for investigating heterogeneity or for test comparisons when the rationale for simplifying hierarchical models is not due to the number of studies or convergence issues. A univariate random-effects logistic meta-regression model that allowed for a separate variance term for the random effects of logit(sensitivity) for each test was used in the main meta-analysis comparing the accuracy of nine first-trimester serum test strategies for Down syndrome screening (Alldred 2015). The analysis

---

Box 10.6.e Simplifying the bivariate model to univariate random-effects logistic regression models for CT and MRI comparative studies (model without covariate)

(i) Model without covariance parameter

Fit Statistics	
-2 Log Likelihood	106.4
AIC (smaller is better)	114.4
AICC (smaller is better)	117.1
BIC (smaller is better)	112.9

		Parameter Estimates							
Parameter	Estimate	Standard Error	DF	t Value	Pr > |t|	95% Confidence Limits		Gradient	Active BC
msens	2.2385	0.1953	3	11.46	0.0014	1.6168	2.8602	0.000407	
mspec	1.3122	0.3363	3	3.90	0.0299	0.2418	2.3825	−0.00025	
s2usens	0	-	3	-	-	-	-	1.81131	Lower BC
s2uspec	0.4111	0.3602	3	1.14	0.3366	−0.7353	1.5575	−8.11E-6	

(ii) Model without covariance parameter and variance parameter for logit (sensitivity)

Fit Statistics	
-2 Log Likelihood	106.4
AIC (smaller is better)	112.4
AICC (smaller is better)	113.9
BIC (smaller is better)	111.3

		Parameter Estimates						
Parameter	Estimate	Standard Error	DF	t Value	Pr > |t|	95% Confidence Limits		Gradient
msens	2.2385	0.1953	4	11.46	0.0003	1.6961	2.7809	0.000012
mspec	1.3122	0.3363	4	3.90	0.0175	0.3784	2.2460	−0.00012
s2uspec	0.4111	0.3602	4	1.14	0.3174	−0.5890	1.4112	−0.00004

---

included all studies that used a 5% FPR threshold. Equation 10.8 expressed only for logit(sensitivity) was thus extended as follows:

$$\left(\mu_{Aik}\right) \sim N\left[\left(\mu_A + v_A Z_k\right), \sigma_{Ak}^2\right].$$ (10.8)

where μ_{Aik} is the logit(sensitivity) for the kth test within the ith study; Z_k represents the kth test; μ_A estimates the mean logit(sensitivity) for the index test used as the referent test (note not the reference standard); $\mu_A + v_A Z_k$ estimates the mean logit(sensitivity) for the kth test; and σ_{Ak}^2 is the variance of logit(sensitivity) for the kth test. The Stata

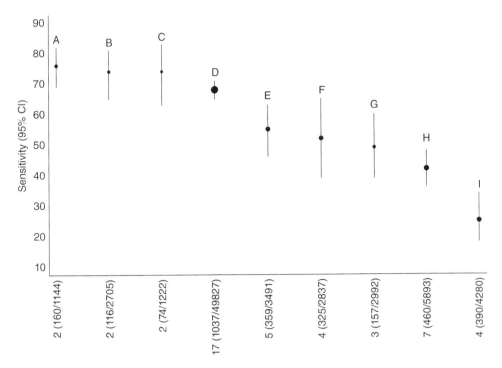

Figure 10.6.d Sensitivity at a 5% false positive rate for nine first-trimester serum test strategies for Down syndrome screening. Sensitivity is presented as percentages. Each circle represents the summary sensitivity for a test strategy and the size of each circle is proportional to the number of Down syndrome cases. The estimates are shown with 95% confidence intervals. The test strategies are ordered on the plot according to decreasing detection rate. The number of studies, cases and women included for each test strategy are shown on the horizontal axis. A = Age, PlGF, PAPP-A and free ßhCG; B = Age, PAPP-A, free ßhCG and AFP; C = Age, ADAM 12, PAPP-A and free ßhCG; D = Age, PAPP-A and free ßhCG; E = Age, PAPP-A; F = PAPP-A; G = Age, free ßhCG and AFP; H = Age, free ßhCG; I = Free ßhCG. Source: Adapted from Alldred 2015

code and output of the parameter estimates are in Appendix 17 of the online supplementary material (10.S1 Code for undertaking meta-analysis). Figure 10.6.d shows the summary estimates of sensitivity obtained, including their 95% confidence intervals, at the 5% FPR. The test combinations were ordered on the plot according to decreasing sensitivity. The plot shows that the single-test strategies with and without maternal age (PAPP-A alone, free βhCG alone, PAPP-A and maternal age, and free βhCG and maternal age) have the worst performance, whereas the triple-test strategies (ADAM 12, PAPP-A, free βhCG and maternal age; PAPP-A, free βhCG, AFP and maternal age) have the highest performance.

10.7   Meta-analysis with multiple thresholds per study

As noted in Chapter 9, Section 9.4.5, some studies may report sensitivity and specificity at more than one threshold, because the results of the index test are ordinal categories or continuous measurements (see Chapter 4). The development of methods that allow for the inclusion of multiple thresholds from each included study is an active area of research (Zapf 2021). This section describes and demonstrates implementation of the Steinhauser (2016) and Jones (2019) approaches introduced in Chapter 9, Section 9.4.5. Both models performed similarly when evaluated empirically using data for a subset of published thresholds as well as all relevant thresholds from an individual participant data set of 45 studies (Benedetti 2020). The models are for tests that produce a continuous, numerical result. It is assumed that each study reports sensitivity and specificity at one or more numerical threshold values.

We first define a common notation for both models. Study $i = 1, \ldots, I$ provides data on sensitivity and specificity at threshold values C_{it}, where $t = 1, \ldots, T_i$. Both models accommodate varying numbers of, and different sets of, thresholds across studies and the possibility that some studies report accuracy data at only a single threshold (i.e. T_i equals 1).

10.7.1 Meta-analysis of multiple thresholds with R

The Steinhauser approach for meta-analysis of multiple thresholds creates a link between the range of thresholds and the respective pairs of sensitivity and specificity (Steinhauser 2016). The model is a two-stage random-effects model. At the study level, the reported specificity estimates across thresholds provide an estimate of the cumulative distribution function (cdf) of continuous test results among individuals without the target condition. Likewise, the set of sensitivity estimates across reported thresholds provides an estimate of the cdf of test results among individuals with the target condition. At the meta-analytical level, the model fits the data for both groups and all available thresholds over all studies. Based on a chosen parametric model, for example a logistic model, it provides estimates of the two cdfs for the two groups across all studies, accounting for the between-study heterogeneity and across-study correlation between groups.

The general model, here assuming an underlying logistic distribution for the log-transformed continuous test results, is given by

$$\text{logit}\left(\widehat{sp}_{it}\right) = \alpha_0 + a_{0i} + \left(\beta_0 + b_{0i}\right)\log\left(C_{it}\right) + \epsilon_{it}$$

$$\text{logit}\left(1 - \widehat{se}_{it}\right) = \alpha_1 + a_{1i} + \left(\beta_1 + b_{1i}\right)\log\left(C_{it}\right) + \delta_{it}$$

where $\widehat{sp}_{it}$ and $\widehat{se}_{it}$ denote the observed values of specificity and sensitivity at threshold C_{it} in study i, α_1 and α_0 are fixed intercepts, and β_1 and β_0 are fixed slopes for the individuals with and without the target condition. The terms $a_{0i}, a_{1i}, b_{0i}, b_{1i}$ denote random intercepts and slopes. These are assumed to follow a multivariate normal distribution, reflecting the correlation across studies. The terms ϵ_{it} and δ_{it} represent within-study random errors. The parameters are estimated using weighted least squares, where each data point is weighted with the inverse variance of the respective logit-transformed proportion.

The model provides estimates of the average distribution functions for both study groups. This allows derivation of a model-based SROC curve. If, in addition, criteria for selecting a threshold can be specified – in this case maximization of the Youden index (defined as sensitivity + specificity − 1), which applies if false negatives and false positives are of equal importance – an estimate of this threshold can be obtained from the model. Alternatively, a larger or smaller weight can be specified (for details, see later), implemented in the R package `diagmeta` (Rücker 2020).

The practical use of `diagmeta version 0.5-0` is demonstrated using an example provided with the diagmeta package. The data are from a meta-analysis of the diagnostic accuracy of fractional exhaled nitric oxide (FeNO) for diagnosis of asthma (Schneider 2017). First, the `diagmeta` package must be installed on the user's platform from the CRAN repository:

```
install.packages("diagmeta")
```

After the package has been installed, it must be made available in the working space using the command `library(diagmeta)`. Load the FENO data using `data(Schneider2017)` and examine the data structure using the command `View(Schneider2017)`, which provides the full data table. Alternatively, the first few lines of the table can be examined using the command `head(Schneider2017)`, which produces the output in Box 10.7.a.

The first number in each row is a row number automatically provided by R (not given in the data set). The second column (study_id) is the study identifier, here a number; the third and fourth columns provide study author and year of publication. All the visible lines belong to the same study, Arora 2006, with a study ID of 1. The 'group' column is empty for this study (it refers to a later study, Malinovschi 2012, which provides data in three sub-studies). The 'cutpoint' column contains the threshold for FeNO measured in ppb. The last four columns (tpos, fneg, fpos and tneg) give the numbers of true positive (TP), false negative (FN), false positive (FP) and true negative (TN) results (2×2 data), if the value in the 'cutpoint' column is used to determine test positivity. Because larger values indicate asthma (the target condition), the numbers of (true or false) positives must decrease with increasing threshold, whereas the numbers of (true or false) negatives increase with the threshold within a study. Note that it is also possible to start from individual participant data with a given study ID, true status of the participant and individual marker value. This type of data can be transformed to the format needed using the function `IPD2diag()`.

The main function of `diagmeta` is also called `diagmeta()`. To see the arguments required by `diagmeta()`, look at the help file using `help(diagmeta)` or look directly at the arguments using `args(diagmeta)` to give the output presented in Box 10.7.b.

Box 10.7.a Subset of fractional exhaled nitric oxide data for diagnosis of asthma

	study_id	author	year	group	cutpoint	tpos	fneg	fpos	tneg
1	1	Arora	2006		6	133	5	34	0
2	1	Arora	2006		7	131	7	33	1
3	1	Arora	2006		8	130	8	31	3
4	1	Arora	2006		9	127	11	30	4
5	1	Arora	2006		10	119	19	28	6
6	1	Arora	2006		11	115	23	26	8

Box 10.7.b Arguments of the function diagmeta()

```
function (TP, FP, TN, FN, cutoff, studlab, data = NULL,
distr = "logistic",
      model = "CICS", equalvar = FALSE, lambda = 0.5, log.
cutoff = FALSE,
      method.weights = "invvar", level = 0.95, incr = 0.5,
      n.iter.max = 1000, tol = 1e-08, silent = TRUE, ...)
```

The first six arguments are mandatory; TP, FP, TN, and FN represent the 2×2 data, `cutoff` represents the threshold and `studlab` the study identifier. The argument `data` refers to the data set used, `distr` is one of "logistic" (default) or "normal", `model` the model used for estimation (see later), and with `equalvar` it can be specified whether the variances of the marker in both groups are assumed to be equal or not (default is FALSE). The argument `log.cutoff` is to specify whether the marker values are to be log-transformed. Here is a typical call for diagmeta():

```
diag1 <- diagmeta(tpos, fpos, tneg, fneg, cutpoint,
                  studlab = paste(author, year, group),
                  data = Schneider2017,
                  model = "CICS", log.cutoff = TRUE)
```

The first five arguments TP, FP, TN, FN, cutoff correspond to the columns tpos, fpos, tneg, fneg, cutpoint for the FeNO dataset. Note that here these arguments are not explicitly written, thus they are interpreted in the fixed order given by args(). It would also be possible to call them in a different order, but then they must be explicitly specified, for example

```
diag1 <- diagmeta(TP = tpos, FP = fpos, TN = tneg, FN = fneg,
                  cutoff = cutpoint, ...)
```

(call truncated). The study label (argument `studlab`) is a combination of author, year and (sub)group (the latter is empty except for one study). Alternatively, the variable `study_id` could be chosen as the study label, as it uniquely characterizes the study or substudy. The dataset is Schneider 2017, the model is "CICS", which stands for "Common Intercept and Common Slope" and refers to the random part of the model. For more details of the modelling, see the original publication (Steinhauser 2016). The argument `log.cutoff` is set to TRUE, which means that the thresholds are log-transformed (because FeNO is known to have a skewed distribution). The call of diagmeta() creates an R object named diag1. Writing print(diag1) gives the output in Box 10.7.c.

The output in Box 10.7.c presents the number of studies (29), the number of data lines (150), the number of unique reported thresholds (53), details of the model and a summary of the results, consisting of the 'optimal' threshold (28.179) – for this example defined as the threshold that maximizes the Youden index – and sensitivity and specificity at this threshold with 95% CIs. Here, sensitivity and specificity are equally weighted. Alternatively, different weights can be specified. If, for example, one is more concerned about false negatives than false positives, one might like to give more weight to

---

Box 10.7.c Output of the R object diag1 after calling diagmeta()

```
*** Results of multiple cutoffs model ***
Total number of studies: 29
Total number of cutoffs: 150
Number of different cutoffs: 53
Model: CICS
Type of distribution: logistic
Cutoffs log transformed: TRUE
The optimal cutoff value: 28.179
Sensitivity and specificity at optimal cutoff:
        Sens: 0.5841 [0.4853; 0.6766]
        Spec: 0.8086 [0.7348; 0.8656]
Area under the curve (AUC):
 0.7342 [0.6667; 0.7938] - confidence region for sensitivity
given specificity
 0.7340 [0.6888; 0.7745] - confidence region for specificity
given sensitivity
```

Box 10.7.d Using function diagstats() to obtain sensitivity and specificity at specified thresholds

---

```
diagstats (diag1, c(25, 30))
cutoff   Sens seSens lower.Sens upper.Sens   Spec seSpec lower.Spec upper.Spec
    25 0.6320 0.1995    0.5374    0.7174 0.7550 0.2110    0.6708    0.8233
    30 0.5583 0.2056    0.4580    0.6541 0.8329 0.2177    0.7649    0.8842
```

---

sensitivity (say, 80%) by setting the weighting parameter lambda of function diag-meta to a different value, say lambda = 0.8.

A more extensive output (not shown) can be obtained using summary(diag1), which lists all thresholds and their frequency, all studies with their number of thresholds, information about the distribution of thresholds, and the summary output from the lmer() function from the lme4 package, which is run in the background. Use function diagstats() to obtain sensitivity and specificity at the chosen thresholds of 25 and 30 shown in Box 10.7.d. For further options of diagstats(), see the help file.

Finally, to create graphical output, use plot(diag1), which provides the four plots (panels a to d) in Figure 10.7.a. Studies on the plots are characterized by different colours. Panel (a) shows 'survival curves' that give the estimated probability for individuals with (solid line, TP) or without (dashed line, FP) the target condition (here asthma) having a positive result, given the threshold. Each circle corresponds to either a true-positive rate (solid circles) or a false positive rate (hollow circles) within a study. Thus, this plot provides the true-positive rate and the false positive rate of the test at each threshold. The vertical line indicates the point where the curves have maximal distance apart (28.179). Panel (b) shows the Youden index (the difference between both curves) as a function of the varying threshold, its maximum (0.393, assumed in 28.179) indicated by the vertical line. Panel (c) shows the study-specific ROC curves and panel (d) shows the model-based SROC curve based on the full data.

Figure 10.7.a was also obtained using the `plot.diagmeta` function as follows:

```
plot(diag1, which = "SROC", mark.optcut = TRUE,
     ciSens = TRUE, ciSpec = TRUE, shading = "hatch",
     ellipse = TRUE)
```

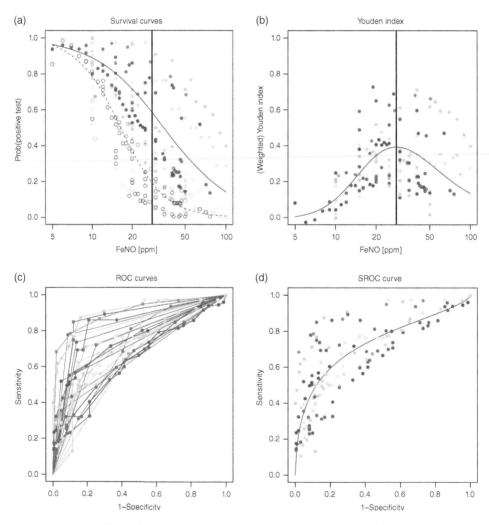

Figure 10.7.a **Graphical output from diagmeta for meta-analysis of multiple thresholds using FeNO data**. (a) Survival plot of positive rates for individuals with and without asthma (solid circles/ hollow circles), varying with the threshold; (b) Youden index, varying with the threshold; (c) study-specific ROC curves; (d) model-based SROC curve. Points or lines of the same colour belong to the same study.

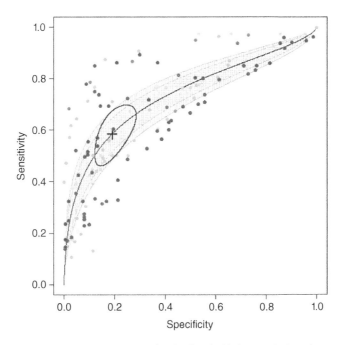

Figure 10.7.b SROC curve and summary point for the threshold that maximizes the Youden index with 95% confidence regions

The generic plot function can be applied to objects of a large number of classes. Here, using function `diagmeta()`, an R object `diag1` of class `"diagmeta"` was created. When the plot function is applied to `diag1`, R recognizes that this is a `diagmeta` object and calls `plot.diagmeta`. Figure 10.7.b shows the model-based SROC curve with two 95% confidence regions (vertical hatching corresponds to pointwise confidence intervals for sensitivity, given specificity; horizontal hatching corresponds to pointwise confidence intervals for specificity, given sensitivity). The cross represents the summary point that corresponds to the threshold that maximizes the Youden index, and the summary point is surrounded by its 95% confidence region. For a full description of possible features, see `help(plot.diagmeta)`.

10.7.2 Meta-analysis of multiple thresholds with rjags

An alternative model, fitted using Bayesian statistical software, was described by Jones (2019). WinBUGS code to fit the model can be found in the article's appendix. This section shows how to fit the model using rjags, with application to the FeNO data introduced in Section 10.7.1. In contrast to the two-stage model described in Section 10.7.1, which requires normal approximations to the likelihood, this model is fitted in a single stage and models the observed count data directly using multinomial likelihoods. In fitting the model, these multinomial distributions are re-parameterized as conditional binomial distributions for computational convenience.

It is assumed that higher values of the numerical test result are associated with increased likelihood of having the target condition, such that test results lying above a threshold are considered positive and those below are considered negative. The populations without and with the target condition are indexed by $j = 1, 2$, respectively. The Jones model is based on the assumption that *some transformation*, $g()$, of the continuous test results in population j of study i has a logistic distribution, with mean μ_{ij} and scale parameter σ_{ij}. The transformation $g()$ can be pre-specified: for example, as the identity function or (if the continuous test results are known to be right skewed) the log transformation. This corresponds to assumptions of underlying logistic or log-logistic distributions, respectively. A much more flexible but more computationally intensive option is to assume only that $g()$ is in the set of Box-Cox transformations, defined by a transformation parameter λ that is estimated alongside the other model parameters. This extended version of the model allows for a wide range of possible distributions for the underlying continuous test results.

The probability of a positive test result at threshold C_{it} in population j of study i is denoted by pf_{ijt}, i.e. FPR ($j = 1$) and TPR ($j = 2$). It follows from the earlier distributional assumption that

$$logit\left(pf_{ijt}\right) = \frac{\mu_{ij} - g\left(C_{it}\right)}{\sigma_{ij}}$$

(10.9)

The study-specific location and scale parameters are modelled as random effects, assumed to be normally distributed across studies, the latter on the log scale (which ensures that fitted scale parameters are always positive, as they must be by definition). Across studies, μ_{ij} has mean $m_{\mu j}$ and standard deviation $\tau_{\mu j}$, while $\log(\sigma_{ij})$ has mean $m_{\sigma j}$ and standard deviation $\tau_{\sigma j}$. Several options for the correlation structure between these four sets of random effects are described in Jones (2019). Prior distributions are required for the hyperparameters: $m_{\mu j}, m_{\sigma j}, \tau_{\mu j}, \tau_{\sigma j} (j = 1, 2)$ and any correlation parameters.

Box 10.7.e shows JAGS model code for the version of the model with $g()$ set to $log()$ and with a structured covariance matrix of the form described in Schneider (2017). This choice of $g()$ may be a reasonable approximation for many positive-valued test results, which are often right skewed. JAGS code for the extended version of the model, with $g()$ not pre-specified, is provided in Appendix 18 of the online supplementary material (10. S1 Code for undertaking meta-analysis).

In the model code, x_{ijt} is used to denote the number of positive test results in study i, population j, at threshold C_{it}. In other words, x_{i1t} denotes numbers of false positives and x_{i2t} denotes numbers of true positives. Binomial likelihoods are assumed for these, similar to Section 10.3.2. For $t > 1$, each binomial likelihood is conditional on the number of positive results at the preceding (next lowest) threshold, x_{ijt-1}. This conditional formulation is equivalent to fitting multinomial likelihoods to full contingency tables of test results.

Note that if there are zero positive test results at threshold $C_{i,t-1}$ in population j (i.e. $x_{ij,t-1} = 0$), then there are, by definition, zero positives at threshold C_{it} in that population. This is the case, for example, in the Woo 2012 study in the FeNO dataset, where there are zero false positive results at the 13th, 14th and 15th thresholds (i.e. $x_{i,1,13} = x_{i,1,14} = x_{i,1,15} = 0$). If fitting the model in WinBUGS, we need to first remove the last two, uninformative, data points, because WinBUGS will not accept binomial observations with a denominator of zero (see Jones 2019). This is not necessary with JAGS, however.

Box 10.7.e Specification of the Jones multiple thresholds model in rjags

```
model{
  #=== LIKELIHOOD ===#
  for(i in 1:I){
   for(j in 1:2){
    for(t in 1:T[i]){
      x[i,j,t] ~ dbin(p[i,j,t], n[i,j,t])
                        }
        # DEFINE CONDITIONAL BINOMIAL ORDER PARAMETERS
        n[i,j,1] <- N[i,j]
        for(t in 2:T[i]){
        n[i,j,t] <- x[i,j,t-1]
        }
        # DEFINE CONDITIONAL BINOMIAL PROBABILITIES
        # IN TERMS OF FPR AND TPR
        p[i,j,1] <- pr[i,j,1]
        for(t in 2:T[i]){
        p[i,j,t] <-  pr[i,j,t] / pr[i,j,t-1]
        }
         # === MODEL FOR STUDY-LEVEL LOGIT(FPR) AND LOGIT(TPR) === #
         for(t in 1:T[i]){
         d[i,j,t] <- (mu[i,j] - log(C[i,t]) ) / s[i,j]
                    pr[i,j,t] <- ilogit(d[i,j,t])
     }
    }
# === 4 SETS OF RANDOM EFFECTS ACROSS STUDIES === #
# COVARIANCE STRUCTURE AS DESCRIBED IN JONES 2019
mu[i,1] ~ dnorm(m_mu[1], prec_mu[1])

mu[i,2] ~ dnorm(cond_mean_mu[i], cond_prec_mu)
cond_mean_mu[i] <- m_mu[2] + (rho_mu*tau_mu[2]/tau_
mu[1]) * (mu[i,1] - m_mu[1])

for(j in 1:2){
     cond_mean_s[i,j] <- m_sigma[j] + (rho_mu_sigma*tau_
     sigma[j]/tau_mu[j]) * (mu[i,j] - m_mu[j])
     logs[i,j] ~ dnorm(cond_mean_s[i,j], cond_prec_s[j])
     s[i,j] <- exp(logs[i,j])
    }
 }
```

```
# DEFINE PRECISION PARAMETERS FOR CONDITIONAL NORMAL DISTRIBUTIONS
  cond_var_mu <- (1- pow(rho_mu,2))*pow(tau_mu[2], 2)
  cond_prec_mu <- 1/cond_var_mu
  for(j in 1:2){
    cond_var_s[j]<- (1- pow(rho_mu_sigma,2))*pow(tau_sigma[j], 2)
    cond_prec_s[j] <- 1/cond_var_s[j]
  }

#=== HYPER PRIOR DISTRIBUTIONS ===#
for(j in 1:2){
    # MEAN LOCATION PARAMETERS OF UNDERLYING LOGISTIC DISTRIBUTIONS
    m_mu[j] ~ dnorm(0, 0.001)
    # MEAN LOG(SCALE) PARAMETERS OF UNDERLYING LOGISTIC DISTRIBUTIONS
    m_sigma[j] ~ dnorm(0, 0.001)
    # BETWEEN-STUDY STANDARD DEVIATION OF LOCATION PARAMETERS
    tau_mu[j] ~ dunif(0,5)
    # BETWEEN-STUDY STANDARD DEVIATION OF LOG(SCALE) PARAMETERS
    tau_sigma[j] ~ dunif(0,5)
    prec_mu[j] <- pow(tau_mu[j], -2)
    prec_sigma[j] <- pow(tau_sigma[j], -2)
  }
  # BETWEEN-STUDY CORRELATIONS
  rho_mu ~ dunif(-1,1)
  rho_mu_sigma ~ dunif(-1,1)
}
```

In Box 10.7.e, we assume vague Normal prior distributions for $m_{\mu j}$, $m_{\sigma j}$ and Uniform priors for the standard deviation parameters $\tau_{\mu j}$, $\tau_{\sigma j}$. As noted in Section 10.2.4.4, other prior distributions are often used for standard deviations of random effects, and sensitivity analyses may be run varying these.

To fit the model, the following data are required to pass to JAGS:

- I: Number of studies.
- N: I by 2 dimensional matrix, with elements N_{ij} denoting the number of individuals in population $j = 1, 2$ of study i.
- T: I dimensional vector, with elements T_i denoting the number of distinct thresholds reported in study i.
- C: I by $max(T_i)$ dimensional matrix, containing the explicit threshold values reported in each study, C_{it}. Elements $C_{it} = NA$ for $t > T_i$.
- x: An array of dimension I by 2 by $max(T_i)$, containing numbers of individuals testing positive at each threshold: x_{ijt} = number of individuals testing positive in study i, population j at threshold C_{it}, $x_{ijt} = NA$ for $t > T_i$.

Code to fit the model to the FeNO data using rjags is provided in Appendix 18 of the online supplementary material (10.S1 Code for undertaking meta-analysis). As with all Bayesian modelling, it is crucial that the analyst checks convergence and mixing of the chains; see Section 10.2.4.2 for details. This is particularly important for the extended ('Box-Cox') version of the model (provided in Appendix 18 of the online supplementary material (10.S1 Code for undertaking meta-analysis)), for which mixing of the chains may be poor, requiring long simulation runs for robust parameter estimation.

The main quantities of interest from this model will usually be the 'summary' estimates of TPR and FPR (or, equivalently, sensitivity and specificity) across a range of possible threshold values. These are estimated by evaluating equation 10.9 at each iteration of the MCMC simulation. This can be done by adding additional lines to the JAGS model code or, alternatively, by post processing of the 'coda' (simulated values from the posterior distributions of each parameter) in R. Post processing of the coda is more computationally efficient. R code to achieve this is provided in Appendix 18 of the online supplementary material (10.S1 Code for undertaking meta-analysis), while the WinBUGS code provided in Jones (2019) can be adapted to perform the calculations within JAGS if preferred. As with all other parameters, we then summarize the chains by the medians (parameter estimates) and 2.5th and 97.5th percentiles (95% credible intervals). As in the other Bayesian models (e.g. Section 10.2.4), it is also straightforward to obtain predicted distributions for the sensitivity and specificity (in this case, for any given threshold value) in a new study. See Jones (2019) for details.

For the FeNO dataset, summary TPR and FPR with 95% credible intervals, across a range of reported threshold values, are shown in Figure 10.7.c, alongside the observed study-level data. R code to generate this plot is provided in Appendix 18 of the online supplementary material (10.S1 Code for undertaking meta-analysis).

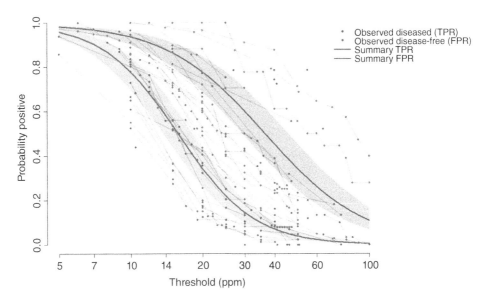

Figure 10.7.c Summary true-positive rate (TPR or sensitivity) and false positive rate (FPR or 1-specificity) across thresholds, with 95% credible intervals, for the FeNO data

10.8 Meta-analysis with imperfect reference standard: latent class meta-analysis

This section illustrates one approach for extending the bivariate model to the situation where the reference standard is not perfect (Xie 2017). The target condition of interest is assumed to be latent, i.e. it cannot be observed. Therefore, a slightly different notation is used. The 2×2 table observed in each study included in the meta-analysis is denoted by (n11, n10, n01, n00), where n_{ij} refers to the number of subjects in the cell where the index test has value i and the reference standard has value j, where i,j have a value of 1 for a positive test result and a value of 0 for a negative test result.

The meta-analysis of the accuracy of the GeneXpert (Xpert) test for tuberculosis (TB) meningitis (Kohli 2018) is used as a motivating example. In each study the index test was Xpert and the reference standard was culture. Both tests have near perfect specificity but suboptimal sensitivity, therefore the true TB meningitis status of each subject is not known with certainty. The likelihood function of an individual study is expressed as follows:

```
(n11,n10,n01,n00) ~ Multinomial((p11,p10,p01,p00), N),        where
p11 = prev*(se1*se2 + covs) + (1-prev)*((1-sp1)*(1-sp2) + covc)
p10 = prev*(se1*(1-se2) - covs) + (1-prev)*((1-sp1)*sp2 - covc)
p01 = prev*((1-se1)*se2 - covs) + (1-prev)*(sp1*(1-sp2) - covc)
p00 = prev*((1-se1)*(1-se2) + covs) + (1-prev)*(sp1*sp2 + covc), where
```

$$- (1 - s1) * (1 - s2) < covs < \max(s1, s2) - s1^* s2$$
$$- (1 - c1) * (1 - c2) < covc < \max(c1, c2) - c1^* c2 \qquad (10.10)$$

where prev denotes the prevalence of the latent target condition, se1 and sp1 denote the sensitivity and specificity of the index test, se2 and sp2 denote the sensitivity and specificity of the reference standard, covs is the covariance between the tests among those who have the target condition, covc is the covariance between the tests among those who do not have the target condition and N is the total sample size in all four cells.

Notice that the probability of each cell of the 2×2 table is the sum of two parts. The latent class model assumes that each observed cell can be further split into those that have the target condition and those that do not have it. The covariance terms adjust for conditional dependence, i.e. the dependence between the index test and reference standard conditional on the target condition. In our example, conditional dependence may arise among patients with the target condition because among individuals with a low bacterial load, the target condition is more likely to be missed (false negative) by both Xpert and culture, whereas among individuals with a high bacterial load, the target condition is more likely to be detected by both tests (true positive). Ignoring the possibility of conditional dependence will lead to biased estimates for test accuracy and prevalence parameters (Vacek 1985, Torrance-Rynard 1997).

10.8.1 Specification of the latent class bivariate meta-analysis model in rjags

This section describes how to extend the rjags model for bivariate meta-analysis introduced in Section 10.2.4 to include the structure of a latent class analysis (see Appendix 6 of the online supplementary material (10.S1 Code for undertaking meta-analysis),

Section A6.5). The likelihood function is replaced by a multinomial likelihood whose probabilities are given in equation 10.10. A prior distribution is needed for each unknown parameter to carry out Bayesian estimation. A hierarchical prior distribution structure is specified for the sensitivity and specificity of the index test to account for both between- and within-study variability and the correlation between sensitivity and specificity across studies. A similar hierarchical prior distribution is specified over the sensitivity and specificity of the reference standard. Additionally, prior distributions must be specified for the prevalence in each study and for the covariance parameters.

10.8.2   Monitoring convergence

When running the jags.model() function in the rjags code, it is possible that a warning message appears about the adaptation phase being incomplete. This is due to the complexity of the latent class meta-analysis model (this message is unlikely to appear for the simpler Bayesian models presented earlier where a perfect reference standard was assumed). After carefully studying convergence, we conclude that this warning has little to no impact on our results and can be ignored. Monitoring the trace plots and density plots of the posterior samples is crucial in the case of a latent class meta-analysis model to determine whether the model has converged. A peculiarity of latent class analysis is that the model may interchange the labels of 'target condition positive' and 'target condition negative'. This results in different MCMC chains reaching apparently different but algebraically identical solutions. For example, one chain may reach the solution for (prev, se1, sp1, se2, sp2), while the other reaches the 'mirror' solution (1-prev, 1-se1, 1-sp1, 1-se2, 1-sp2). Consequently, the average results across chains may not be very meaningful. This problem is magnified in the case of latent class meta-analysis, as it can happen separately for each study. The plots in Figure 10.8.a illustrate the problem using the example of the posterior distribution of the disease prevalence and specificity of the Xpert test for the study by Bahr 2015 from the TB meningitis meta-analysis. The individual chains converge to a solution, but the blue chain reaches one solution while the red chain reaches another. Which of these solutions is correct?

For this particular example, from prior experience it is known that Xpert has very high specificity and that the solution attained by the red curve (posterior median = 0.99) is the correct one, while the solution attained by the blue curve (posterior median = 0.15) is not sensible. This implies that the correct solution for the prevalence is also that obtained by the red line (posterior median = 0.24) and not the solution obtained by the blue line (posterior median = 0.88). An appropriate selection of initial values closer to the solution with the desired labelling will usually avoid the problem. In some cases, redefining the prior distribution so that its domain only covers plausible values is helpful. In this example, a prior distribution for the logit specificity of Xpert that is truncated at the lower limit of 0 could be used to ensure that specificity is always above 50%. Alternatively, an informative prior distribution may be used.

10.8.3   Summary statistics and summary ROC plot

The results of summary statistics for the bivariate latent class meta-analysis model are compared here to those obtained from the Bayesian estimation of the standard bivariate meta-analysis model for the same data (Box 10.8.a). Figure 10.8.b compares the SROC plots obtained from the two methods.

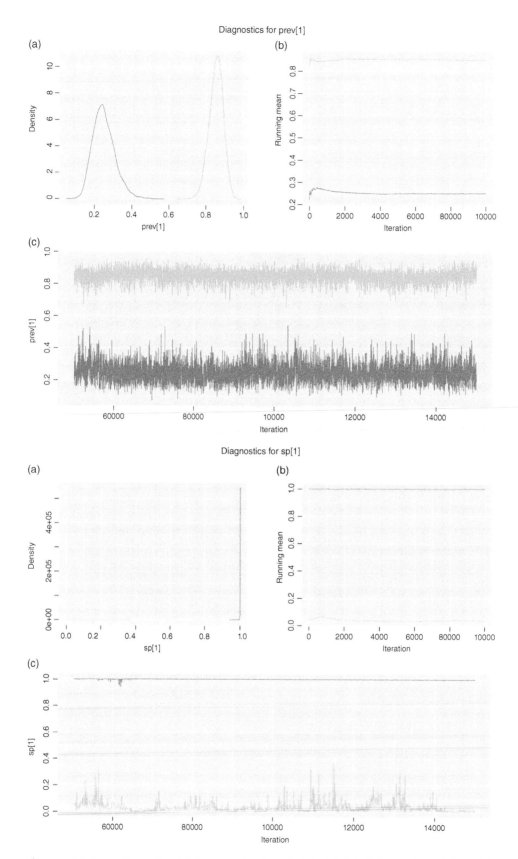

Figure 10.8.a MCMC diagnostics plots for parameters from the bivariate latent class meta-analysis model

Box 10.8.a Comparison of results from Bayesian bivariate latent class and standard bivariate meta-analysis models

Bivariate latent class meta-analysis model

```
Iterations = 31010:331000
Thinning interval = 10
Number of chains = 5
Sample size per chain = 30000
```

1. Empirical mean and standard deviation for each variable, plus standard error of the mean:

	Mean	SD	Naive SE	Time-series SE
Summary_Se	0.6465190	0.051066	1.319e-04	8.234e-04
Summary_Se2	0.7000913	0.052723	1.361e-04	8.537e-04
Summary_Sp	0.9942673	0.003753	9.690e-06	9.778e-05
Summary_Sp2	0.9914815	0.004494	1.160e-05	1.053e-04
Predicted_Se	0.6397513	0.111522	2.879e-04	7.782e-04
Predicted_Sp	0.9930580	0.008756	2.261e-05	1.129e-04
rho	0.0530568	0.571872	1.477e-03	7.836e-03
tau.sq[1]	0.2191830	0.135772	3.506e-04	1.329e-03
tau.sq[2]	0.3822149	0.385743	9.960e-04	4.324e-03

2. Quantiles for each variable:

	2.5%	25%	50%	75%	97.5%
Summary_S	5.496e-01	6.119e-01	0.645373	0.6799865	0.750382
Summaryan_S2	5.975e-01	6.650e-01	0.699523	0.7345158	0.806461
Summary_C	9.850e-01	9.923e-01	0.995022	0.9970767	0.999236
Summary_C2	9.811e-01	9.888e-01	0.992067	0.9948021	0.998417
Predicted_Se	4.060e-01	5.679e-01	0.644651	0.7171661	0.844417
Predicted_Sp	9.748e-01	9.913e-01	0.995149	0.9974802	0.999469
rho	-9.374e-01	-4.321e-01	0.080262	0.5518103	0.951745
tau.sq[1]	7.387e-02	1.312e-01	0.184130	0.2650333	0.575089
tau.sq[2]	8.752e-02	1.764e-01	0.273575	0.4494636	1.325901

Standard bivariate meta-analysis model

```
Iterations = 6001:16000
Thinning interval = 1
Number of chains = 3
Sample size per chain = 10000
```

1. Empirical mean and standard deviation for each variable, plus standard error of the mean:

	Mean	SD	Naive SE	Time-series SE
Summary_Se	0.7143	0.048716	2.813e-04	9.707e-04
Summary_Sp	0.9812	0.004695	2.710e-05	1.045e-04
Predicted_Se	0.6862	0.175487	1.013e-03	1.219e-03
Predicted_Sp	0.9713	0.035431	2.046e-04	2.314e-04
rho	0.2989	0.263569	1.522e-03	7.750e-03
tau.sq[1]	0.8680	0.463325	2.675e-03	1.495e-02
tau.sq[2]	0.9229	0.439277	2.536e-03	1.285e-02

2. Quantiles for each variable:

	2.5%	25%	50%	75%	97.5%
Summary_Se	0.6154	0.6830	0.7157	0.7470	0.8076
Summary_Sp	0.9711	0.9783	0.9815	0.9844	0.9894
Predicted_Se	0.2766	0.5801	0.7136	0.8203	0.9454
Predicted_Sp	0.8832	0.9658	0.9813	0.9899	0.9976
rho	-0.2517	0.1221	0.3144	0.4925	0.7631
tau.sq[1]	0.2828	0.5468	0.7657	1.0756	2.0372
tau.sq[2]	0.3354	0.6122	0.8350	1.1386	2.0107

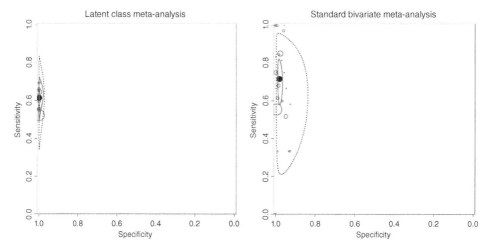

Figure 10.8.b Comparison of credible and prediction regions from bivariate latent class and standard bivariate meta-analysis models

The box shows that the latent class meta-analysis model resulted in a lower estimate of the sensitivity of the index test (Summary_S = 0.645373) than the standard bivariate meta-analysis (Summary_Se = 0.7157). The summary specificity of the index test was slightly higher in the latent class meta-analysis model (Summary_C = 0.995022 versus Summary_Sp = 0.9815). Of course, the standard bivariate meta-analysis does not provide any estimates for the sensitivity and specificity of the reference standard, which are assumed to be 100%. Under the latent class meta-analysis model, the posterior median estimates of the summary sensitivity and specificity of the reference standard were Summary_S2 = 0.699523 and Summary_C2 = 0.992067, respectively. An important consequence of adjusting for the imperfect nature of the reference standard is that the apparent heterogeneity in the accuracy of the index test is reduced. We can see this reflected in the parameters tau.sq[1] and tau.sq[2], which are much higher in the standard bivariate meta-analysis, and also in the standard deviations of the predicted sensitivity and specificity in a future study. Furthermore, the correlation parameter (rho) is practically zero in the latent class meta-analysis, removing the apparent positive correlation suggested by the standard bivariate meta-analysis. This is confirmed by a comparison of the credible and prediction regions on the SROC plot (Figure 10.8.b).

10.8.4 Sensitivity analyses

Sensitivity analyses are particularly important for latent class models, as the number of unknown parameters is very large and the model can encounter identifiability problems (i.e. where there are multiple solutions). In such situations, informative prior distributions may be necessary over some parameters, e.g. the sensitivity and specificity of the reference standard. In this situation it would be important to carry out sensitivity analyses to see whether the results are robust to the form of the prior distribution. As with any bivariate meta-analysis, it is important to examine the impact of changing the form of the vague prior distributions over the parameters capturing the between-study variability, as the results are known to be sensitive to this choice, particularly when the number of studies is small.

10.9   Concluding remarks

Prior to 2008, only one user-written program (metandi) was available for fitting the bivariate model for meta-analysis of test accuracy. Since then considerable progress has been made and there is now a plethora of user-written programs for fitting bivariate or HSROC models for meta-analysis of test accuracy. Using software packages frequently used for frequentist analyses and different published systematic reviews, this chapter has illustrated how to fit standard bivariate and HSROC models. The chapter also illustrated analyses within a Bayesian framework for the standard models as well as when there is an imperfect reference standard. Many tests are measured on a continuum and so a threshold is needed for defining test positivity. Studies may report one or more thresholds, and this chapter has also shown how to perform meta-analysis that allows for multiple thresholds from the included studies.

When performing hierarchical meta-regression for investigating heterogeneity and test comparisons, it is often assumed that the variances of the respective model parameters are identical across subgroups or tests (i.e. equal variances). A similar assumption is commonly made about between-study variances for treatment effects in multiple treatment comparisons (network meta-analysis). While this assumption has the advantage of simplifying estimation of the models and may be appropriate for treatment effects, it is not generalizable, as shown by examples in this chapter and empirically by Takwoingi (2016). The complexity of models and/or the number of tests or subgroups in relation to the number of studies available pose a challenge. Therefore, the chapter also addressed how to facilitate convergence, and how to simplify hierarchical models if appropriate.

This chapter has provided several examples and guidance on fitting meta-analysis models, but the expertise of a statistician or methodologist familiar with these methods may still be required. Commercial software packages like Stata and SAS require purchase of a user licence and this may limit software options available to some meta-analysts. SAS has a free package (SAS on demand for academics; www.sas.com/en_gb/software/on-demand-for-academics.html) for academic, non-commercial use. Additional resources such as tutorials and user guides that provide step-by-step guidance for both novice and experienced meta-analysts of test accuracy are available on the Cochrane Screening and Diagnostic Tests Methods Group website (methods.cochrane.org/sdt). The resources also include other programs and macros not covered in this chapter.

10.10   Chapter information

Authors: Yemisi Takwoingi (*Institute of Applied Health Research, University of Birmingham, UK*), Nandini Dendukuri (*McGill University, Montreal, Canada*), Ian Schiller (*Centre for Outcomes Research, McGill University Health Centre – Research Institute, Canada*), Gerta Rücker (*Institute of Medical Biometry and Statistics, University of Freiburg, Germany*), Hayley E. Jones (*Population Health Sciences, University of Bristol, UK*),

Christopher Partlett (*Nottingham Clinical Trials Unit, University of Nottingham, UK*), Petra Macaskill (*Sydney School of Public Health, University of Sydney, Australia*).

Sources of support: Yemisi Takwoingi is funded by a UK National Institute for Health Research (NIHR) Postdoctoral Fellowship. Yemisi Takwoingi is supported by the NIHR Birmingham Biomedical Research Centre at the University Hospitals Birmingham NHS Foundation Trust and the University of Birmingham. The views expressed are those of the authors and not necessarily those of the NHS, the NIHR or the Department of Health and Social Care. Ian Schiller was supported by a grant from the Canadian Institutes of Health Research (PJT-156039). Gerta Rücker was supported by the German Research Foundation (DFG), grant RU 1747/1-2. Hayley E. Jones was supported by an MRC-NIHR New Investigator Research Grant (MR/T044594/1). No other authors declare sources of support for writing this chapter.

Declarations of interest: Yemisi Takwoingi, Nandini Dendukuri and Petra Macaskill are members of Cochrane's Diagnostic Test Accuracy Editorial Team. Yemisi Takwoingi and Petra Macaskill are co-convenors of the Cochrane Screening and Diagnostic Tests Methods Group. Yemisi Takwoingi created the MetaDAS SAS macro and wrote the Stata tutorial for fitting the bivariate model. Yemisi Takwoingi and Christopher Partlett co-authored the R tutorial for fitting the bivariate model. Gerta Rücker is the first author of the R package diagmeta. Hayley E. Jones led development of the multiple thresholds model described in Section 10.7.2. The authors declare no other potential conflicts of interest relevant to the topic of this chapter.

Acknowledgements: The authors would like to thank Sarah Berhane, Kurinchi Gurusamy, Alex Sutton and Bada Yang for useful comments.

10.11   References

Alldred SK, Takwoingi Y, Guo B, Pennant M, Deeks JJ, Neilson JP, Alfirevic Z. First trimester serum tests for Down's syndrome screening. *Cochrane Database of Systematic Reviews* 2015; **11**: CD011975.

Allen VB, Gurusamy KS, Takwoingi Y, Kalia A, Davidson BR. Diagnostic accuracy of laparoscopy following computed tomography (CT) scanning for assessing the resectability with curative intent in pancreatic and periampullary cancer. *Cochrane Database of Systematic Reviews* 2016; **7**: CD009323.

Bates D, Maechler M, Bolker B, Walker S, Christensen RHB, Singmann H, Dai B, Grothendieck G, Green P. lme4: linear mixed-effects models using 'Eigen' and S4; 2016. cran.r-project.org/web/packages/lme4/index.html.

Benedetti A, Levis B, Rücker G, Jones HE, Schumacher M, Ioannidis JPA, Thombs B. An empirical comparison of three methods for multiple cutoff diagnostic test meta-analysis of the Patient Health Questionnaire-9 (PHQ-9) depression screening tool using published data vs individual level data. *Research Synthesis Methods* 2020; **11**: 833-848.

Chu H, Cole SR. Bivariate meta-analysis of sensitivity and specificity with sparse data: a generalized linear mixed model approach. *Journal of Clinical Epidemiology* 2006; **59**: 1331-1332; author reply 1332-1333.

Chung Y, Rabe-Hesketh S, Choi IH. Avoiding zero between-study variance estimates in random-effects meta-analysis. *Statistics in Medicine* 2013; **32**: 4071-4089.

Dewey M. CRAN Task View: Meta-Analysis version 2018-05-10; 2018. CRAN.R-project.org/view=MetaAnalysis.

Doebler P. mada: Meta-Analysis of Diagnostic Accuracy; 2015. cran.r-project.org/web/packages/mada/index.html.

Dwamena B. midas: Stata module for meta-analytical integration of diagnostic test accuracy studies. Statistical Software Components S456880. Department of Economics, Boston College; 2007. ideas.repec.org/c/boc/bocode/s456880.html.

Freeman SC, Kerby CR, Patel A, Cooper NJ, Quinn T, Sutton AJ. Development of an interactive web-based tool to conduct and interrogate meta-analysis of diagnostic test accuracy studies: MetaDTA. *BMC Medical Research Methodology* 2019; **19**: 81.

Gasparrini A. mvmeta: multivariate and univariate meta-analysis and meta-regression; 2015. cran.r-project.org/web/packages/mvmeta/index.html.

Gelman A, Carlin JB, Stern HS, Dunson DB, Vehtari A, Rubin DB. *Bayesian data analysis*. 3rd ed. Boca Raton (FL): Chapman and Hall-CRC; 2013.

Guo J, Riebler A. meta4diag: Bayesian bivariate meta-analysis of diagnostic test studies for routine practice; 2015. arxiv.org/abs/1512.06220.

Gurusamy KS, Giljaca V, Takwoingi Y, Higgie D, Poropat G, Štimac D, Davidson BR. Endoscopic retrograde cholangiopancreatography versus intraoperative cholangiography for diagnosis of common bile duct stones. *Cochrane Database of Systematic Reviews* 2015; **2**: Cd010339.

Harbord RM, Deeks JJ, Egger M, Whiting PF, Sterne JA. A unification of models for meta-analysis of diagnostic accuracy studies. *Biostatistics* 2007; **8**: 239-251.

Harbord R. metandi: Stata module for meta-analysis of diagnostic accuracy. Revised 15 Apr 2008. Statistical Software Components, Boston College Department of Economics; 2008.

Harbord RM, Whiting P. Metandi: meta-analysis of diagnostic accuracy using hierarchical logistic regression. *Stata Journal* 2009; **9**: 211-229.

Jones HE, Gatsonis CA, Trikalinos TA, Welton NJ, Ades AE. Quantifying how diagnostic test accuracy depends on threshold in a meta-analysis. *Statistics in Medicine* 2019; **38**: 4789-4803.

Kay AW, Gonzalez Fernandez L, Takwoingi Y, Eisenhut M, Detjen AK, Steingart KR, Mandalakas AM. Xpert MTB/RIF and Xpert MTB/RIF Ultra assays for active tuberculosis and rifampicin resistance in children. *Cochrane Database of Systematic Reviews* 2020; **8**: CD013359.

Kohli M, Schiller I, Dendukuri N, Dheda K, Denkinger CM, Schumacher SG, Steingart KR. Xpert® MTB/RIF assay for extrapulmonary tuberculosis and rifampicin resistance. *Cochrane Database of Systematic Reviews* 2018; **8**: CD012768.

Kruschke J. *Doing Bayesian data analysis: a tutorial with R, JAGS, and Stan*. 2nd ed. Cambridge, MA: Academic Press; 2015.

Lambert PC, Sutton AJ, Burton PR, Abrams KR, Jones DR. How vague is vague? A simulation study of the impact of the use of vague prior distributions in MCMC using WinBUGS. *Statistics in Medicine* 2005; **24**: 2401-2428.

Lu B, Lian Q, Hodges J, Chen Y, Chu H. NMADiagT: network meta-analysis of multiple diagnostic tests. Version 0.1.2; February 2020. cran.r-project.org/web/packages/NMADiagT/index.html.

Lunn D, Spiegelhalter D, Thomas A, Best N. The BUGS project: evolution, critique and future directions. *Statistics in Medicine* 2009; **28**: 3049-3067.

Macaskill P. Contributions to the analysis and meta-analysis of diagnostic test comparisons. Sydney: University of Sydney; 2003.

Nikoloulopoulos A. CopulaREMADA: Copula mixed effect models for bivariate and trivariate meta-analysis of diagnostic test accuracy studies; 2015. cran.r-project.org/web// packages//CopulaREMADA/CopulaREMADA.pdf.

Nishimura K, Sugiyama D, Kogata Y, Tsuji G, Nakazawa T, Kawano S, Saigo K, Morinobu A, Koshiba M, Kuntz KM, Kamae I, Kumagai S. Meta-analysis: diagnostic accuracy of anti-cyclic citrullinated peptide antibody and rheumatoid factor for rheumatoid arthritis. *Annals of Internal Medicine* 2007; **146**: 797-808.

Nyaga VN, Arbyn M, Aerts M. CopulaDTA: an R package for Copula-based bivariate beta-binomial models for diagnostic test accuracy studies in a Bayesian framework. *Journal of Statistical Software, Code Snippets* 2017; **82**: 27.

Partlett C, Takwoingi Y. Meta-analysis of test accuracy studies in R: a summary of user-written programs and step-by-step guide to using glmer. Version 2.0; August 2021. methods.cochrane.org/sdt/.

Patel A, Cooper N, Freeman S, Sutton A. Graphical enhancements to summary receiver operating characteristic plots to facilitate the analysis and reporting of meta-analysis of diagnostic test accuracy data. *Research Synthesis Methods* 2021; **12**: 34-44.

Plummer M. rjags: Bayesian graphical models using MCMC. R package version 4-10; 2019. CRAN.R-project.org/package=rjags.

Reitsma JB, Glas AS, Rutjes AW, Scholten RJ, Bossuyt PM, Zwinderman AH. Bivariate analysis of sensitivity and specificity produces informative summary measures in diagnostic reviews. *Journal of Clinical Epidemiology* 2005; **58**: 982-990.

Riley RD, Abrams KR, Sutton AJ, Lambert PC, Thompson JR. Bivariate random-effects meta-analysis and the estimation of between-study correlation. *BMC Medical Research Methodology* 2007; **7**: 3.

Rücker G, Steinhauser S, Kolampally S, Schwarzer G. diagmeta: meta-analysis of diagnostic accuracy studies with several cutpoints. R package version 0.4-0; 2020. CRAN.R-project. org/package=diagmeta.

Schneider A, Linde K, Reitsma JB, Steinhauser S, Rücker G. A novel statistical model for analyzing data of a systematic review generates optimal cutoff values for fractional exhaled nitric oxide for asthma diagnosis. *Journal of Clinical Epidemiology* 2017; **92**: 69-78.

Schuetz GM, Zacharopoulou NM, Schlattmann P, Dewey M. Meta-analysis: noninvasive coronary angiography using computed tomography versus magnetic resonance imaging. *Annals of Internal Medicine* 2010; **152**: 167-177.

Spiegelhalter DJ, Abrams KR, Myles JP. *Bayesian approaches to clinical trials and healthcare evaluation.* New York (NY): John Wiley & Sons; 2004.

Steinhauser S, Schumacher M, Rücker G. Modelling multiple thresholds in meta-analysis of diagnostic test accuracy studies. *BMC Medical Research Methodology* 2016; **16**: 97.

Takwoingi Y, Deeks J. MetaDAS: A SAS macro for meta-analysis of diagnostic accuracy studies. User Guide Version 1.3; 2010. methods.cochrane.org/sdt/ software-meta-analysis-dta-studies.

Takwoingi Y. Meta-analytic approaches for summarising and comparing the accuracy of medical tests [PhD]. Birmingham: University of Birmingham; 2016.

Takwoingi Y, Guo B, Riley RD, Deeks JJ. Performance of methods for meta-analysis of diagnostic test accuracy with few studies or sparse data. *Statistical Methods in Medical Research* 2017; **26**: 1896-1911.

Takwoingi Y. Meta-analysis of test accuracy studies in Stata: a bivariate model approach. Version 2.01; February 2023. methods.cochrane.org/sdt/.

Torrance-Rynard VL, Walter SD. Effects of dependent errors in the assessment of diagnostic test performance. *Statistics in Medicine* 1997; **16**: 2157-2175.

Vacek PM. The effect of conditional dependence on the evaluation of diagnostic tests. *Biometrics* 1985; **41**: 959-968.

Verde PE. bamdit: an R package for Bayesian meta-analysis of diagnostic test data. *Journal of Statistical Software* 2018; **86**: 32.

Xie X, Sinclair A, Dendukuri N. Evaluating the accuracy and economic value of a new test in the absence of a perfect reference test. *Research Synthesis Methods* 2017; **8**: 321-332.

Zapf A, Albert C, Frömke C, Haase M, Hoyer A, Jones HE, Rücker G. Meta-analysis of diagnostic accuracy studies with multiple thresholds: comparison of different approaches. *Biom J* 2021; **63**: 699-711.

11

Presenting findings

Jonathan J. Deeks, Patrick M. Bossuyt, Mariska M. Leeflang and Yemisi Takwoingi

---

KEY POINTS

- Results of the search, characteristics of the included studies and methodological quality assessment should be summarized to provide the reader with an overview of the evidence.
- For each objective, the review should present the relevant evidence and the findings, such as results from individual studies and from meta-analyses to enable conclusions to be drawn about the accuracy of the index test(s).
- When summarizing findings from a comparison of two tests, review authors should focus on describing the magnitude and direction of the difference between tests, the uncertainty in the estimates and the degree of heterogeneity.
- Review authors should express the degree of statistical uncertainty associated with summary estimates of test accuracy and consider the between-study variability.
- When investigations of sources of heterogeneity were made, the results should be cautiously interpreted.
- Presenting summary estimates of sensitivity, specificity and predictive values as frequencies has been shown to helpful for readers and is strongly encouraged.
- Tables, forest plots and/or summary receiver operating characteristic (SROC) plots are valuable tools for presenting findings in reviews with and without meta-analysis.

11.1   Introduction

The potential to inform readers of a systematic review not only depends on the quality of the search and other steps of the systematic review process, but also on the review authors' ability to present the key findings of the review in a valid and informative way.

This chapter should be cited as: Deeks JJ, Bossuyt PM, Leeflang MM, Takwoingi Y. Chapter 11: Presenting findings. In: Deeks JJ, Bossuyt PM, Leeflang MM, Takwoingi Y, editors. *Cochrane Handbook for Systematic Reviews of Diagnostic Test Accuracy*. 1st edition. Chichester (UK): John Wiley & Sons, 2023: 327–348.

Cochrane Handbook for Systematic Reviews of Diagnostic Test Accuracy, First Edition. Edited by Jonathan J. Deeks, Patrick M. Bossuyt, Mariska M. Leeflang and Yemisi Takwoingi.
© 2023 The Cochrane Collaboration. Published 2023 by John Wiley & Sons Ltd.

This chapter focuses on the contents of the results section of a review. It describes what is expected in such a report and how to report the findings to ensure that they are adequately presented in an accessible manner to readers.

Reporting the results of a review requires judicious use of text, tables and figures to produce a full description of the included evidence and the associated analyses. The results section of the review will summarize the following.

- The results of the search.
- Key characteristics and the methodological quality of the included studies.
- Key findings about test accuracy.
- Findings for secondary objectives, including investigations of heterogeneity.
- Findings for any additional analyses, such as sensitivity analyses.

Unlike Cochrane Reviews of interventions, Cochrane Reviews of diagnostic test accuracy allow more flexibility in how the findings can be presented. These reviews invite authors to construct tables and select figures to report results as they think most appropriate. Review authors need to thoughtfully consider what evidence to include in the results section of the main report and the supporting material that should be presented in appendices.

11.2   Results of the search

This section will typically report the number of records that were screened for inclusion, the number of titles that were retained, the number of full-text reports screened for eligibility, the number of studies excluded and the number of studies eventually included. The search and selection process will be clarified by including a PRISMA-style flow diagram, summarizing the numbers of studies initially retrieved, excluded and included in the review and eventual meta-analyses. For further information, see Chapter 6, Section 6.4.2.

If additional efforts beyond searching bibliographic databases to identify studies were stated as part of the search methods (such as screening reference lists, citing articles, conference proceedings or trial registries) review authors should also report the outcome of these searches.

11.3   Description of included studies

In reviews with a very small number of studies, the description of included studies can be structured as a summary of each study. For larger reviews this will not be possible, and the description can be phrased in terms of the overall composition of studies included in the review.

Describing the evidence base requires summarizing key characteristics across the included studies. This may include sample sizes and number of participants with the target condition, key characteristics of the participants (typically summarizing both demographic and clinical characteristics), the numbers of studies evaluating each index test, variations in the testing processes, reference standards used and study designs.

Details for the included studies may best be reported in a 'Characteristics of included studies' table. Such a table may present at a glance key details for each study. Chapter 7 details the characteristics that should be extracted from each study to populate a 'Characteristics of included studies' table. Careful planning of the data extraction form can help ensure that items are recorded in a manner that allows their direct incorporation in the table. This saves time, particularly in reviews with substantial numbers of included studies.

11.4   Methodological quality of included studies

This section describes the methodological quality of studies included in the systematic review. For most systematic reviews of test accuracy, the QUADAS-2 tool will be used to evaluate methodological quality in terms of risk of bias and concerns regarding applicability (see Chapter 8).

The results of the assessment are usually presented in a table or figure. A figure may show the results for individual studies or across studies. For reviews with multiple target conditions or index tests, figures may also be presented separately for each target condition or test. If there are several tables or figures, review authors should carefully consider which ones to include in the main text and which ones to include in an appendix.

An informative description of the assessments of risk of bias would indicate, for each domain, whether studies were considered at risk of producing biased results, and why they were classified as such. Readers would also like to know to what extent an included study helped to answer the review question, i.e. whether there were concerns regarding applicability. Here also, it is informative to indicate whether such concerns arose, and why.

If studies were potentially eligible but excluded after an evaluation of their risk of bias or applicability, they should not be reported here. The characteristics of studies excluded because of risk of bias or concerns regarding applicability should be reported elsewhere, in a separate table or supplementary file.

If the review addresses comparisons of test accuracy between two or more index tests, the results of the assessment with the QUADAS-C tool will be presented next. The QUADAS-C results are typically specific to a comparison of two tests within the review. If there are two or more such comparisons, separate QUADAS-C assessments need to be reported.

11.5   Individual and summary estimates of test accuracy

For each objective, the review should present the relevant evidence and the findings, to enable conclusions to be drawn. For primary objectives this typically requires presentation of results from individual studies as well as from meta-analyses, if such analyses were performed. Meta-analyses may produce summary estimates of sensitivity and specificity or SROC curves (see Chapter 9, Section 9.2.2 and Section 9.3). If no meta-analysis could be performed, a different approach to summarizing the results of individual studies will be adopted (see Section 11.9).

11.5.1   Presenting results from included studies

It will be informative to present test accuracy results from the individual studies. Such overviews typically include the study identifier, year of publication, total number of participants, number of participants with the target condition, number of true and false positives, number of true and false negatives, estimates of test accuracy, as defined in the protocol, and expressions of statistical imprecision (typically as 95% confidence intervals). These overviews may be presented in tables or, more succinctly, on coupled forest plots of sensitivity and specificity (see Chapter 9, Section 9.2.1 and example Figure 9.2.a).

For pairwise comparisons of accuracy, individual studies will present multiple pairs of estimates of sensitivity and specificity. In that case, it is helpful to structure the table or graph in such a way that the link between these pairs is obvious. This can be done by presenting a linked SROC plot showing the multiple estimates from each study (one for each test), connected by a line (see Chapter 9, Figure 9.4.g, for an example).

11.5.2   Presenting summary estimates of sensitivity and specificity

Review authors should carefully consider the summary measures that are relevant and appropriate to present for a given analysis, rather than compute and report all possible measures of test accuracy. Many systematic reviews of test accuracy present summary estimates of sensitivity and specificity.

Other summary estimates, like positive and negative predictive values, may also be produced. The selection of appropriate summary estimates will also depend on the design of the primary studies. For example, if one reference standard is always used in index test positives and a different one in index test negatives, it will be more meaningful to present summary estimates of the negative and predictive values. The use of different reference standards is known to introduce bias in estimates of sensitivity and specificity.

A review may include multiple meta-analyses and corresponding summary estimates. These estimates can be summarized in one or more tables as appropriate. The table(s) should include the number of studies, participants and participants with and without the target condition on which each analysis is based (see an example in Table 11.5.a).

When summary estimates of sensitivity and specificity are reported as an output of meta-analysis, they need to be interpreted as expressions of a central tendency of estimates across the included studies. There may be considerable uncertainty in these summary estimates and substantial variability in accuracy across studies.

11.5.3   Presenting SROC curves

Including a 2×2 table of the number of true positives, false positives, false negatives and true negatives from each study regardless of threshold value allows estimation of an SROC curve. If an SROC curve is assumed to be symmetrical (i.e. the shape parameter in the HSROC model is assumed to be zero), then accuracy does not depend on threshold. In that case, the SROC curve can be described by a constant diagnostic odds ratio (DOR) (see Chapter 4, Section 4.5.7). A DOR of 1 represents an uninformative test (the upward diagonal in Figure 11.5.a). SROC curves closer to the top left-hand corner of the SROC plot represent tests with a higher DOR, hence more discriminatory power.

Table 11.5.a Accuracy of Xpert MTB/RIF for detection of extrapulmonary tuberculosis

Type of specimen	Reference standard	Number of studies (participants)	Number with TB (%)	Summary sensitivity % (95% credible interval)	Summary specificity % (95% credible interval)
CSF	Culture	30 (3395)	571 (16.8)	71.1 (62.8 to 79.1)	96.9 (95.4 to 98.0)
CSF	Composite	14 (2203)	862 (39.1)	42.3 (32.1 to 52.8)	99.8 (99.3 to 100.0)
Pleural fluid	Culture	25 (3065)	644 (21.0)	49.5 (39.8 to 59.9)	98.9 (97.6 to 99.7)
Pleural fluid	Composite	10 (1024)	616 (60.1)	18.9 (11.5 to 27.9)	99.3 (98.1 to 99.8)
Lymph node aspirate	Culture	14 (1588)	627 (39.5)	88.9 (82.7 to 93.6)	86.2 (78.0 to 92.3)
Lymph node aspirate	Composite	4 (679)	377 (55.5)	81.6 (61.9 to 93.3)	96.4 (91.3 to 98.6)

CSF, cerebrospinal fluid; TB, tuberculosis.
Source: Adapted from Table 2 in Kohli 2021.

When interpreting DORs, review authors should note that the same DOR may be achieved by different combinations of sensitivity and specificity (see Chapter 4, Section 4.5.7). In addition, single measures of test accuracy, like the DOR, are often not clinically informative, because of a lack of information on errors in those with the target condition (false negatives) and those without the condition (false positives). The relative

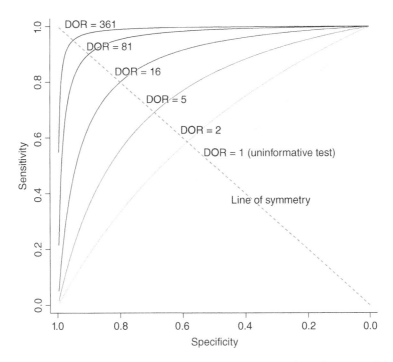

Figure 11.5.a   Symmetrical summary receiver operating characteristic (SROC) curves and diagnostic odds ratios (DORs)

331

magnitude of such errors is essential for judging the extent and likely impact of consequences of positive and negative test results.

DORs are probably most useful in meta-analysis when making comparisons between
tests or between subgroups (see Chapter 9, Section 9.4.6.4, and Section 11.6.2). For
these comparisons, if two curves are symmetrical or have the same shape, then the
relative accuracy of the two curves can be summarized using the ratio of the DORs or
relative DOR (RDOR).

It may be challenging to describe an SROC curve that is not symmetrical, either ver-
bally or numerically. As explained in Chapter 10 (Section 10.3.1), the anticipated sensitivity at a given value of specificity (or the other way round) can be computed from the
SROC curve to illustrate test performance in such cases. If review authors choose to
report such sensitivity and specificity pairs from an SROC curve, then the most informative estimates will be points on the curve that lie within the range of the sensitivity and
specificity estimates reported by the included studies. For example, these could be values that represent the median and interquartile range from the studies included in the
meta-analysis (see Chapter 10, Box 10.3.b).

Alternatively, if minimizing false positives – therefore maximizing specificity – in a
particular testing context is desired, the sensitivity of the test could be reported at the
minimally acceptable specificity (for example, a specificity of 95%).

Whatever the approach taken to select sensitivity and specificity pairs, the values and
corresponding estimates can be presented in a table, as shown in the example in
Table 11.5.b. Likelihood ratios can also be estimated at such fixed values.

11.5.4   Describing uncertainty in summary statistics

The summary sensitivity and specificity are estimates based on the included studies
and there will always be statistical uncertainty about their true value. Review authors
should express the degree of statistical uncertainty associated with summary estimates
of test accuracy, irrespective of the metric used. Confidence intervals or credible intervals should therefore be reported alongside the point estimates of summary sensitivity
and specificity in text and tables. For summary points on SROC plots, confidence regions
should also be presented (see Chapter 9, Figure 9.4.a).

Table 11.5.b Sensitivity and likelihood ratios for 11C-PIB-PET at fixed values of specificity
for Alzheimer's dementia

Statistic	Fixed value of specificity %	Estimated sensitivity % (95% CI)	Positive likelihood ratio (95% CI)	Negative likelihood ratio (95% CI)
Lower quartile	56	96 (88 to 99)	2.19 (2.09 to 2.29)	0.07 (0.02 to 0.23)
Median	58	96 (87 to 99)	2.29 (2.17 to 2.41)	0.07 (0.02 to 0.24)
Upper quartile	81	89 (68 to 97)	4.66 (4.03 to 5.39)	0.14 (0.05 to 0.44)

CI, confidence interval. Nine studies (n: 112 with dementia; 162 without dementia)
Source: Adapted from Table 4 in Zhang 2014.

11.5.5   Describing heterogeneity in summary statistics

Statistical heterogeneity (referred to simply as heterogeneity) exists whenever estimates of test accuracy vary between studies, more than would be expected from within-study sampling error (chance) alone. This is extremely common in systematic reviews of test accuracy. Prediction intervals and prediction regions give an indication of heterogeneity. Prediction regions plotted around summary points in ROC space represent the area where the sensitivity and specificity estimates from a future test accuracy study are expected to lie (see Chapter 9, Section 9.3.2, Section 9.4.1 and Section 9.4.2).

Systematic reviews of test accuracy studies can include prediction regions with coverage probabilities of 50%, 90% or 95%. The 95% prediction regions often cover large areas of ROC space because of the presence of substantial heterogeneity common in many systematic reviews of test accuracy. While the confidence region depicts uncertainty in the summary estimates of sensitivity and specificity due to within-study variability, the prediction region depicts the uncertainty due to both within- and between-study variability (see Chapter 9, Figure 9.4.a). As such, when heterogeneity is high, the 95% prediction region will be much larger than the 95% confidence region.

As stated in Chapter 9, estimation of a prediction interval or region relies on the assumption of normal distributions for the effects across studies. This may be very problematic when the number of studies is small and can lead to spuriously large (or small) regions (Deeks 2019). In addition, if the variance parameters and the correlation (or covariance) between logit sensitivity and specificity in a bivariate model cannot be reliably estimated, a prediction region will be misleading. Therefore, when there are few studies (e.g. fewer than 10) in the meta-analysis of a single test, review authors should carefully consider the appropriateness of presenting a prediction region around the summary point.

11.6   Comparisons of test accuracy

Review authors should consider two issues in reviews that compare the accuracy of multiple tests: (1) the statistical measures that can be used; and (2) the strength of the evidence for the comparison. The strength primarily relates to whether the meta-analysis is based on within-study (direct) or between-study (indirect) comparisons of tests (see Chapter 9, Section 9.1.4.3). This will be considered in Chapter 12 (Section 12.1.3.5 and Section 12.6.2.4). The appropriate statistical measures are not affected by this issue.

When summarizing findings from a comparison of two tests, review authors should focus on describing (1) the magnitude and direction of the difference between tests; (2) the uncertainty in the estimates; and (3) the degree of heterogeneity. Presentation of test comparisons can be facilitated by summaries of test accuracy in ROC space, which allow readers to compare test performance in one SROC plot. This may be in the form of summary estimates of sensitivity and specificity or SROC curves (shape and relative position). In addition, within-study test comparisons can be annotated to distinguish them from between-study comparisons.

11.6.1   Comparing tests using summary points

The magnitude and direction of the difference between tests can be summarized by reporting point estimates of the summary sensitivity and specificity for each test

Table 11.6.a Accuracy of chest ultrasonography and chest radiography for diagnosis of pneumothorax

Test	Studies	Participants (with pneumothorax)	Summary sensitivity (95% CI)	Summary specificity (95% CI)
CUS	9	1271 (410)	0.91 (0.85 to 0.94)	0.99 (0.97 to 1.00)
CXR	9	1271 (410)	0.47 (0.31 to 0.63)	1.00 (0.97 to 1.00)
Absolute difference			0.44 (0.27 to 0.61) $P < 0.001$	−0.007 (−0.018 to 0.005) $P = 0.26$

CUS, chest ultrasonography; CXR, chest radiography. The P values are from Wald tests.
Source: Adapted from Table 2 in Chan 2020.

and by measures of absolute or relative differences in sensitivity and specificity (see Table 11.6.a). Focusing on the size and the uncertainty in the estimated difference in summary sensitivity and specificity between tests illustrates the potential impact of using one test or the other.

For the example in Table 11.6.a, the summary sensitivities of 0.91 for chest ultrasonography and 0.47 for chest radiography indicate that chest ultrasonography can be expected to correctly detect 44 more patients out of every 100 with pneumothorax, compared to chest radiography. The 95% confidence interval translates into a difference that lies between 27 and 61 more patients out of every 100 with pneumothorax. A similar approach can be used if predictive values are being compared.

11.6.2   Comparing tests using SROC curves

When SROC curves of two or more tests are compared, it matters whether or not the SROC curves for the tests have the same shape. If they do, the value of the RDOR will be constant all the way along the curve. In those situations, the RDOR is a valid reflection of the difference in accuracy between tests. In that case, it will be informative to report the summary DOR for each test and estimates of the RDOR, with expressions of statistical uncertainty and heterogeneity.

Table 11.6.b presents the results of an indirect comparison of the accuracy of urea breath test, serology and stool antigen test for detecting a *Helicobacter pylori* infection. It is based on an HSROC model with symmetrical shape for the curves (Best 2018). The RDOR of 3.22 (95% CI 1.24 to 8.37, P = 0.017) indicates that the DOR for the urea breath-^{13}C test is about three times that of serology, and that we are 95% confident that this ratio lies between 1.24 and 8.37 times higher.

A higher DOR means that, for any selected positivity threshold for the inferior test, we can find a positivity threshold for the superior test that produces higher sensitivity for the same specificity, higher specificity for the same sensitivity, or both higher sensitivity and specificity. We cannot, however, identify the positivity thresholds on the SROC curve that correspond to specific sensitivity–specificity pairs.

Where tests have been compared using SROC curves, it may nevertheless be informative to report selected sensitivity–specificity pairs on each of the curves, to facilitate test comparisons. For example, the sensitivity of each test at the same fixed specificity could be reported, or the other way round. Review authors should be cautious when choosing

Table 11.6.b Comparison of the accuracy of non-invasive tests for *Helicobacter pylori* infection

Index test	Studies; participants (with *H. pylori*)	DOR (95% CI)	Relative diagnostic odds ratios (95% CI), P value		
			Urea breath test-^{13}C	Urea breath test-^{14}C	Serology
Urea breath test-^{13}C	34; 3139 (1526)	153 (73.7 to 316)			
Urea breath test-^{14}C	21; 1810 (1018)	105 (74.0 to 150)	1.45 (0.65 to 3.26) P = 0.36		
Serology	34; 4242 (2477)	47.4 (25.5 to 88.1)	3.22 (1.24 to 8.37) P = 0.017	2.22 (1.09 to 4.51) P = 0.028	
Stool antigen test	29; 2988 (1311)	45.1 (24.2 to 84.1)	3.39 (1.30 to 8.83) P = 0.013	2.33 (1.14 to 4.76) P = 0.020	1.05 (0.44 to 2.53) P = 0.91

CI, confidence interval. The indirect comparison included all studies that evaluated at least one of the four tests, i.e. all available data. The RDOR is the diagnostic odds ratio (DOR) of the test in the column relative to the DOR of the test in the row. If the RDOR is greater than one, then the test in the column is more accurate than the test in the row. The P values are from Wald tests.
Source: Adapted from Table 2 in Best 2018.

pairs for comparison. To be valid, the pairs should be based on the results in the review: they should lie within the range of observed sensitivity and specificity estimates from the included studies.

If the SROC curves for two or more tests differ in shape, the ratio of the corresponding DOR will not be constant along the entire length of the curve. In these situations, comparisons are challenging and interpretation of meta-analysis results needs to be done carefully, similarly considering the observed range of sensitivity and specificity estimates in individual studies. Here also, selecting pairs on the fitted curves may assist in interpretation, provided that these lie within the range of estimates reported by the included studies.

11.6.3   Interpretation of confidence intervals for differences in test accuracy

It has been shown that some readers wrongly apply heuristics about ratio measures, as used in systematic reviews of interventions (Zhelev 2013). In comparing interventions, they know that a confidence interval including unity indicates no significant difference in outcomes between the interventions. Readers should not interpret confidence intervals for sensitivity and specificity in a similar way. A confidence interval for sensitivity and specificity that includes unity (1.00, or 100%) does not reflect poor test performance but rather the opposite: the possibility of perfect performance. Review authors should therefore consider supplementing numerical presentation of statistical uncertainty in confidence intervals with verbal explanations. A natural frequency presentation format may additionally help (see Box 11.6.a and Section 11.8), particularly if a systematic review of test accuracy includes both estimates of the accuracy of single tests and a comparison of test accuracy.

When interpreting confidence intervals associated with comparisons, confidence intervals that do not overlap can be assumed to represent statistically significant differences. Confidence intervals that overlap may or may not reflect statistically significant differences; P values will be required to draw conclusions about statistical significance. Interpretation of a test comparison is illustrated in Box 11.6.a.

11.7   Investigations of sources of heterogeneity

Investigations of heterogeneity aim to assess whether test accuracy tends to vary with identifiable features, such as the characteristics of the participants, settings, tests, reference standards or others. As explained in Chapter 9 and Chapter 10, hierarchical meta-regression models can estimate differences in accuracy between subgroups (or the association of accuracy with a continuous measure) and formally test differences and associations for statistical significance.

Comparisons of subgroups based solely on studies that report data for subgroups within studies provide more valid evidence of sources of heterogeneity than comparisons between studies. For example, a Cochrane Review on Down syndrome screening explored the effect of advanced maternal age (< 35 years versus ≥ 35 years) on test performance. Of the 69 studies for one of the index tests assessed in the review, 5 provided data to compare the performance of the test between women younger than 35 years and those 35 years or more within the same study (Alldred 2017). The 5 studies all showed a higher sensitivity and higher false positive fraction for the ≥ 35 years compared to the < 35 years subgroup, as shown in Figure 11.7.a. Such analyses are

Box 11.6.a   Interpretation of confidence intervals and P values for comparisons of test performance

A Cochrane Review compared the accuracy of rapid diagnostic tests (RDTs) for detecting *Plasmodium falciparum* malaria (Abba 2011). RDTs use different types of antibody or antibody combinations to detect *Plasmodium* antigens. Two RDT types, type 1 and type 4, were compared in one of the meta-analyses in the review.

RDT type	Summary sensitivity % (95% CI)	Summary specificity % (95% CI)
Type 1: HRP-2 antibody-based tests	94.8 (93.0 to 96.1)	95.2 (93.2 to 96.7)
Type 4: pLDH antibody-based tests	91.5 (84.7 to 95.3)	98.6 (96.9 to 99.5)
Relative difference (type 1/type 4)	0.96 (0.91 to 1.02) P = 0.20	1.04 (1.02 to 1.06) P < 0.001

CI, confidence interval. P values were obtained from likelihood ratio tests.
Source: Adapted from Table 6 in Abba 2011.

The results can be interpreted as follows:

- The summary sensitivity of type 1 is 94.8%. We are 95% confident that the true value of sensitivity lies between 93.0% and 96.1%.
- The summary specificity of type 1 is 95.2%. We are 95% confident that the true value of specificity lies between 93.2% and 96.7%.
- The summary sensitivity of type 4 is 91.5%. We are 95% confident that the true value of sensitivity lies between 84.7% and 95.3%.
- The summary specificity of type 4 is 98.6%. We are 95% confident that the true value of specificity lies between 96.9% and 99.5%.
- Relative difference in sensitivity of type 4 and type 1 RDTs: the relative sensitivity of 0.96 indicates that the sensitivity of type 4 RDTs is 4% lower than the sensitivity of type 1 RDTs, in terms of the corresponding summary estimates. We are 95% confident that this difference lies between 9% lower and 2% higher. This difference is not statistically significant (P = 0.20).
- Relative difference in specificity of type 1 and type 4 RDTs: the relative specificity of 1.04 indicates that the specificity of type 4 RDTs is 4% higher than that of type 1 RDTs. We are 95% confident that this difference lies between 2% higher and 6% higher. This difference is statistically significant (P < 0.001).

NT, PAPP-A, free βhCG and maternal age-maternal age < 35 years

Study	TP	FP	FN	TN	Sensitivity (95% CI)	Specificity (95% CI)	Sensitivity (95% CI)	Specificity (95% CI)
Hadlow 2005	14	165	3	8042	0.82 [0.57, 0.96]	0.98 [0.98, 0.98]		
Krantz 2000	7	169	1	3589	0.88 [0.47, 1.00]	0.96 [0.95, 0.96]		
Marchini 2010	2	35	1	1200	0.67 [0.09, 0.99]	0.97 [0.96, 0.98]		
Schielen 2006	1	27	1	1704	0.50 [0.01, 0.99]	0.98 [0.98, 0.99]		
Wapner 2003	8	151	4	3933	0.67 [0.35, 0.90]	0.96 [0.96, 0.97]		

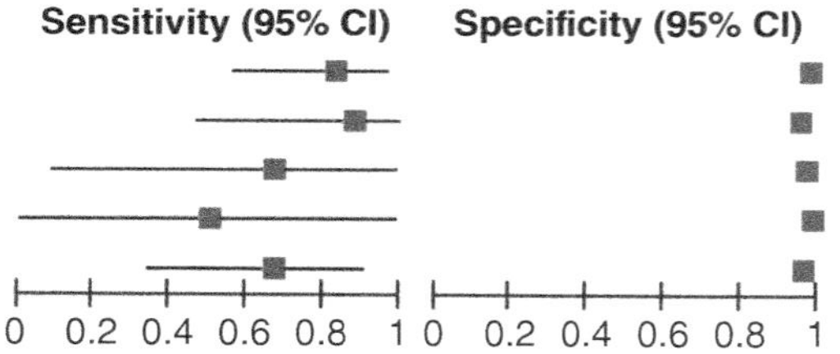

NT, PAPP-A, free βhCG and maternal age-maternal age ≥ 35 years

Study	TP	FP	FN	TN	Sensitivity (95% CI)	Specificity (95% CI)	Sensitivity (95% CI)	Specificity (95% CI)
Hadlow 2005	15	209	0	1988	1.00 [0.78, 1.00]	0.90 [0.89, 0.92]		
Krantz 2000	23	289	2	1729	0.92 [0.74, 0.99]	0.86 [0.84, 0.87]		
Marchini 2010	4	39	1	261	0.80 [0.28, 0.99]	0.87 [0.83, 0.911]		
Schielen 2006	14	163	5	2118	0.74 [0.49, 0.91]	0.93 [0.92, 0.94]		
Wapner 2003	44	619	5	3452	0.90 [0.78, 0.97]	0.85 [0.84, 0.86]		

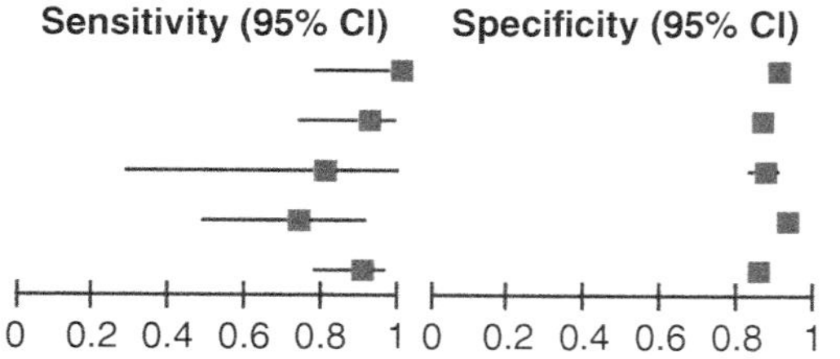

Figure 11.7.a Forest plot of the NT, PAPP-A, free βhCG and maternal age test strategy by maternal age group (< 35 years versus ≥ 35 years). βhCG, beta human chorionic gonadotrophin; FN, false negative; FP, false positive; NT, nuchal translucency; PAPP-A, pregnancy-associated plasma protein A; TN, true negative; TP, true positive. Source: Adapted from Figure 6 in Alldred 2017

uncommon in systematic reviews because data needed for such comparisons are often not reported in the included studies. In this Cochrane Review the subgroups were not formally compared using meta-regression due to the small number of studies and different test positivity thresholds used in the studies.

Meta-analytical results from heterogeneity analyses are often presented in a table and graphically in SROC plots displaying summary points or SROC curves for each category. The investigation of heterogeneity presented in Table 11.7.a compared studies of type 1 rapid diagnostic tests for *Plasmodium falciparum* malaria performed in Africa and studies performed in Asia.

Care should be exercised in interpreting the results of heterogeneity investigations. There are several points that should be considered.

First, subgroup findings are more credible if they have a scientific rationale. Ideally, selection of characteristics for investigation should be motivated by biological, clinical and methodological hypotheses supported by evidence from other sources. Subgroup analyses based on characteristics that are implausible or irrelevant are unlikely to be useful and should be avoided.

Second, exploratory heterogeneity investigations are less trustworthy than those that were pre-specified in the protocol. Review authors are expected to report whether heterogeneity investigations were pre-specified or data driven. Exploratory analyses are often data driven and prompted by observations made in informal data analyses, rather than by carefully crafted research hypotheses, supported by prior evidence. Pre-specification of investigations of heterogeneity in systematic reviews is often difficult, as review authors can be aware of some of the results in the included studies before they start the review.

Third, the chance of obtaining spurious significant results increases with the number of statistical comparisons that are undertaken. There is no formal rule on the maximum number of investigations that can be undertaken. The total number of hypotheses investigated must be kept in mind when interpreting the significance of the results. Adjustments to P values using rules for multiple testing are not encouraged, as they will be overly conservative due to the inevitable correlations between the factors investigated.

Fourth, heterogeneity investigations based on small numbers of studies are unlikely to produce useful findings and should be avoided. The statistical power of a comparison depends on the number of studies as well as on the precision of the test accuracy estimates from each study. When the characteristic is unevenly distributed across

Table 11.7.a Investigation of heterogeneity between studies of type 1 rapid diagnostic tests for *Plasmodium falciparum* malaria

Continent	Studies	Patients	Malaria cases	Summary sensitivity % (95% CI)	Summary specificity % (95% CI)	P value
Africa	39	21,958	7445	94.0 (91.2 to 96.0)	93.1 (89.7 to 95.3)	P = 0.03
Asia	24	15,810	4060	96.4 (93.7 to 97.9)	96.6 (94.0 to 98.1)	

CI, confidence interval. P value obtained from a likelihood ratio test comparing models with and without the covariate.
Source: Adapted from Table 7 in Abba 2011.

groups, it is possible that important differences may be missed. Since most comparisons will not be made within study participants, or based on randomization, statistically significant differences may not reflect the actual cause of the difference.

Fifth, only characteristics that were reported at study level or in subgroups defined within studies can be investigated. This limits the ability to detect relevant associations with test accuracy on an individual level. For example, if accuracy varies with age but study groups are similar in mean age, no association will be detected in a systematic review that relies on aggregate data. This problem is known as aggregation or ecological bias: the failure of ecological (aggregate)-level associations to properly reflect individual-level associations.

Sixth, it should be remembered that most subgroup comparisons are observational, and suffer from the same limitations as other comparisons in observational research. It may not be appropriate to make a causal interpretation of observed differences, although causal effects may have the greatest relevance for clinical practice. Confounding has to be considered: a difference between subgroups may be influenced by other factors that are also associated with differences in test accuracy. For example, if reference standards varied over time, but there were also changes over time in the composition of the study groups, it will not be possible to identify which, if either, is the cause of observed differences in test accuracy. Multivariable analysis, investigating multiple sources of heterogeneity in parallel, is usually infeasible due to the limited number of studies available (Takwoingi 2020).

Many review authors discover sooner or later that their plans for investigating heterogeneity are infeasible, either because of there being too few studies, or because studies do not report the desired information. Cochrane Reviews of diagnostic test accuracy contain a dedicated section to describe how the review differs from the protocol, where these issues can be described.

11.8 Re-expressing summary estimates numerically

11.8.1 Frequencies

Sensitivity and specificity are typically presented as proportions or percentages, and so are positive and negative predictive values. Presenting probabilities as frequencies has been shown to help readers understand their relative magnitude (Hoffrage 1998, Evans 2000, Zhelev 2013), and this approach is encouraged both in the 'Summary of main results' section of the review and in the 'Summary of findings' table.

A natural frequency description expresses a proportion as the number of individuals out of a group (typically 10, 100 or 1000) in whom an event or outcome is observed. A 95% sensitivity can be presented as a group of 100 persons with the target condition, of which 95 test positive.

As with conditional probabilities, one should be explicit about the group to which natural frequencies refer. For example, they may refer to all those tested, those with or without the target condition, or those with positive or with negative index test results.

Although sensitivity and specificity do not provide information on the absolute impact of a test at a particular prevalence of the target condition, expressing them as natural frequencies may help readers to interpret them. In addition, natural frequencies explicitly illustrate that sensitivity provides information on the false negatives and specificity on the false positives.

For example:

- For a test with a sensitivity of 90%: the index test will detect 90 out of every 100 with the target condition, but 10 will be missed (i.e. will be false negatives).
- For a test with a specificity of 80%: of every 100 individuals without the target condition, 20 will be wrongly diagnosed as having it (i.e. will be false positives).

11.8.2 Predictive values

There is a considerable body of empirical evidence demonstrating that sensitivity and specificity can be difficult to interpret for many clinicians and patients (Steurer 2002, Puhan 2005). Some researchers have argued that probabilities conditional on index test results (predictive values) rather than actual disease status (sensitivity and specificity) may be more intuitive to decision makers (Reid 1998).

Historically the use of predictive values has been discouraged, because sensitivity and specificity were assumed to be statistically independent of the proportion of participants with the target condition in the study group. If there are more study participants with the target condition, and sensitivity and specificity do not change, positive predictive values will be higher and negative predictive values lower. We now know that this is a simplification, as we are becoming increasingly aware of the variation in sensitivity and specificity caused by differences in the setting, previous testing and severity of disease (spectrum of disease) (Leeflang 2012). Review authors should therefore be mindful of the transferability of any accuracy measures, regardless of the type of summary statistic used.

Meta-analysis of predictive values is possible and sometimes necessary (Leeflang 2012), but it is not recommended to perform two meta-analyses in parallel: one of sensitivity and specificity and a second, separate meta-analysis of positive and negative predictive values. If review authors wish to use predictive values as a means of expressing test accuracy from a meta-analysis producing summary estimates of sensitivity and specificity, they should compute predictive values based on these estimates for a representative proportion of those with the target condition.

Predictive values are most simply obtained from summary estimates of sensitivity and specificity by creating an illustrative 2×2 table and computing predictive values directly (the simple equations to do this are in Chapter 4). This exercise can be done on paper, using a spreadsheet or a calculator tool (see Figure 11.8.a).

To compute predictive values manually or using a calculator, one needs a fictional group size (say, 1000), the proportion with the target condition ('prevalence' in the calculator), and the summary estimates of sensitivity and specificity of the test – i.e. the boxes in green in Figure 11.8.a. For example, a test that has sensitivity of 0.9 and specificity of 0.8 yields the values in Figure 11.8.a if 0.25 (25%) have the target condition. This computes the positive predictive value to be 0.60 and the negative predictive value to be 0.96. The same computations can be done using Bayes equation, as shown in Box 11.8.a.

Natural frequencies can be used to describe the absolute impact of a test in a population with a given prevalence (25% in Figure 11.8.a and Box 11.8.a).

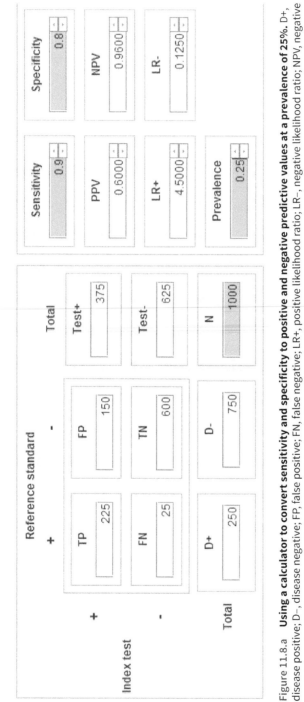

Figure 11.8.a   **Using a calculator to convert sensitivity and specificity to positive and negative predictive values at a prevalence of 25%.** D+, disease positive; D−, disease negative; FP, false positive; FN, false negative; LR+, positive likelihood ratio; LR−, negative likelihood ratio; NPV, negative predictive value; PPV, positive predictive value; TN, true negative; TP, true positive.

Box 11.8.a Calculation of predictive values using Bayes equation and estimates of sensitivity, specificity and prevalence

$$PPV = \frac{\text{sensitivity} \times \text{prevalence}}{\left[\text{sensitivity} \times \text{prevalence}\right] + \left[(1 - \text{specificity})(1 - \text{prevalence})\right]}$$

$$PPV = \frac{0.9 \times 0.25}{\left[0.9 \times 0.25\right] + \left[(1 - 0.8)(1 - 0.25)\right]}$$

$$PPV = 0.6$$

$$NPV = \frac{\text{specificity} \times (1 - \text{prevalence})}{\left[(1 - \text{sensitivity}) \times \text{prevalence}\right] + \left[\text{specificity} \times (1 - \text{prevalence})\right]}$$

$$NPV = \frac{0.8 \times (1 - 0.25)}{\left[(1 - 0.9) \times 0.25\right] + \left[0.8 \times (1 - 0.25)\right]}$$

$$NPV = 0.96$$

NPV, negative predictive value; PPV, positive predictive value.

- For a test with a positive predictive value of 60%: 60 out of every 100 positive index test results will have the target condition, but 40 will not (i.e. will be false positives). In a group in which 25% have the target condition, this will result in 150 false positive test results for every 1000 people tested.
- For a test with a negative predictive value of 96%: 96 out of every 100 negative index test results will not have the target condition, but 4 will (i.e. will be false negatives). In a group in which 25% have the target condition, this will result in 25 false negative test results for every 1000 people tested.

Although predictive values may be intuitive summary metrics, choosing the proportion of those with the target condition (prevalence) is not straightforward. The term 'prevalence' is often used to refer to the proportion of those with the target condition, for lack of a better term, but the proportion of those with the target condition in the population being tested will rarely be equal to the prevalence of the target condition in the population. In testing for SARS-CoV-2 infection, for example, the proportion with the SARS-CoV-2 virus in symptomatic persons undergoing testing will be substantially higher than the population prevalence. Similarly, the proportion with the virus in asymptomatic contacts of persons who recently tested positive will also be higher than the population prevalence, but lower than the proportion in symptomatic persons.

To select a proportion for the conversion to predictive values, the median value for the proportion of those with the target condition might be used, if that median is calculated from studies that relied on consecutive or random sampling of participants in the intended-use setting. Because of their design, studies that separately recruited participants with the target condition and healthy controls should be excluded from calculating the median proportion. Alternatively, review authors may consider computing predictive values across a range of plausible values for the intended-use setting. In some circumstances, estimates of disease prevalence may be more reliably obtained from other data sources, such as disease registries that correspond to the settings in which the studies in the meta-analysis were conducted.

The proportion of those with the target condition selected for presenting predictive values usually falls in the range of corresponding proportions observed in the studies included in the meta-analysis. The selection of a value outside that range would be an extrapolation, and should be done with caution.

11.8.3   Likelihood ratios

The use of likelihood ratios to express test performance (see Chapter 4) has been promoted by some as a metric that facilitates Bayesian probability updating: the calculation of post-test probabilities for specific pre-test probabilities (Straus 2019). Actual evidence that likelihood ratios improve diagnostic decision-making in groups of clinicians is lacking.

Parallel or separate meta-analysis of likelihood ratios is not recommended (see Chapter 9, Section 9.3). Summary estimates of the positive and negative likelihood ratios can be calculated from the summary estimates of sensitivity and specificity. These summary positive and negative likelihood ratios (and their 95% confidence intervals) can be obtained as additional estimates, as indicated in Chapter 9, Section 9.3, and illustrated in the software code in the appendices of Chapter 10.

Ideally, the confidence intervals for likelihood ratios should be used to calculate confidence intervals for predictive values because, unlike sensitivity and specificity, the positive likelihood ratio jointly considers the number of true and false positives and the negative likelihood ratio jointly considers the number of true and false negatives. Using likelihood ratio outputs from SAS and Stata, the lower and upper confidence limits of the positive likelihood ratio can be converted into lower and upper confidence limits of the positive predictive value, at a stated proportion with the target condition. Likewise, confidence limits of the negative likelihood ratio can be converted into confidence limits of the negative predictive value.

The simplest approach for deriving predictive values from likelihood ratios is to use a calculator tool, similar to the one for deriving point estimates of the predictive values (see Figure 11.8.a). Alternatively, predictive values can be calculated using the equations in Box 11.8.b.

Only the uncertainty in the summary estimates of sensitivity and specificity as expressions of test accuracy is captured in these 95% confidence intervals, not the uncertainty in the proportion with the target condition. This uncertainty could be explored by computing point estimates and 95% confidence intervals for predictive values across a range of plausible values for the proportion with the target condition (see Chapter 12).

11.9   Presenting findings when meta-analysis cannot be performed

Meta-analysis is not always possible due to few studies, convergence issues with the analysis (see Chapter 10, Section 10.6), clinical heterogeneity or other factors. Such situations are common. Of the 135 Cochrane Reviews of diagnostic test accuracy published up to 31 July 2020, 32 (24%) did not include a meta-analysis. In the 32 reviews,

---

Box 11.8.b Calculation of predictive values using post-test odds and likelihood ratios

---

Pre-test odds = pre-test probability/(1 − pre-test probability)
Post-test odds of disease given positive test result = pre-test odds of disease × LR+
Post-test odds of disease given negative test result = pre-test odds of disease × LR−
Post-test probability = Post-test odds/(1 + post-test odds)
Post-test probability of disease given a positive test result = PPV
Post-test probability of disease given a negative test result = 1 − NPV

Repeating the example shown in Figure 11.8.a, a test that has a positive likelihood ratio (LR+) of 4.5 and negative likelihood (LR−) of 0.125 will give a positive predictive value (PPV) of 0.60 and negative predictive value (NPV) of 0.96 using the previous equations as follows.

Pre-test odds = 0.25/(1 − 0.25) = 1/3
Post-test odds of disease given positive test result = (1/3) × 4.5 = 1.5
Post-test odds of disease given negative test result = (1/3) × 0.125 = 0.0417
Post-test probability of disease given a positive test result = 1.5/(1 + 1.5) = 0.60
Post-test probability of disease given a negative test result = 0.0417/(1 + 0.0417) = 0.04, therefore NPV = 1 − 0.04 = 0.96

---

the number of included studies ranged between 1 and 33; the median was 4 (inter-quartile range 3 to 9). A frequent reason for not performing meta-analysis was considerable between-study variation in clinical and methodological characteristics. For example, Chan (2019) did not perform meta-analysis due to risk-of-bias concerns and heterogeneity.

Tables, forest plots and/or SROC plots are valuable tools for presenting findings in reviews without meta-analysis. Plots provide a visual summary across studies and are more readily accessible to readers than listing many results from individual studies in the text. When there are few included studies, an SROC plot showing point estimates of sensitivity and specificity and their confidence intervals can be an effective display if study points and confidence interval lines do not overlap considerably (see Figure 11.9.a).

Review authors may also want to present and describe the results of individual studies. For example, Crawford (2016) included four studies and described the results of each study in the text and outlined key findings from the studies in the 'Summary of findings' table. Describing the results of individual studies will be impractical when there are many studies. Instead, review authors could provide a narrative summary that includes the ranges of reported estimates of sensitivity and specificity and the body of evidence (number of studies, number of participants, number with the target condition).

Presenting findings in the absence of a meta-analysis becomes even more challenging when there are multiple index tests, target conditions or reference standards. In such situations, review authors should carefully consider how best to present the findings, using text, tables and figures as appropriate.

For example, a Cochrane Review reported that the 33 included studies evaluated a myriad of index tests against different reference standards (Hanchard 2013). In addition, there were five categories of the target condition. Altogether, there were 170 combinations of target condition and index test. None of these combinations was assessed in a similar manner by more than two studies. The review authors concluded that

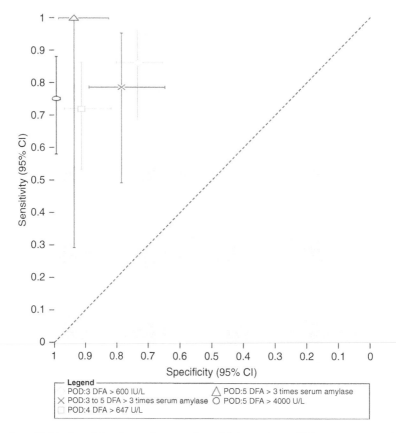

Figure 11.9.a   **SROC plot with point estimates of sensitivity and specificity and 95% confidence intervals**. The Cochrane Review assessed amylase in drain fluid for detecting pancreatic leak in post-pancreatic resection. In the five included studies, drain fluid amylase was measured on different days and at different thresholds. A meta-analysis was not performed. The numbers following POD (postoperative day) indicate the number of the postoperative day. The numbers or text following DFA (drain fluid amylase) indicate the threshold. Source: Adapted from Davidson 2017

meta-analysis was inappropriate because of substantial clinical heterogeneity and a limited number of studies for each combination. To keep the number of forest plots to a minimum and to enhance readability, the review authors presented estimates of sensitivity and specificity on forest plots grouped according to target condition. A narrative summary with a similar structure accompanied the forest plots.

11.10   Chapter information

Authors: Jonathan J. Deeks (Institute of Applied Health Research, University of Birmingham, UK), Patrick M. Bossuyt (*Department of Epidemiology and Data Science, University of Amsterdam, The Netherlands*), Mariska M. Leeflang (*Department of Epidemiology and Data Science, University of Amsterdam, The Netherlands*), Yemisi Takwoingi (*Institute of Applied Health Research, University of Birmingham, UK*).

Sources of support: Jonathan J. Deeks is a UK National Institute for Health Research (NIHR) Senior Investigator Emeritus. Yemisi Takwoingi is funded by a UK National Institute for Health Research (NIHR) Postdoctoral Fellowship. Jonathan J. Deeks and Yemisi Takwoingi are supported by the NIHR Birmingham Biomedical Research Centre at the University Hospitals Birmingham NHS Foundation Trust and the University of Birmingham. The views expressed are those of the authors and not necessarily those of the NHS, the NIHR or the Department of Health and Social Care. The authors declare no sources of support for writing this chapter.

Declarations of interest: Jonathan J. Deeks, Yemisi Takwoingi and Mariska M. Leeflang are members of Cochrane's Diagnostic Test Accuracy Editorial Team. Yemisi Takwoingi and Mariska M. Leeflang are co-convenors of the Cochrane Screening and Diagnostic Tests Methods Group. The authors declare no other potential conflicts of interest relevant to the topic of this chapter.

Acknowledgements: The authors would like to thank Karen R. Steingart, Marta Roque and Daniël Korevaar for helpful peer review comments.

11.11   References

Abba K, Deeks JJ, Olliaro P, Naing CM, Jackson SM, Takwoingi Y, Donegan S, Garner P. Rapid diagnostic tests for diagnosing uncomplicated P. falciparum malaria in endemic countries. *Cochrane Database of Systematic Reviews* 2011; **7**: CD008122.

Alldred SK, Takwoingi Y, Guo B, Pennant M, Deeks JJ, Neilson JP, Alfirevic Z. First trimester ultrasound tests alone or in combination with first trimester serum tests for Down's syndrome screening. *Cochrane Database of Systematic Reviews* 2017; **3**: CD012600.

Best LM, Takwoingi Y, Siddique S, Selladurai A, Gandhi A, Low B, Yaghoobi M, Gurusamy KS. Non-invasive diagnostic tests for Helicobacter pylori infection. *Cochrane Database of Systematic Reviews* 2018; **3**: CD012080.

Chan CC, Fage BA, Burton JK, Smailagic N, Gill SS, Herrmann N, Nikolaou V, Quinn TJ, Noel-Storr AH, Seitz DP. Mini-Cog for the diagnosis of Alzheimer's disease dementia and other dementias within a secondary care setting. *Cochrane Database of Systematic Reviews* 2019; **9**: CD011414.

Chan KK, Joo DA, McRae AD, Takwoingi Y, Premji ZA, Lang E, Wakai A. Chest ultrasonography versus supine chest radiography for diagnosis of pneumothorax in trauma patients in the emergency department. *Cochrane Database of Systematic Reviews* 2020; **7**: CD013031.

Crawford F, Andras A, Welch K, Sheares K, Keeling D, Chappell FM. D-dimer test for excluding the diagnosis of pulmonary embolism. *Cochrane Database of Systematic Reviews* 2016; **8**: CD010864.

Davidson TB, Yaghoobi M, Davidson BR, Gurusamy KS. Amylase in drain fluid for the diagnosis of pancreatic leak in post-pancreatic resection. *Cochrane Database of Systematic Reviews* 2017; **4**: CD012009.

Deeks JJ, Higgins JPT, Altman DG. Chapter 10: Analysing data and undertaking meta-analyses. In: Higgins JPT, Thomas J, Chandler J, Cumpston M, Li T, Page MJ, Welch VA, editors. *Cochrane Handbook for Systematic Reviews of Interventions* version 6.0. Cochrane, 2019.

Evans JS, Handley SJ, Perham N, Over DE, Thompson VA. Frequency versus probability formats in statistical word problems. *Cognition* 2000; **77**: 197–213.

Hanchard NC, Lenza M, Handoll HH, Takwoingi Y. Physical tests for shoulder impingements and local lesions of bursa, tendon or labrum that may accompany impingement. *Cochrane Database of Systematic Reviews* 2013; **4**: CD007427.

Hoffrage U, Gigerenzer G. Using natural frequencies to improve diagnostic inferences. *Academic Medicine* 1998; **73**: 538–540.

Kohli M, Schiller I, Dendukuri N, Yao M, Dheda K, Denkinger CM, Schumacher SG, Steingart KR. Xpert MTB/RIF Ultra and Xpert MTB/RIF assays for extrapulmonary tuberculosis and rifampicin resistance in adults. *Cochrane Database of Systematic Reviews* 2021; **1**: CD012768.

Leeflang MM, Deeks JJ, Rutjes AW, Reitsma JB, Bossuyt PM. Bivariate meta-analysis of predictive values of diagnostic tests can be an alternative to bivariate meta-analysis of sensitivity and specificity. *Journal of Clinical Epidemiology* 2012; **65**: 1088–1097.

Puhan MA, Steurer J, Bachmann LM, ter Riet G. A randomized trial of ways to describe test accuracy: the effect on physicians' post-test probability estimates. *Annals of Internal Medicine* 2005; **143**: 184–189.

Reid MC, Lane DA, Feinstein AR. Academic calculations versus clinical judgments: practicing physicians' use of quantitative measures of test accuracy. *American Journal of Medicine* 1998; **104**: 374–380.

Steurer J, Fischer JE, Bachmann LM, Koller M, ter Riet G. Communicating accuracy of tests to general practitioners: a controlled study. *BMJ* 2002; **324**: 824–826.

Straus SE, Glasziou P, Richardson WS, Haynes RB. *Evidence-based medicine: how to practice and teach EBM.* 5th ed. Philadelphia (PA): Elsevier; 2019.

Takwoingi Y, Partlett C, Riley RD, Hyde C, Deeks JJ. Methods and reporting of systematic reviews of comparative accuracy were deficient: a methodological survey and proposed guidance. *Journal of Clinical Epidemiology* 2020; **121**: 1–14.

Zhang S, Smailagic N, Hyde C, Noel-Storr AH, Takwoingi Y, McShane R, Feng J. (11)C-PIB-PET for the early diagnosis of Alzheimer's disease dementia and other dementias in people with mild cognitive impairment (MCI). *Cochrane Database of Systematic Reviews* 2014; **7**: CD010386.

Zhelev Z, Garside R, Hyde C. A qualitative study into the difficulties experienced by healthcare decision makers when reading a Cochrane diagnostic test accuracy review. *Systematic Reviews* 2013; **2**: 32.

12

Drawing conclusions

Mariska M. Leeflang, Karen R. Steingart, Rob J. Scholten and Clare Davenport

---

KEY POINTS

- Key issues threatening the strength of the evidence in a review are risk of bias, concerns regarding applicability, heterogeneity, imprecision, and completeness of the body of evidence.
- When using the GRADE approach for assessing the certainty of the evidence, these key issues can be translated to the five GRADE domains: risk of bias, indirectness, inconsistency, imprecision, and publication bias. These key issues also should be addressed in the Discussion section and Authors' conclusion section of the review, together with an explanation of what the results practically mean.
- A 'Summary of findings' table can present the findings of the review in a clear, transparent and structured format, as well as key information regarding the overall strength or certainty of the evidence.
- When discussing the implications of the review's findings for practice, the potential consequences of testing should be considered. Such a discussion should take into account the fact that evidence of consequences is typically not documented in the studies included in the review.

12.1   Introduction

The purpose of Cochrane Reviews is to facilitate healthcare decision-making by patients and the general public, by clinicians or other healthcare workers, administrators and policy makers. Such people will rely on the 'Summary of findings' tables, Discussion and Authors' conclusions to make sense of the information in the review and to help them to interpret the results and the strength of the available evidence. Owing to the importance of the discussion and conclusions sections, review authors should take great care that these sections accurately reflect the data and information contained in the review.

For systematic reviews of test accuracy, the key results are usually summary estimates of sensitivity and specificity from meta-analysis, or summary estimates of differences in accuracy between tests. The risk of bias and concerns regarding applicability of the accuracy estimates from an individual study should be assessed in the methodological quality assessment stage of a systematic review, as explained in Chapter 5. The included studies contribute to the overall body of evidence for a specific review question.

How much confidence we have in the overall body of evidence is referred to as the strength of the evidence, or certainty in the evidence. Several alternative terms, such as quality, have been used. Throughout this chapter we use 'strength of the evidence' as the broader term, to distinguish it from methodological quality, which covers risk of bias and concerns regarding applicability. Review authors who use the GRADE (Grading of Recommendations Assessment, Development and Evaluation) framework will come across the term 'certainty of the evidence'. In this *Handbook*, we only use the term 'certainty of the evidence' when we refer specifically to GRADE guidance.

In addition to the strength of the evidence, the contribution of test accuracy to evidence-based decision-making needs to be made explicit. Accuracy results usually do not provide readers with clear answers about whether to buy, reimburse, implement or order tests. Such decisions usually need more evidence concerning the potential consequences of index test-positive results and index test-negative results, and other ways in which tests have an impact on patients. The Discussion section of a systematic review of test accuracy should at least alert readers to this and indicate where additional information might be found.

Above all, readers should weigh the results and their implications against the risk of bias and concerns regarding applicability of the body of evidence from which they stem, to know how confident they can be that the results are valid and applicable to the review question. In addition, one should take into account how large and complete the body of evidence is, and likely heterogeneity in accuracy. The following sections in a Cochrane Review of diagnostic test accuracy facilitate interpretation of the review findings.

The **'Summary of findings' table** presents a summary of the review findings in a clear, transparent, and structured format, as well as key information about the strength of the evidence.

The **Discussion** section usually starts with a summary of the main findings from the review, placed in the context of other research and knowledge. This section should be followed by an explanation of the strengths and weaknesses of the review, and a section about the applicability of findings to the review question.

Finally, the **Authors' conclusions** section should explain the implications of the review findings for practice and for research. In this chapter we provide suggestions on how to approach each of these sections.

12.2 'Summary of findings' tables

Similar to 'Summary of findings' tables in systematic reviews of interventions, it is important that the main findings of a systematic review of test accuracy are presented in a transparent and simple tabular format. The 'Summary of findings' tables should provide key information on the accuracy of the index test(s) under consideration (and the difference in accuracy when index tests are being compared), and important limitations arising from the assessment of the strength of the evidence.

A 'Summary of findings' table appears at the beginning of a Cochrane Review, before the Background section. Cochrane Reviews of diagnostic test accuracy should have at least one 'Summary of findings' table representing the primary review question. Some reviews may include more than one 'Summary of findings' table if, for example, the review addresses more than one primary objective (Kohli 2021).

In this section we outline the key features that should be included in a 'Summary of findings' table. One method to create a 'Summary of findings' table is using the GRADE approach for assessing the certainty in the evidence (templates available through the software package GRADEpro GDT (GRADEpro 2020)). However, unlike for Cochrane Reviews of interventions, this is not a requirement for Cochrane Reviews of diagnostic test accuracy, and review authors may prefer to summarize using their own structure.

The following essential features should be included in a 'Summary of findings' table, irrespective of which approach is used.

1) The review question and its components, i.e. population, (prior tests), setting, index test(s) and reference standard(s), should be described in full at the head of the table.
2) A brief description of how these components were addressed by the included studies, to facilitate the assessment of whether the included studies are applicable to the review question.
3) The results for each index test should, at a minimum, include:
   a) the number of included studies;
   b) the number of participants, in sufficient detail to calculate the numbers of participants with and without the target condition;
   c) the accuracy of the index test(s). This is usually reported as summary estimates of sensitivity and specificity. For comparative accuracy reviews, the estimates of absolute or relative differences in accuracy may also be reported. In situations where it is not considered meaningful to provide summary estimates, review authors may want to provide the range of reported estimates of sensitivity and specificity. With multiple test positivity thresholds and estimation of a summary receiver operating characteristic (ROC) curve, it may not be meaningful to provide a summary sensitivity and specificity. In these cases, a summary diagnostic odds ratio or summary estimates of sensitivity at certain values of specificity (or the other way round) may be reported (see Chapter 9, Section 9.4 and Chapter 10, Section 10.3); and
   d) the statistical uncertainty around any summary measure of test accuracy used (e.g. 95% confidence interval or 95% credible interval).
4) There should be an explanation of what the results mean when applied to a hypothetical cohort of people who will in practice undergo the index test(s). This means that the absolute numbers of true and false positive and negative test results should be stated (with accompanying confidence intervals), so that the reader gets a sense of what the practical implications may be of using the index test(s). How to derive these numbers is explained in Chapter 11.
5) There should be a clear statement about the strength or certainty of the evidence, including risk of bias, concerns regarding applicability, and between-study variability.

Beyond these essential features, review authors may identify other aspects of the results to include in the 'Summary of findings' table, such as variation in results by cut-off, prevalence or any other important potential source of heterogeneity. If desirable, other accuracy measures may also be stated, such as predictive values or likelihood ratios. However, review authors should be aware that using different metrics to report the same information may be confusing for readers.

Although not essential, review authors could also explain the potential consequences of test results, for example that people with a false positive test result may undergo further, unnecessary testing.

Explanations may be provided about the results presented in the table as comments or as footnotes. These may include, for example, reasons for downgrading the certainty of evidence when the GRADE approach is used. In some reviews, review authors may be concerned that the 'Summary of findings' table for the test cannot be safely interpreted in isolation from the original data presented in the main body of the review, particularly where there is substantial heterogeneity and where prevalence estimates used to derive absolute numbers differ from the proportion with the target condition in included studies.

Here we present four examples of 'Summary of findings' tables that illustrate the points outlined. Table 12.2.a shows a review of a single index test using a structure created by the review authors. The authors did not follow the GRADE approach and did not rate the certainty of the evidence as high, moderate, low or very low. They narratively described the strength of the evidence.

Table 12.2.b shows a 'Summary of findings' table for a review without a meta-analysis, addressing multiplicity in the target condition. The review authors did not use the GRADE approach and the explanation of the strength of the evidence could have been more explicit and detailed. However, this 'Summary of findings' table is an example of how to present the results in the absence of a meta-analysis.

Table 12.2.c shows a review of multiple index tests using the GRADE approach (this format can also be applied to a single index test). Table 12.2.d shows a review comparing two index tests using the GRADE approach. A further explanation of the GRADE approach can be found in Section 12.4. Review authors should be explicit about whether they used the GRADE approach or not.

12.3 Assessing the strength of the evidence

12.3.1 Key issues to consider when assessing the strength of the evidence

In this section, we first introduce the key issues that should be considered when assessing the strength of the overall body of evidence in a systematic review of test accuracy. In section 12.4, we explain the GRADE approach to assessing the certainty in the evidence.

Most systematic reviews will contain one or multiple meta-analyses and provide summary sensitivity and specificity. However, some reviews may have estimated a summary ROC curve and presented a summary diagnostic odds ratio. In other reviews the body of evidence may have been insufficient or too heterogeneous to justify a meta-analysis. In these cases, the assessment of the strength of the evidence may differ. Where applicable, guidance is provided for these situations.

Table 12.2.a **'Summary of findings' table:** What is the diagnostic accuracy of serum galactomannan for invasive aspergillosis in immunocompromised patients?

Population: immunocompromised patients, mostly haematology patients; applicable to the review question
Prior testing: varied, mostly physical examination and history (fever, neutropenia); applicable to the review question
Setting: mostly inpatients in haematology or cancer departments; applicable to the review question
Index test: Platelia Aspergillus test, which measures galactomannan, an Aspergillus antigen
Importance: depends on the time-gain the test may provide
Reference standard: a composite reference standard of clinical and microbiological criteria; the reference standard classifies the patients in four groups: no – possible – probable – proven invasive aspergillosis (IA). In this 'Summary of findings' table, sensitivity refers to the proven or probable IA patients and specificity to the patients with possible or no IA
Studies: 29 cross-sectional studies; two-group designs and studies excluding patients with possible IA were not included; studies had to report cut-off values that were used and some studies reported more than one cut-off

Cut-off value	Summary sensitivity (95% CI)	Summary specificity (95% CI)	No. of participants (studies)	Median proportion with target condition (interquartile range)	What do the results mean? With a prevalence of 11%*, 11 out of 100 patients will have IA	Strength of the evidence
0.5	0.78 (0.70 to 0.85)	0.85 (0.78 to 0.91)	394 proven or probable IA 3549 possible or no IA (27)	11% (6.5% to 16%)	2 (95% CI 2 to 3) IA patients will be missed, but will be tested again. 13 (8 to 20) out of 89 patients without IA will be unnecessarily referred for CT scanning	Risk of bias was unclear for most domains in most studies, due to poor reporting. Three studies had concerns regarding applicability of the included patients. Low numbers of diseased patients (1 to 20). Much between-study variability, with sensitivity ranging from 0% to 100%
1.0	0.71 (0.63 to 0.78)	0.90 (0.86 to 0.93)	145 proven or probable IA 1246 possible or no IA (8)	13% (4.2% to 31%)	3 (95% CI 2 to 4) IA patients will be missed, but will be tested again 9 (6 to 12) out of 89 patients without IA will be unnecessarily referred for CT scanning	Risk of bias was unclear for most studies, due to poor reporting. No concerns regarding applicability for any of the QUADAS-2 domains. Low numbers of diseased patients (1 to 34)
1.5	0.63 (0.49 to 0.77)	0.93 (0.89 to 0.97)	209 proven or probable IA 2412 possible or no IA (15)	7.4% (4.3% to 16%)	4 (95% CI 2 to 5) IA patients will be missed, but will be tested again 6 (2 to 10) out of 89 patients without IA will be unnecessarily referred for CT scanning	Low numbers of diseased patients (1 to 17), except one study (98 IA patients). One study had high risk of bias in the patient domain and three studies in the reference standard domain One study had high concerns regarding applicability of the patients

* Median proportion with target condition over all studies was 11% (range 0.8% to 56%). CI, confidence interval; CT, computed tomography.
Comment: The results in this table should not be interpreted in isolation from the results of the individual included studies contributing to each summary test accuracy measure. These are reported in the main body of the text of the review.
Source: Adapted from Leeflang 2015.

Table 12.2.b **'Summary of findings' table:** What is the diagnostic accuracy of physical tests for various causes of shoulder impingements in people whose symptoms, history or both suggest impingement?

Setting: most people with shoulder pain symptomatic of impingements and related pathologies are diagnosed and managed in the primary care setting; this is applicable to the review question

Index tests: physical tests used singly or in combination to identify shoulder impingement and related pathologies

Importance: accurate diagnosis using readily applied, convenient, low-cost physical tests would enable appropriate and well-timed management of these common causes of shoulder pain

Reference standard: while a definitive reference standard is lacking, surgery, whether open or arthroscopic, is generally regarded as the best available; Non-invasive contenders include ultrasound and magnetic resonance imaging (MRI)

Studies: 33 studies including 4002 shoulders in 3852 patients; These incorporated numerous standard, modified or combinations of index tests and 14 novel index tests

Methodological quality: methodological quality was generally poor; All but two studies failed to meet the criteria for having a representative spectrum of patients

Data analysis: the studies assessed 170 target condition/index test combinations, with only six instances of any index test being performed and interpreted similarly in two studies; Meta-analysis of the latter was considered to be inappropriate, however

Target condition*	Subcategory of target condition, if applicable	Studies	Shoulders/ patients	Tests or variants evaluated
Subacromial and internal impingement	Subacromial impingement	5	361/356	13
	Subacromial versus internal impingement	1	110/110	1
	Internal impingement	0	0	0
LHB tendinopathy or tears	LHB/labral pathology; LHB/SLAP lesions; SA-SD bursitis/ bursal-side degeneration of supraspinatus; and SIS/rotator cuff tendinitis or tear	3	660/557	10
Multiple, undifferentiated target conditions		4	201/200	10

LHB, long head of biceps; SA-SD, subacromial-subdeltoid bursa; SIS, subacromial impingement syndrome; SLAP lesions, Superior Labrum Anterior to Posterior lesions.
* A selection of target conditions as presented in the original review is presented here.
Note that methodological quality assessment was performed using QUADAS, hence the reason there is no explicit mention of risk of bias and applicability.
Source: Adapted from Hanchard 2013.

Table 12.2.c **'Summary of findings' table:** What is the diagnostic accuracy of rapid diagnostic tests (RDTs) for detecting *Plasmodium vivax* malaria parasitaemia in people living in malaria-endemic areas who present to ambulatory healthcare facilities with symptoms suggestive of malaria?

Population: people presenting with symptoms of uncomplicated malaria

Prior testing: none

Setting: ambulatory healthcare settings in *P vivax*-endemic areas

Index tests: immunochromatography-based RDTs for *P vivax* malaria that meet the World Health Organization (WHO) malaria RDT performance criteria (WHO 2017a); This table presents the results for the CareStart Malaria Pf/Pv Combo test

Reference standards: conventional microscopy, polymerase chain reaction

Target condition: *P vivax* malaria

Importance: accurate and fast diagnosis of *P vivax* from other malaria species allows appropriate treatment to be provided quickly

Study design: all cross-sectional studies

Findings: 10 studies of six different RDT brands; Only two brands (CareStart Malaria Pf/Pv Combo test and Falcivax Device Rapid test) were evaluated against the same reference standard by more than one study

Limitations: a small number of studies were included in the analyses and meta-analyses were only possible for two RDT brands; Studies often did not report how patients were selected, blinding of the RDT results to the reference standard, and the storage conditions and lot testing of RDTs

Outcome	Number of studies	Number of patients	Numbers in a cohort of 1000 patients tested (95% confidence interval (CI))[a]			Certainty of the evidence (GRADE)
			Prevalence of 0.5%	Prevalence of 5%	Prevalence of 20%	
CareStart Malaria Pf/Pv Combo test against microscopy: summary sensitivity (95% CI) = 99% (94% to 100%) and summary specificity (95% CI) = 99% (99% to 100%), summary positive likelihood ratio (95% CI) = 141.1 (68.2 to 292.0) and summary negative likelihood ratio (95% CI) = 0.01 (0.00 to 0.06)						
True positives (patients with *P vivax* malaria)	4	251	5 (5 to 10)	50 (47 to 50)	198 (188 to 200)	⊕⊕⊕⊖ MODERATE[1]
False negatives (patients incorrectly classified as not having *P vivax* malaria)			0 (0 to 0)	0 (0 to 3)	2 (0 to 12)	
True negatives (patients without *P vivax* malaria)	4	2147	985 (980 to 995)	941 (941 to 950)	792 (792 to 800)	⊕⊕⊕⊖ MODERATE[1]
False positives (patients incorrectly classified as having *P vivax* malaria)			10 (0 to 10)	9 (0 to 9)	8 (0 to 8)	

(Continued)

Table 12.2.c (Continued)

Outcome	Number of studies	Number of patients	Numbers in a cohort of 1000 patients tested (95% confidence interval (CI))[a]			Certainty of the evidence (GRADE)
			Prevalence of 0.5%	Prevalence of 5%	Prevalence of 20%	
Falcivax Device Rapid test against microscopy: summary sensitivity (95% CI) = 77% (53% to 91%) and summary specificity (95% CI) = 99% (98% to 100%), summary positive likelihood ratio (95% CI) = 120.3 (43.1 to 335.9) and summary negative likelihood ratio (95% CI) = 0.23 (0.10 to 0.53)						
True positives (patients with *P vivax* malaria)	2	89	4 (3 to 5)	50 (47 to 50)	198 (188 to 200)	⊕⊕◯◯ LOW[1,2]
False negatives (patients incorrectly classified as not having *P vivax* malaria)			1 (0 to 2)	11 (4 to 23)	46 (18 to 94)	
True negatives (patients without *P vivax* malaria)		2621	985 (975 to 995)	941 (931 to 950)	792 (784 to 800)	⊕⊕⊕◯ MODERATE[1]
False positives (patients incorrectly classified as having *P vivax* malaria)			10 (0 to 10)	9 (0 to 19)	8 (0 to 16)	

[a] Median values were chosen from ranges of prevalence considered to be moderate, low and very low transmission settings for *P vivax* (WHO 2017b).

[1] Downgraded for risk of bias by one.

[2] Downgraded for imprecision by one due to wide confidence intervals.

GRADE Certainty of the evidence

High: we are very confident that the true effect lies close to that of the estimate of the effect.

Moderate: we are moderately confident in the effect estimate: the true effect is likely to be close to the estimate of the effect, but there is a possibility that it is substantially different.

Low: our confidence in the effect estimate is limited: the true effect may be substantially different from the estimate of the effect.

Very low: we have very little confidence in the effect estimate: the true effect is likely to be substantially different from the estimate of effect.

Source: Adapted from Agarwal 2020.

Table 12.2.d **'Summary of findings' table:** What is the diagnostic accuracy of Xpert Ultra versus Xpert MTB/RIF for the detection of pulmonary tuberculosis in adults with presumptive pulmonary tuberculosis?

Population: adults with presumptive pulmonary tuberculosis; participants were unselected, meaning they were not enrolled in a study based on prior testing with microscopy examination (smear results) or a history of tuberculosis
Role: an initial test
Setting: primary care facilities and local hospitals
Index tests: Xpert Ultra and Xpert MTB/RIF on sputum
Threshold for index tests: an automated binary result is provided
Reference standards: solid or liquid culture
Studies: 7 cross-sectional and cohort studies that directly compared the accuracy of Xpert Ultra and Xpert MTB/RIF were included
Xpert Ultra summary sensitivity 90.9% (95% credible interval (CrI) 86.2 to 94.7) and summary specificity 95.6% (95% CrI 93.0 to 97.4)
Xpert MTB/RIF summary sensitivity 84.7% (95% CrI 78.6 to 89.9) and summary specificity 98.4% (95% CrI 97.0 to 99.3)

| | Number of results per 1000 patients tested (95% CrI)* | | | | | | | |
| | Prevalence 2.5% | | Prevalence 10% | | Prevalence 30% | | | |
Test result	Xpert Ultra	Xpert MTB/RIF	Xpert Ultra	Xpert MTB/RIF	Xpert Ultra	Xpert MTB/RIF	Number of participants	Certainty of the evidence (GRADE)
True positives (TP)	23 (22 to 24)	21 (20 to 22)#	91 (86 to 95)	85 (79 to 90)	273 (259 to 284)	254 (236 to 270)	983	⊕⊕⊕⊕ High
	2 more TP in Xpert Ultra#		6 more TP in Xpert Ultra		19 more TP in Xpert Ultra			
False negatives (FN)	2 (1 to 3)	4 (3 to 5)	9 (5 to 14)	15 (10 to 21)	27 (16 to 41)	46 (30 to 64)		
	2 fewer FN in Xpert Ultra		6 fewer TN in Xpert Ultra		19 fewer TP in Xpert Ultra			

(Continued)

Table 12.2.d (Continued)

| | Number of results per 1000 patients tested (95% CrI)* | | | | | | | |
| | Prevalence 2.5% | | Prevalence 10% | | Prevalence 30% | | | |
Test result	Xpert Ultra	Xpert MTB/RIF	Xpert Ultra	Xpert MTB/RIF	Xpert Ultra	Xpert MTB/RIF	Number of participants	Certainty of the evidence (GRADE)
True negatives (TN)	932 (907 to 950)	959 (946 to 968)	860 (837 to 877)	886 (873 to 894)	669 (651 to 682)	689 (679 to 695)	1852	⊕⊕⊕⊕ High
	27 fewer TN in Xpert Ultra		26 fewer TN in Xpert Ultra		20 fewer TN in Xpert Ultra			
False positives (FP)	43 (25 to 68)	16 (7 to 29)	40 (23 to 63)	14 (6 to 27)	31 (18 to 49)	11 (5 to 21)		
	27 more FP in Xpert Ultra		26 more FP in Xpert Ultra		20 more FP in Xpert Ultra			

* 95% credible limits were estimated based on those around the point estimates for summary sensitivity and specificity; 95% confidence intervals were estimated for true positives, false negatives, true negatives and false positives. Prevalence estimates were suggested by the World Health Organization Global Tuberculosis Programme. The median proportion with tuberculosis in the included studies was 30.1% (range 12.8% to 72.2%).

These differences have been derived using GRADEpro, which does not provide credible or confidence intervals for the difference between tests.

GRADE Certainty of the evidence

High: we are very confident that the true effect lies close to that of the estimate of the effect.

Moderate: we are moderately confident in the effect estimate: the true effect is likely to be close to the estimate of the effect, but there is a possibility that it is substantially different.

Low: our confidence in the effect estimate is limited: the true effect may be substantially different from the estimate of the effect.

Very low: we have very little confidence in the effect estimate: the true effect is likely to be substantially different from the estimate of effect.

Source: Adapted from Zifodya 2021.

12.3.1.1 How valid are the summary estimates?

Validity here refers to low risk of bias. The QUADAS-2 tool and QUADAS-C (its extension for comparative accuracy studies) are recommended for assessing risk of bias and applicability of test accuracy studies (see Chapter 8). High risk of bias caused by participant selection, conduct of the index test, conduct and nature of the reference standard or flaws in the flow of participants, including timing of tests or missing values, may have a negative impact on the findings of a systematic review.

Just stating that the findings may come from studies with a high risk of bias is insufficient; review authors should judge to what extent included studies with a high risk of bias may lead to bias in the summary estimates or affect the findings of the systematic review otherwise. For example, one or two studies at high risk of bias in a large number of included studies will have a different impact on estimates compared to one or two studies at high risk of bias in a review containing a small number of included studies. One way to gain some insight into the effect of studies with high or unclear risk of bias is to perform sensitivity analyses by excluding such studies (see Chapter 9, Section 9.4.9). If the results of the sensitivity analyses indicate that such studies greatly influence the findings of the review and thus question the robustness of the findings, then this should be explicitly noted.

12.3.1.2 How applicable are the summary estimates?

A study can be at low risk of bias but, because of the included participants, test or reference standard, may nevertheless not apply well to the review question. Concerns regarding the applicability of the individual studies to the review question can be assessed using QUADAS-2. Review authors should judge to what extent studies with some concerns regarding applicability may affect the strength of the results in the whole body of evidence. The results of sensitivity analyses may support these judgements.

A specific concern regarding applicability may occur in comparative accuracy studies. As stated in Chapter 5, studies that directly compare two tests could have recruited a study group that is unrepresentative of the patient population in whom the tests will be used in clinical practice. For example, a systematic review assessed whether exercise electrocardiography (ECG) may be replaced with computed tomography (CT) coronary angiography to detect coronary stenosis in patients with stable angina pectoris suspected of coronary disease (Nielsen 2014). The review authors only included studies that directly compared the two index tests. The exercise ECG test is usually done in patients with less severe coronary disease, whereas CT coronary angiography is used in more advanced cases. Therefore, only including studies of patients who received both tests in the past decreases the confidence in the applicability of the resulting comparative accuracy estimates, even though the risk of bias for estimates of accuracy generated by studies that directly compared the two index tests may be low.

12.3.1.3 How heterogeneous are the individual study estimates?

Variability in the study results may be explained by chance variation, if small and few studies have been included. Alternatively, it may be explained by the recruitment from different study populations, differences in the use and/or definition of the index tests, the use of different thresholds for test positivity, or variation in study methods. In Chapter 9, heterogeneity is defined as variation that goes beyond what may be expected by chance. Chapter 9 also explains how potential sources of heterogeneity can be investigated.

In the Discussion section of a review and in the 'Summary of findings' tables, review authors should comment not only on the effect of possible sources of heterogeneity, but also on the consequences of heterogeneity for the interpretation of the findings.

The accuracy of a test is not a fixed property; it is likely to vary across populations and settings. Hence, heterogeneity is expected in systematic reviews of diagnostic accuracy. Whether heterogeneity exists may be difficult to assess in systematic reviews of a single test. If the sensitivity and specificity estimates of all studies in a review lie within a relatively narrow space in the ROC space, then one could claim little or no heterogeneity. When the estimates of sensitivity and specificity vary between 0% and 100%, the variation is likely to go beyond chance variation. However, the situations in between are more difficult to assess, especially when the study results are also imprecise and the role of chance may be considerable.

One way to communicate heterogeneity is to report a prediction region. As explained in Chapter 9, a 95% prediction region represents the region within which one has 95% confidence that the true sensitivity and specificity of any future study (resembling the studies included in the review) should lie (Harbord 2007). The greater the between-study heterogeneity, the larger this region will be.

Another way to communicate heterogeneity may be to focus on a minimally required estimate for sensitivity, specificity or another outcome measure. One could then explain to what extent the studies provide point estimates above this minimally required estimate, and how the confidence intervals of the studies relate to this point.

Little evidence and guidance have been developed to assess and communicate inconsistency when summary receiver operating characteristic (SROC) curves and odds ratios are presented. In those situations, review authors may comment on the SROC plots and how the study estimates are visually distinct from the summary curve.

Assessment of heterogeneity in comparative studies may be focused on the difference in sensitivity or specificity between the tests evaluated, in case of binary test results. For example, if some of the included studies indicate that test A has a much higher sensitivity than test B, while other studies report that test B has a higher sensitivity, then these studies contradict one another, which may indicate heterogeneity.

12.3.1.4   How precise are the summary estimates?

If only one small study was found that assessed the accuracy of an index test, then the estimates of sensitivity and specificity will be very imprecise. If a systematic review contains many large studies with a considerable number of both people with and those without the target condition, then the summary estimates will be a more precise reflection of the sensitivity and specificity over all the included studies.

Review authors are therefore expected to report:

- the number of included studies;
- the number of included participants with the target condition, which informs estimation of sensitivity;
- the number of included participants without the target condition, which informs estimation of specificity; and
- the statistical uncertainty around the summary estimates (e.g. 95% confidence interval).

These may be used to provide a judgement about the precision of the estimates.

The example of only one small study versus many large studies illustrates two extremes. The judgement of imprecision is subjective, but one could pre-specify a required width of the confidence interval (e.g. maximum 10 percentage points wide) to support this judgement.

Another way to address imprecision is to check whether the confidence interval crosses a pre-specified lower or upper bound of sensitivity or specificity. For example, if the test needs to be at least 70% sensitive and the lower 95% confidence interval is 65%, then one could decide that the point estimate was not sufficiently precise to judge whether the test is at least 70% sensitive. Such a pre-specification requires judgement about the potential for a test to have clinical utility based on the role of the test in the clinical pathway.

If no meta-analysis can be done, review authors may report the individual study estimates of test accuracy, including information about the imprecision of these estimates (e.g. confidence intervals). These findings may be summarized by providing a range of estimates across included studies in the 'Summary of findings' table. In those situations, it should be made clear that a summary estimate cannot be provided.

12.3.1.5 How complete is the body of evidence?

One of the most prominent threats to the validity of a meta-analysis is the omission of certain results from the available literature. Even with the most comprehensive search strategy, reporting bias may occur. This could result from selective reporting of results within a study, from selective publication of studies, or from excluding reports in specific languages.

The most obvious form of this omission manifests as publication bias: studies with promising or favourable results are more likely to be published and thus included in a systematic review, which may bias the summary estimates towards more favourable numbers (Simes 1986).

Chapter 9, Section 9.5.3, addressed investigation and handling of publication bias. Although an appropriate test for detecting funnel plot asymmetry in systematic reviews of test accuracy that may indicate publication bias exists, it has limitations (Deeks 2005). Therefore, review authors are encouraged to explore how mechanisms underpinning reporting bias may operate in their clinical area and to inform the reader about the potential for reporting bias whenever possible. For example, review authors with knowledge about clinical testing pathways may be able to comment on the potential for selective reporting of results in studies that describe patients undergoing 'multiple index tests' as part of their routine care, but report the results of only some or one of these tests.

Some decisions made in the review methods may also lead to more favourable results than are justified. An example is language bias, caused by a restriction to reports in English and the phenomenon that larger and more positive studies may be more frequently published in English-language journals. Another example is missing studies due to flawed search strategies.

More information about the effects of choices in the search strategy and about publication bias can be found in Chapter 6. Review authors should judge to what extent any of these effects may be present and, if so, what their potential effect on the summary estimates would be. Expressing concerns about missing evidence and explaining why review authors think this may be problematic is more informative than merely stating that 'there is publication bias'.

12.3.1.6   Were index test comparisons made between or *within* primary studies?

Many comparative accuracy reviews include studies assessing the accuracy of only one of the index tests in the comparison. Estimates of accuracy from these single index test accuracy studies may be at low risk of bias, with low concerns regarding applicability, but estimates of comparative accuracy will then be based on an indirect comparison (see Chapter 9, Section 9.1.4.3) and may be susceptible to bias. Indirect comparisons are at higher risk of bias than direct comparisons made using studies that have compared tests head to head.

   With an indirect comparison, an observed difference in the accuracy of the index tests may be confounded by the test settings, or by the difference in participants included in the respective studies for each of the tests. If all exercise ECG studies in the example in Section 12.3.1.2 were done in patients with less severe coronary disease and all CT angiography studies were done in patients with more severe coronary disease, then the observed difference in accuracy between the two tests may be due to differences in disease severity rather than a genuine difference in accuracy.

12.4   GRADE approach for assessing the certainty of evidence

The GRADE Working Group developed a comprehensive and transparent system for grading the certainty of evidence and subsequently for grading the strength of recommendations following from evidence. As more recent GRADE guidance uses the term 'certainty of the evidence' instead of 'quality of the evidence' or 'strength of the evidence', we also use the term 'certainty' in this section. In systematic reviews, the certainty in evidence reflects the extent to which we are confident that estimates are close to the truth. GRADE publications of particular relevance to systematic reviews of test accuracy include Schünemann (2008), Schünemann (2020a) and Schünemann (2020b).

   The GRADE approach assesses certainty of evidence using the following five domains that are described in detail in Section 12.4.1.

- Risk of bias
- Indirectness (applicability)
- Inconsistency (heterogeneity)
- Imprecision
- Publication bias

   These domains overlap and correspond with the key features presented in Section 12.3.1, but may be used and named slightly differently within the GRADE framework. The certainty of the evidence starts as high when there are appropriate test accuracy studies that recruit a group of participants with an uncertain diagnosis and who are representative of the target population. If a reason is found for downgrading, systematic review authors should use their judgement to classify the reason as either serious (e.g. downgraded by one level for serious imprecision) or very serious (e.g.

downgraded by two levels for very serious imprecision). The overall certainty of the evidence for a given outcome can then range from high to very low. Review authors should be transparent about their judgements by explicitly stating the reason for downgrading in footnotes (labelled as 'Explanations' in the GRADE 'Summary of findings' table), so that the reader can understand the reason for the decision. See Table 12.2.c and Table 12.2.d for examples of 'Summary of findings' tables using the GRADE framework.

In addition, the GRADE approach for systematic reviews of interventions uses three reasons to upgrade the certainty of the evidence from a lower to a higher level of certainty. These reasons are (1) a large effect; (2) any plausible confounding that would reduce the effects found; and (3) a dose-response gradient. However, these reasons are difficult to translate to systematic reviews of test accuracy. As clear guidance for upgrading diagnostic accuracy evidence is lacking, we do not advise upgrading.

Review authors using GRADE (or any other formal method) to assess the certainty of the evidence should make this explicit in the Methods section of the review. The description of the application of GRADE should include how judgements were made and whether the software package GRADEpro GDT was used to build the 'Summary of findings' tables (GRADEpro 2020).

The GRADE guidance for diagnostic accuracy questions is mainly based on summary estimates of the sensitivity and specificity of a single test, or the summary estimates of the difference in sensitivity and specificity of two tests (Yang 2021).

12.4.1 GRADE domains for assessing certainty of evidence for test accuracy

Using the GRADE approach, the five domains are assessed separately for participants with the target condition (sensitivity estimates, true positive and false negative) and those without the target condition (specificity estimates, true negative and false positive). The five domains are described in detail in the following sections (Schünemann 2008, Schünemann 2020a, Schünemann 2020b).

12.4.1.1 Risk of bias

Review authors may downgrade the certainty of evidence by one or two levels depending on the number (percentage) of included studies considered to have a high or unclear risk of bias for one or more of the QUADAS-2 domains (see Section 12.3.1.1 and Chapter 8). Moving from risk-of-bias judgements of individual studies to an overall judgement about downgrading the body of evidence, however, can be challenging and relies on subjective judgement.

In a systematic review on tests for identifying people with glaucoma, the review authors downgraded the certainty of the evidence for four of the five tests they assessed due to risk of bias. For example, the certainty of the evidence for the sensitivity and specificity of the Oblique flashlight test was downgraded one level because 40% of studies had a high risk of bias in one or more QUADAS-2 domains.

12.4.1.2 Indirectness (applicability)

Indirectness can be regarded as a synonym for applicability and can be assessed by judging whether concerns regarding applicability, as identified with QUADAS-2, justify downgrading the certainty of evidence.

Review authors may downgrade the certainty of evidence for indirectness if there are important differences between the participants in the studies and the population stated in the review question, with respect to either prior testing, spectrum of disease or comorbidities, or settings.

They may also downgrade if there are important differences between the characteristics of the index test(s) and/or the expertise of the people applying the test(s) in the studies compared to the characteristics of the test(s) and/or users in real-world settings.

They may downgrade in case of comparative questions if the index tests were not directly compared in each of the studies included in the test comparison (i.e. indirect comparisons).

A systematic review of tests for plague downgraded the certainty of the evidence for specificity one level for indirectness: there was a high concern about applicability due to exclusion of people who received antibiotics prior to sample collection. The index test was performed in a central laboratory, which may not reflect the field conditions in case of an outbreak (Jullien 2020).

12.4.1.3 Inconsistency (heterogeneity)

Inconsistency can be caused by identifiable clinical heterogeneity, or it may remain unexplained. As GRADE recommends downgrading for *unexplained* inconsistency in sensitivity and specificity estimates, review authors should state whether they carried out pre-specified analyses to investigate potential sources of heterogeneity and consider downgrading when they cannot explain inconsistency in the accuracy estimates. Downgrading is not necessary if the inconsistency can be explained, for example due to differences in setting or population or index test execution. If that is the case, the 'Summary of findings' tables should report the results per subgroup.

For example, in a systematic review about Xpert MTB/RIF Ultra and Xpert MTB/RIF assays for extrapulmonary tuberculosis and rifampicin resistance in adults (Kohli 2021), the review authors performed sensitivity analyses based on selected QUADAS-2 items and found that they could not explain the heterogeneity. The review authors then downgraded one level for inconsistency.

Questions to consider are 'Are the individual point estimates in the forest plots more or less the same?' and, more importantly, 'How much do confidence intervals overlap?' A scatter plot of sensitivity and specificity (i.e. an SROC plot) is helpful for visual assessment of heterogeneity ('Are the sensitivity–specificity pairs clustered closely together or are they spread all over the ROC space?'). In addition, the size of the 95% prediction region (if presented) can assist in this assessment, particularly when there are many studies.

Downgrading for inconsistency may also be warranted when the differences between two tests differ too much. What is regarded to be 'too much' should then be specified. For example, one could decide – based on expected consequences of testing – that test A is chosen over test B when the sensitivity of test A is at least 10 percentage points higher than test B. When the review then includes studies that show much larger differences, studies showing no difference and studies with a difference the other way (i.e. test B being more sensitive than test A), this may be a reason to downgrade for inconsistency (Hultcrantz 2020).

12.4.1.4 Imprecision

Efforts to provide guidance on how to operationalize the assessments of imprecision for diagnostic test accuracy are ongoing. As per GRADE for systematic reviews of interventions and the explanation in Section 12.3.1.1, one could look at the width of the 95% confidence intervals of the summary estimates of sensitivity and specificity and assess whether they cross a certain clinically acceptable lower limit (for which we would downgrade) or not. This clinically acceptable lower limit should depend on the clinical context and the potential consequences of testing, as explained in the clinical pathway (see Chapter 5, Section 5.3.1).

The systematic review of tests for plague, mentioned earlier, downgraded the certainty of the evidence for specificity one level for imprecision. The review authors based this judgement on the 95% confidence intervals around the proportion of false positives and the proportion of false negatives: the lower limit of these confidence intervals would lead to a different decision than the upper limit of the confidence intervals (Jullien 2020).

12.4.1.5 Publication bias

Publication bias may occur when the body of evidence is incomplete. It can lower certainty of evidence, mainly because studies with favourable results tend to be published more often than those with less favourable results. Although test accuracy studies with promising results about the performance of tests seem to be published more rapidly compared to those reporting lower estimates, there is no strong evidence that specific results, either favourable or unfavourable, end up less frequently in meta-analyses (Korevaar 2016). Still, review authors should be aware of the possibility of publication bias (see Section 12.3.1.5).

Downgrading may be considered when published evidence is limited to a few small studies, in particular if they support a pre-existing hypothesis and were funded by a body with a vested interest in a specific test (Schünemann 2020b). In some situations, there may be direct evidence that results of particular studies have been withheld or that studies are reporting partial findings, for example reporting only the sensitivity or specificity of the test, or reporting only particular subgroups of patients. All these examples are publication and reporting practices that should be reported in the review. Alternatively, if few concerns were identified, review authors may judge that publication bias was undetected.

The systematic review about Xpert MTB/RIF Ultra and Xpert MTB/RIF assays (Kohli 2021) included studies with for-profit interest and small studies, which were thought to be an indication of potential publication bias. However, the review authors did not downgrade for publication bias, as the literature search was thought to be comprehensive and the review authors contacted researchers of primary studies to identify unpublished studies.

12.5 Summary of main results in the Discussion section

The Discussion section should begin with a restatement of the clinical question or questions that the review is attempting to answer. It should then give a summary of the results that provide answers to these questions. As a starting point, the number of included studies, total number of participants with and without the target condition, results of the risk of bias and applicability assessments, and consistency of findings should be summarized. This summary should be consistent with what was reported in the 'Summary of findings' table and may be an elaboration or explanation of the information in the table.

If meta-analysis was performed, appropriate summary statistics from estimation of summary points or summary curves should be reported (see Chapter 11). Although sensitivity and specificity are the most frequent measures in test accuracy studies, there is some evidence that predictive values are better understood (Whiting 2015). We therefore recommend that review authors present potential consequences of testing by applying the summary estimates to a hypothetical cohort of persons to be tested.

If meta-analysis was not possible, review authors should provide a narrative summary of the review findings, if possible, combined with the range of estimates of test accuracy from the included studies. Review authors should also summarize the relevance of the findings from investigations of heterogeneity, if such analyses were feasible. This section should be consistent with and link to the 'Summary of findings' table(s), including the assessment of the certainty of the body of evidence, as outlined in Chapter 13, Section 13.3, or using the GRADE approach, as outlined in Section 12.4. Many of the issues discussed in previous sections may be briefly but clearly mentioned in the Discussion section to provide a complete picture of the evidence.

12.6   Strengths and weaknesses of the review

In this section we focus on a narrative of the strengths and weaknesses of the primary studies, the strengths and weaknesses of the systematic review methods and the consequences these may have for the interpretation of the review's results and conclusions. If review authors are aware of key issues that potentially limit or bias the results of their review, such as those considered when assessing the certainty of evidence for the 'Summary of findings' table, then these should be pointed out to readers. Review authors could consider using the following subheadings, when appropriate: 'Strengths and weaknesses of the included studies' (or 'Certainty of the evidence') and 'Strengths and weaknesses of the review process'.

Review authors should discuss the strengths and weaknesses of the review with regard to accuracy estimates, not the strengths and weaknesses of the evidence with regard to policy-making decisions, which would rely on other considerations, such as the acceptability or feasibility of the test, the impact of the test on people-important outcomes, and resource requirements (costs).

12.6.1   Strengths and weaknesses of included studies

This section narratively summarizes assessments made about the strength or certainty of the evidence. It is important to highlight the strength of the evidence, including its potential limitations, not only in the 'Summary of findings' tables but also in the main text of the review.

Relative strengths of the included studies may be highlighted here, without overstating the implications. For example, it may be good to know that a review contained many large studies with very similar results. For comparative questions, it may be important to highlight that results were obtained from fully paired (within-participant or head-to-head) comparative accuracy studies in the relevant population, and if the superiority of one test over another was consistent across the included studies.

Relative weaknesses of the included studies should at least be summarized with reference to each of the four QUADAS-2 domains (patient selection, index test(s), reference standard, and flow and timing), highlighting items particularly relevant to the review question, as reflected by the tailoring of QUADAS-2 or QUADAS-C to the review topic. A detailed discussion of the types of bias that might occur in test accuracy studies, including comparative test accuracy studies, can be found in Chapter 8.

Review authors should be mindful that readers of systematic reviews of test accuracy are likely to be less familiar with the types of bias that are encountered in test accuracy research (Zhelev 2013) and that descriptions of the mechanisms underlying important potential sources of bias may facilitate understanding.

Assessing the impact of bias on estimates of accuracy can be challenging, especially as an overall quality score is discouraged (Whiting 2005). Assessment should include consideration of the relative importance of the four QUADAS-2 domains to the review topic and the proportion and size of studies at risk of bias. The assessment of the strength of the evidence can be helpful for such a summary, as described in Section 12.4.

12.6.2 Strengths and weaknesses of the review

Limitations of the review focus on the review *process* and may include shortcomings in the search strategy, selection of studies, data extraction and analyses. This section should summarize the potential implications of these limitations on the strength of the conclusions. Review authors may not have been able to conduct their review as originally intended in the protocol. For example, paucity of studies may have precluded planned investigations of heterogeneity. Limitations of the search strategy should be addressed as a shortcoming and the potential for bias caused by failure to retrieve or to translate reports should be discussed.

12.6.2.1 Strengths and weaknesses due to the search and selection process

Some decisions made in the retrieval process may lead to omissions in the body of evidence that may be relevant for its interpretation; for example, excluding certain languages or only searching in a limited number of databases. The potential consequences of these choices should be addressed in this section.

Lack of consensus in the selection of included studies is another potential limitation of the review process. If there has been substantial disagreement between review authors about the inclusion of studies, there is a risk of including less appropriate studies or of excluding studies from which it is more difficult to extract data. Although the effects of these shortcomings may be limited, they are still potential sources of bias.

12.6.2.2 Strengths and weaknesses due to methodological quality assessment and data extraction

Information about the characteristics of participants, setting, study design and other key information may be missing in reports of primary studies and, therefore, limit assessment of the methodological quality of included studies. The potential impact of 'unclear' assessments of risk of bias will depend on how these 'unclear' assessments have been judged or interpreted when assessing risk of bias or concerns regarding applicability. For example, if all 'unclear' assessments were ignored when judging risk of bias, then the risk of bias for the whole body of evidence may be judged to be overly optimistic.

Although contacting study authors is not a requirement of the review process, the successful identification of additional data can be regarded as a strength of the review process.

12.6.2.3   Weaknesses due to the review analyses

Although meta-analysis in general may result in more precise estimates than analysis of individual primary studies, a small number of included studies or small number of participants may still jeopardize the precision of the results of the review. This especially holds when substantial heterogeneity is observed, and when sources of heterogeneity cannot be explored, let alone explained. In the assessment of the strength of the evidence, this is taken into account when considering imprecision and inconsistency.

With respect to heterogeneity and spectrum effects, review authors should make a priori hypotheses about possible differences in accuracy between subgroups. The Discussion section is the place to put these differences into context. Review authors may be able to discuss how consistent results are across different clinical settings and in different groups of individuals. This allows readers to judge to what extent summary estimates of test accuracy can be applied to different clinical settings.

If review authors find apparent differences in accuracy between subgroups, they should decide whether or not these effects are credible and relevant to readers. These differences should be considered carefully, as variation in results due to chance may play a role. It may be important to consider whether the variable was defined a priori; whether the difference in subgroups was seen within studies rather than between studies; and whether there is additional evidence to support the relevance of findings in a specific subgroup. Cochrane Reviews are written for an international audience, and the discussion should not be limited to the applicability of results to a single healthcare organization or country.

12.6.2.4   Direct and indirect comparisons

Reviews with a comparative question may base their conclusions on direct comparisons (the studies included in the review all directly compare the accuracy of different index tests) or on indirect comparisons (primary studies evaluated one of the index tests) or on both. As explained in Section 12.3.1.6, direct comparisons are ideal because they are less prone to bias due to confounding.

When both direct and indirect comparisons are included in the same review, it should be clear that they are separate analyses and review authors should discuss any differences in results. In addition to potential for bias associated with indirect comparisons (Takwoingi 2013), review authors should acknowledge that estimates of test accuracy derived from indirect comparisons are typically based on a greater number of studies than direct comparisons, leading to more statistical power to detect differences between tests, if such differences exist, and to generate more precise estimates.

12.6.3   Comparisons with previous research

Cochrane Review authors are advised to put their research in the context of what previous reviews and other research have shown. In many cases, a Cochrane Review of diagnostic test accuracy may not be the first review to address the review question. It may also be possible that other systematic reviews have been published for the same test, but for different yet related target conditions. If so, the review authors should discuss any differences between their review and the previously published reviews. These could be differences in the search dates, the number and designs of the studies included, or a different statistical approach for the meta-analysis. Sometimes multiple (related) reviews stem from one generic protocol. If that is the case, review authors should state this and put their particular review in the context of the related reviews.

   If a review is based on an update of an existing review, the review authors may want to point out key differences in the results from those in the previous review, in particular if test features or important technical aspects of an index test or reference standard have changed over time or if, for example, the use of an index test is extended to a new target population.

12.7   Applicability of findings to the review question

Review authors should discuss the applicability of the results of the review: the degree to which the studies in the review correspond to the review objectives. For intervention reviews, this is described as 'indirectness': the extent to which a review is relevant for the purpose to which it is being put (Higgins 2019). Indirectness is also the term that is used in the GRADE approach for both systematic reviews of interventions and test accuracy.

   Assessment of applicability is particularly important for systematic reviews of test accuracy because of the degree to which setting, patient spectrum, index test and definition of the target condition (as defined by the reference standard) can affect test accuracy estimates. Therefore, estimates and judgements of their applicability should be discussed with respect to these characteristics.

   Two scenarios can be distinguished with different implications for assessing the applicability of review findings. A systematic review of test accuracy may be general, with broad eligibility criteria, which complicates investigation of heterogeneity but allows exploration of differences in accuracy across settings, patient groups or applications or versions of the index test (see Chapter 5, Section 5.4.6). Alternatively, having a narrowly focused question, with restricted review eligibility criteria, may simplify the interpretation of the applicability of findings and avoid investigation of heterogeneity, but the review may end up with very few studies and imprecise summary estimates.

12.8   Drawing conclusions

At this point in the review, the results of the meta-analysis – or the narrative summary of key findings if meta-analysis was not performed – and the strength of the evidence have been considered. The next step is to explain to readers how these results can be used to draw conclusions. The Authors' conclusions section in systematic reviews should discuss both the implications of the findings for practice and the implications for research.

12.8.1 Implications for practice

Implications for practice should be as practical and unambiguous as possible. They should not go beyond the evidence that was reviewed and should be justifiable by the data presented in the review. However, the decision to use a medical test will often be based on the accuracy of other tests not included in the review, and on evidence about the effectiveness of downstream actions, such as starting or withholding therapy to patients with specific test results.

Because Cochrane Reviews have an international audience, the implications for practice should, as far as possible, assume a broad international perspective, rather than addressing specific national or local circumstances. Review authors should be aware that different people might make different decisions based on the same evidence. The primary purpose of the review should be to present information rather than to offer advice. The implications for practice should help readers understand the implications of the evidence in relation to practical decisions.

Therefore, recommendations that depend on assumptions about costs, resources and values should be avoided. A common mistake is for review authors to confuse facts and judgements. For example, if the summary sensitivity is 80%, this is a fact. To describe this as 'high sensitivity' would be a judgement. Review authors need also to bear in mind that the potential consequences of introducing test(s) in practice may vary greatly between countries and that costs in their local area may not be applicable to other localities (see for example Box 12.8.a).

Box 12.8.a An example of implications for practice in a comparative review of chest ultrasonography (CUS) versus supine chest radiography (CXR) for diagnosis of pneumothorax in trauma patients in the emergency department

"The diagnostic accuracy of CUS performed by frontline non-radiologist physicians for the diagnosis of pneumothorax in ED trauma patients is superior to supine CXR. Regardless of type of trauma, type of CUS operator, or type of CUS probe used, the overall sensitivity of CUS is superior to supine CXR and their specificities are similar. While many frontline physicians already use US for FAST scans as 'standard of care' to identify intra-abdominal injuries, this review provides evidence that CUS is an accurate diagnostic tool compared to CXR for ED patients with traumatic pneumothorax. Rapid detection of traumatic pneumothorax with CUS may lead to more timely therapeutic intervention with tube thoracostomy, reducing the incidence of pneumothorax-related complications, and thus improving outcomes in ED trauma patients. The findings of this review provide evidence to suggest that CUS could be incorporated into trauma (e.g. advanced trauma life support, ATLS) protocols and algorithms in future medical training programmes. In addition, CUS may beneficially change routine management of trauma."

Source: Chan 2020

However, if one test is found to have superior accuracy to another and known to have no drawbacks (for example, by being less invasive, cheaper, quicker and easier to deliver), the review may provide adequate evidence to support its use (Lord 2006). In contrast, estimates of accuracy for some tests may be so low as to indicate that conclusions can be drawn that a test has no useful role in diagnosis.

In other situations, the implications for practice may not be so clear. For example, if one test has higher sensitivity but lower specificity than another, which test produces better patient outcomes will not be discernible from evidence about test accuracy alone. The potential consequences of false positives and false negatives need to be known, and their trade-off assessed.

Sometimes the difference is large enough to be clear as to which test is better; other times identifying the preferred test will require decision modelling. In this case, it should be made clear that while a Cochrane Review of diagnostic test accuracy can provide important information to use in the model, it cannot answer the question by itself.

Similarly, if there are other aspects of the test that differ (for example, its invasiveness, cost, speed, acceptability and ease of delivery), the relative importance of accuracy compared to these other features should be assessed. Again, this will require research outside of the review, perhaps synthesized in a decision model, or even requiring a randomized controlled trial comparing testing strategies. In such circumstances, the review authors should point out the key factors involved in assessing the value of the test, and the further research that would be needed to provide an answer, under future research recommendations (see Box 12.8.b).

We suggest that review authors consider the following issues when addressing implications for practice.

Box 12.8.b An example of implications for practice for a review about computed tomography (CT) for diagnosis of acute appendicitis in adults

---

"Sensitivity and specificity of CT for diagnosing acute appendicitis in adults are high, hence the use of CT is likely to assist clinicians in treating persons with possible appendicitis. Unenhanced standard-dose CT appears to have lower sensitivity than standard-dose CT with IV, rectal, or oral and IV contrast enhancement. Use of different types of contrast enhancement or no enhancement does not appear to affect specificity. Differences in sensitivity and specificity between low-dose and standard-dose CT appear to be negligible. In adult persons, it seems that low-dose CT should be preferred over standard-dose CT as a first-line imaging test, with standard-dose CT reserved for persons with inconclusive findings on low-dose CT. To minimise radiation exposure, clinicians should critically assess whether additional information from CT imaging is needed for decision-making about surgery, watchful waiting, or discharge. Results of this review should be interpreted with caution for two reasons. First, the results are based on studies of low methodological quality. Second, the comparisons between types of contrast enhancement and radiation dose may be unreliable because they are based on indirect comparisons that may be confounded by other factors."

Source: Rud 2019

How is the test positioned in the clinical pathway?

The position of the index test in a clinical pathway will affect the absolute numbers of true positives, false positives, true negatives and false negatives and their potential consequences. Tests used early in a clinical pathway where the prevalence of the target condition is often at its lowest (for example, screening asymptomatic individuals) are likely to result in a relatively high absolute number of false positives at any given specificity, and a relatively low absolute number of false negatives at any given sensitivity. A higher prevalence of the target condition is likely to decrease the absolute number of false positives at any given specificity and increase the number of false negatives at any given sensitivity.

How does the index perform in relation to its intended role (e.g. add-on, replacement, triage)?

Chapter 5 outlined the different roles that index tests might have in a clinical testing pathway, such as: Can an index replace another test? Can an index test be added after another test? Can an index test be used to triage individuals, to prevent some from receiving another test? (Bossuyt 2006). Review authors should consider whether the performance characteristics of the test(s) evaluated in the review are consistent with its intended role in practice.

For example, a new test intended to triage individuals for a more invasive test, referring only new test positives to the second test, can be expected to have high sensitivity, to ensure that introduction of the new triage test will not result in cases being missed. It is acceptable for the new triage test to have a relatively low specificity, as introducing the test will still lead to a reduction in the number of individuals having to undergo the more invasive test.

There may be issues in addition to accuracy that should be highlighted by review authors when considering the consequences of introducing the test in its intended role (Ferrante di Ruffano 2012). For example, for a test replacement question, consideration of whether test A should replace test B may not rely solely on evidence of improved accuracy of test A compared to test B. If test B is less costly or less invasive than test A, then evidence of comparable accuracy of the two tests may be considered sufficient.

What are the potential consequences of introducing the index test(s), for the intended use, in the intended role, for patient outcomes?

This refers to the potential consequences of testing, using a hypothetical cohort of people, as explained in Chapter 11 and Chapter 13. Evaluating the potential consequences of introducing the index test(s) into practice requires comparison with other tests – prior tests or additional tests – that are available for the same target condition, and for the same intended use. In addition to the implications of test errors associated with the intended use and the role of the index test, review authors may want to highlight other issues that may be relevant for readers in reaching a decision about the potential benefits and harms of adopting the index test(s). Costs, organizational outcomes, uninterpretable results, acceptability, uptake and direct harms and benefits of tests (physical and psychological) are examples of such issues (Ferrante di Ruffano 2012, Schünemann 2016). Information on these issues may come from other (not systematically searched and assessed) sources.

Review authors should be cautious when providing additional information that has not been gathered in a systematic way and that may therefore be dependent on interpretation, or even be prone to bias. However, information about test features can assist decision-makers assessing the value and use of the test and should be provided where available.

Explorations of heterogeneity may return in the implications for practice. It is possible that the analyses of heterogeneity have pointed to significant and consistent differences in test performance associated with differences in patient selection criteria, setting or prior testing in such a way that this has implications for practice: the test has the desired diagnostic accuracy in some conditions, but not in others. The same could apply to subtypes of the index tests: some assays, for example, may have superior accuracy than others, possibly leading to recommendations for practice.

Finally, the strength of the evidence should also be mentioned in the Authors' conclusions. It may be impossible to draw conclusions, because of all the shortcomings of the included studies and the body of evidence as a whole. This should be made explicit in such a case (see Box 12.8.c).

12.8.2 Implications for research

Implications for research may cover two broad areas: further studies of test accuracy that should be undertaken and additional research needed on aspects of tests beyond their accuracy. Researchers, research funders and commissioners will read this section of the review to help inform decisions about the design and funding of future studies.

Where the evidence on test accuracy is inconclusive, review authors may recommend future test accuracy studies. This may involve stating that similar but better-reported studies are needed, accuracy studies of better methodological quality, done in the appropriate patient population, at the right point in the clinical pathway, or setting, or comparative head-to-head accuracy studies. Review authors should provide as much detail about the design of future studies as possible. If better comparative accuracy studies are needed, it is important to describe the important comparisons that should be made. If there are issues that should be resolved before future accuracy studies are commissioned, such as obtaining consensus on the best reference standard or the delivery method for the new index test, suggestions of how to achieve this could be stated.

Box 12.8.c An example of implications for practice in a situation where there was a very low certainty of the evidence. The review authors used GRADE to assess the certainty of the evidence

---

"Based on the very low certainty of the evidence and the low number of included studies there is little evidence in this review to support the widespread introduction of electrical conductance devices as an adjunct to clinical examination."

Source: Macey 2021

If the review revealed new questions or generated hypotheses, then this is the place to discuss them. This may be particularly important where review authors have disclosed conclusions from investigations of between-study heterogeneity, or where heterogeneity exists but cannot be explained.

Evidence about other routes (such as increased access or benefits of point-of-care testing) by which tests have an impact on patients should be taken into account to assess the potential of tests to improve patient outcomes in clinical practice (Ferrante di Ruffano 2012). Review authors should specify the characteristics of the tests to be assessed and the method by which this should be done (i.e. from other systematic reviews, routine data sources, new primary studies and qualitative research). Additionally, they should indicate whether decision modelling or randomized trials comparing different diagnostic pathways should be undertaken, and comment on the key design features of the studies required.

12.9   Chapter information

Authors: Mariska M. Leeflang (*Department of Epidemiology and Data Science, University of Amsterdam, The Netherlands*), Karen R. Steingart (*Department of Clinical Sciences, Liverpool School of Tropical Medicine, UK*), Rob J. Scholten (*Cochrane Netherlands, Utrecht University, The Netherlands*), Clare Davenport (*Institute of Applied Health Research, University of Birmingham, UK*).

Sources of support: The authors declare no sources of support for writing this chapter.

Declarations of interest: Mariska Leeflang, Karen R. Steingart and Clare Davenport are members of Cochrane's Diagnostic Test Accuracy Editorial Team. Mariska Leeflang is co-convenor of the Cochrane Screening and Diagnostic Tests Methods Group. Rob J. Scholten is a past member of Cochrane's Diagnostic Test Accuracy Editorial Team and the GRADE Working Group. The authors declare no other potential conflicts of interest relevant to the topic of this chapter.

Acknowledgements: The authors would like to thank Mia Schmidt-Hansen, Miranda Langendam and Jérémie Cohen for helpful peer review comments.

12.10   References

Agarwal R, Choi L, Johnson S, Takwoingi Y. Rapid diagnostic tests for Plasmodium vivax malaria in endemic countries. *Cochrane Database of Systematic Reviews* 2020; **11**: CD013218.

Bossuyt PM, Irwig L, Craig J, Glasziou P. Comparative accuracy: assessing new tests against existing diagnostic pathways. *BMJ* 2006; **332**: 1089–1092.

Chan KK, Joo DA, McRae AD, Takwoingi Y, Premji ZA, Lang E, Wakai A. Chest ultrasonography versus supine chest radiography for diagnosis of pneumothorax in trauma patients in the emergency department. *Cochrane Database of Systematic Reviews* 2020; **7**: CD013031.

Deeks JJ, Macaskill P, Irwig L. The performance of tests of publication bias and other sample size effects in systematic reviews of diagnostic test accuracy was assessed. *Journal of Clinical Epidemiology* 2005; **58**: 882–893.

Ferrante di Ruffano L, Hyde CJ, McCaffery KJ, Bossuyt PMM, Deeks JJ. Assessing the value of diagnostic tests: a framework for designing and evaluating trials. *BMJ* 2012; **344**: e686.

GRADEpro. GRADEpro Guideline Development Tool [Software]. Available from gradepro. org. McMaster University (developed by Evidence Prime, Inc.); 2020. www.gradepro.org.

Hanchard NC, Lenza M, Handoll HH, Takwoingi Y. Physical tests for shoulder impingements and local lesions of bursa, tendon or labrum that may accompany impingement. *Cochrane Database of Systematic Reviews* 2013; **4**: CD007427.

Harbord RM, Deeks JJ, Egger M, Whiting PF, Sterne JA. A unification of models for meta-analysis of diagnostic accuracy studies. *Biostatistics* 2007; **8**: 239–251.

Higgins J, Thomas J, Chandler J, Cumpston M, Li T, Page M, Welch V. *Cochrane Handbook for Systematic Reviews of Interventions*. 2nd ed. Chichester (UK): John Wiley & Sons; 2019.

Hultcrantz M, Mustafa RA, Leeflang MMG, Lavergne V, Estrada-Orozco K, Ansari MT, Izcovich A, Singh J, Chong LY, Rutjes A, Steingart K, Stein A, Sekercioglu N, Arevalo-Rodriguez I, Morgan RL, Guyatt G, Bossuyt P, Langendam MW, Schünemann HJ. Defining ranges for certainty ratings of diagnostic accuracy: a GRADE concept paper. *Journal of Clinical Epidemiology* 2020; **117**: 138–148.

Jullien S, Dissanayake HA, Chaplin M. Rapid diagnostic tests for plague. *Cochrane Database of Systematic Reviews* 2020; **6**: CD013459.

Kohli M, Schiller I, Dendukuri N, Yao M, Dheda K, Denkinger CM, Schumacher SG, Steingart KR. Xpert MTB/RIF Ultra and Xpert MTB/RIF assays for extrapulmonary tuberculosis and rifampicin resistance in adults. *Cochrane Database of Systematic Reviews* 2021; **1**: CD012768.

Korevaar DA, Cohen JF, Spijker R, Saldanha IJ, Dickersin K, Virgili G, Hooft L, Bossuyt PM. Reported estimates of diagnostic accuracy in ophthalmology conference abstracts were not associated with full-text publication. *Journal of Clinical Epidemiology* 2016; **79**: 96–103.

Leeflang MM, Debets-Ossenkopp YJ, Wang J, Visser CE, Scholten RJ, Hooft L, Bijlmer HA, Reitsma JB, Zhang M, Bossuyt PM, Vandenbroucke-Grauls CM. Galactomannan detection for invasive aspergillosis in immunocompromised patients. *Cochrane Database of Systematic Reviews* 2015; **12**: CD007394.

Lord SJ, Irwig L, Simes RJ. When is measuring sensitivity and specificity sufficient to evaluate a diagnostic test, and when do we need randomized trials? *Annals of Internal Medicine* 2006; **144**: 850–855.

Macey R, Walsh T, Riley P, Glenny AM, Worthington HV, Clarkson JE, Ricketts D. Electrical conductance for the detection of dental caries. *Cochrane Database of Systematic Reviews* 2021; **3**: CD014547.

Nielsen LH, Ortner N, Nørgaard BL, Achenbach S, Leipsic J, Abdulla J. The diagnostic accuracy and outcomes after coronary computed tomography angiography vs. conventional functional testing in patients with stable angina pectoris: a systematic review and meta-analysis. *European Heart Journal Cardiovascular Imaging* 2014; **15**: 961–971.

Rud B, Vejborg TS, Rappeport ED, Reitsma JB, Wille-Jørgensen P. Computed tomography for diagnosis of acute appendicitis in adults. *Cochrane Database of Systematic Reviews* 2019; **11**: CD009977.

Schünemann HJ, Oxman AD, Brozek J, Glasziou P, Jaeschke R, Vist GE, Williams JW, Jr., Kunz R, Craig J, Montori VM, Bossuyt P, Guyatt GH. Grading quality of evidence and strength of recommendations for diagnostic tests and strategies. *BMJ* 2008; **336**: 1106–1110.

Schünemann HJ, Mustafa R, Brozek J, Santesso N, Alonso-Coello P, Guyatt G, Scholten R, Langendam M, Leeflang MM, Akl EA, Singh JA, Meerpohl J, Hultcrantz M, Bossuyt P, Oxman AD. GRADE Guidelines: 16. GRADE evidence to decision frameworks for tests in clinical practice and public health. *Journal of Clinical Epidemiology* 2016; **76**: 89–98.

Schünemann HJ, Mustafa RA, Brozek J, Steingart KR, Leeflang M, Murad MH, Bossuyt P, Glasziou P, Jaeschke R, Lange S, Meerpohl J, Langendam M, Hultcrantz M, Vist GE, Akl EA, Helfand M, Santesso N, Hooft L, Scholten R, Rosen M, Rutjes A, Crowther M, Muti P, Raatz H, Ansari MT, Williams J, Kunz R, Harris J, Rodriguez IA, Kohli M, Guyatt GH. GRADE guidelines: 21 part 1. Study design, risk of bias, and indirectness in rating the certainty across a body of evidence for test accuracy. *Journal of Clinical Epidemiology* 2020a; **122**: 129–141.

Schünemann HJ, Mustafa RA, Brozek J, Steingart KR, Leeflang M, Murad MH, Bossuyt P, Glasziou P, Jaeschke R, Lange S, Meerpohl J, Langendam M, Hultcrantz M, Vist GE, Akl EA, Helfand M, Santesso N, Hooft L, Scholten R, Rosen M, Rutjes A, Crowther M, Muti P, Raatz H, Ansari MT, Williams J, Kunz R, Harris J, Rodriguez IA, Kohli M, Guyatt GH. GRADE guidelines: 21 part 2. Test accuracy: inconsistency, imprecision, publication bias, and other domains for rating the certainty of evidence and presenting it in evidence profiles and summary of findings tables. *Journal of Clinical Epidemiology* 2020b; **122**: 142–152.

Simes RJ. Publication bias: the case for an international registry of clinical trials. *Journal of Clinical Oncology* 1986; **4**: 1529–1541.

Takwoingi Y, Leeflang MM, Deeks JJ. Empirical evidence of the importance of comparative studies of diagnostic test accuracy. *Annals of Internal Medicine* 2013; **158**: 544–554.

Whiting PF, Harbord R, Kleijnen J. No role for quality scores in systematic reviews of diagnostic accuracy studies. *BMC Medical Research Methodology* 2005; **5**: 19.

Whiting PF, Davenport C, Jameson C, Burke M, Sterne JA, Hyde C, Ben-Shlomo Y. How well do health professionals interpret diagnostic information? A systematic review. *BMJ Open* 2015; **5**: e008155.

World Health Organization. WHO-FIND malaria RDT evaluation programme. Last update 10 July 2017a. Available at www.who.int/malaria/areas/diagnosis/rapid-diagnostic-tests/rdt-evaluation-programme/en.

World Health Organization. A framework for malaria elimination. Last update March 2017b. Available at www.who.int/malaria/publications/atoz/9789241511988/en.

Yang B, Mustafa RA, Bossuyt PM, Brozek J, Hultcrantz M, Leeflang MMG, Schünemann HJ, Langendam MW. GRADE Guidance: 31. Assessing the certainty across a body of evidence for comparative test accuracy. *Journal of Clinical Epidemiology* 2021; **136**: 146–156.

Zhelev Z, Garside R, Hyde C. A qualitative study into the difficulties experienced by healthcare decision makers when reading a Cochrane diagnostic test accuracy review. *Systematic Reviews* 2013; **2**: 32.

Zifodya JS, Kreniske JS, Schiller I, Kohli M, Dendukuri N, Schumacher SG, Ochodo EA, Haraka F, Zwerling AA, Pai M, Steingart KR, Horne DJ. Xpert Ultra versus Xpert MTB/RIF for pulmonary tuberculosis and rifampicin resistance in adults with presumptive pulmonary tuberculosis. *Cochrane Database of Systematic Reviews* 2021; **2**: CD009593.

13

Writing a plain language summary

Penny Whiting and Clare Davenport

KEY POINTS

- A plain language summary is a standalone summary of a Cochrane systematic review written in plain English. It provides rapid access to the contents of the review.
- Measures of accuracy such as sensitivity and specificity are poorly understood, both by lay audiences and by health professionals.
- Explaining the results of a systematic review of test accuracy in plain language is challenging, particularly the numerical findings of the review.
- Reporting test accuracy measures using natural frequencies and linking test results to the potential consequences of testing for patients can improve understanding.
- Generic guidance for writing a Cochrane plain language summary exists and can be applied to a Cochrane Review of diagnostic test accuracy.

13.1 Introduction

A plain language summary is a standalone summary of a Cochrane systematic review written in plain language. It provides rapid access to the contents of the review. Plain language summaries can be used to facilitate shared decision-making between individuals and their healthcare providers. The plain language summary aims to summarize the review in a straightforward style that can be understood by consumers of health care. Because of the lack of familiarity with test accuracy methods and measures, the potential plain language summary audience for a systematic review of test accuracy is likely to be broad and include policy makers, doctors, nurses and journalists. Cochrane plain language summaries are made freely available on the internet, so will often be read as standalone documents.

This chapter should be cited as: Whiting P, Davenport C. Chapter 13: Writing a plain language summary. In: Deeks JJ, Bossuyt PM, Leeflang MM, Takwoingi Y, editors. *Cochrane Handbook for Systematic Reviews of Diagnostic Test Accuracy*. 1st edition. Chichester (UK): John Wiley & Sons, 2023: 377–398.

Cochrane Handbook for Systematic Reviews of Diagnostic Test Accuracy, First Edition. Edited by Jonathan J. Deeks, Patrick M. Bossuyt, Mariska M. Leeflang and Yemisi Takwoingi.
© 2023 The Cochrane Collaboration. Published 2023 by John Wiley & Sons Ltd.

A clear plain language summary is essential to ensure that a systematic review is useful to users who are not familiar with the more technical content of the review. Plain language summaries are mandatory for all Cochrane systematic reviews. The generic guidance for writing a Cochrane plain language summary guides review authors through the steps of preparing the summary with advice on how to write in plain language (Pitcher 2021). The guidance also includes a template that can be used for all types of Cochrane Reviews and explains what to include in each section of the summary, with examples. We recommend that review authors consult the guidance and use it in conjunction with this chapter.

Explaining the results of a systematic review of test accuracy in plain language is challenging. The review methodology and results are less familiar than reviews of interventions. The two-dimensional nature of common measures of a test's accuracy (e.g. sensitivity and specificity) introduces further complexity (Leeflang 2008). Research has shown that even readers familiar with systematic review methods and interpretation of results have difficulties understanding test accuracy reviews and that experience with intervention reviews may even be a disadvantage (Zhelev 2013).

Commonly used measures of test accuracy are often poorly understood by health professionals (Whiting 2015). For example, sensitivity and specificity are not easily translated into the proportion of test results that are correct (true positives and true negatives) and those that are incorrect (false positives and false negatives).

Reporting test accuracy using natural frequencies and visual aids may facilitate improved understanding. Additionally, test accuracy reviews are characterized by a large degree of heterogeneity in results across studies. The reason for this variation is not always clear and explaining this to readers, especially lay readers, is difficult. Ideally, a plain language summary should be easily understandable to all target audiences and provide the information they need to understand the findings of the review.

The recommended structure, content and writing style for a plain language summary for a Cochrane Review of diagnostic test accuracy described in this chapter are based primarily on research undertaken with patient, media and health professional representatives (Whiting 2018a) and guidance on how to structure a plain language summary for Cochrane Reviews (Pitcher 2021). Drawing on this guidance, we discuss the challenges and suggested approaches for writing plain language summaries for different types of systematic review of test accuracy questions (for example, multiple index tests or multiple population subgroups).

13.2   Audience and writing style

Because of the difficulties in understanding measures of test accuracy, the potential audience for a plain language summary for a systematic review of test accuracy is likely to be wide, including the public, policy makers and anyone who talks to the public about health, for example doctors, nurses, journalists and patient groups. The guidance for writing plain language summaries for Cochrane Reviews includes helpful guidance on how to approach writing a Cochrane plain language summary, including general advice on writing in plain language (Pitcher 2021).

Key points include:

- use everyday language;
- avoid long words, research jargon, and words or phrases with dual or nuanced meanings;
- explain 'common' medical words and technical medical terms;
- avoid acronyms and abbreviations;
- write for an international audience;
- keep paragraphs and sentences short (average of 20 words);
- use the active voice;
- use pronouns;
- use good verbs;
- write numbers as numerals rather than words;
- be concise; and
- use subheadings and bullet points.

Research involving a range of user groups (Whiting 2018a) suggested that the following terms and technical language should be avoided in plain language summaries of test accuracy reviews:

- sensitivity and specificity;
- positive and negative likelihood ratio;
- positive and negative predictive value; and
- risk of bias, verification bias, review bias, spectrum bias.

The term bias is not well understood by lay audiences and sources of bias specific to test accuracy reviews are unlikely to be familiar to lay audiences or health professionals. Bias can be explained in terms of its impact on test accuracy estimates and suggested language is provided in Section 13.3.8. Terms such as positive test result, negative test result and reference standard require explanation in plain language summaries. Positive and negative test results are sometimes associated by lay audiences with good and bad outcomes, respectively. Therefore, these terms require explanation in terms of their potential implications for patient outcomes.

Textual and graphical approaches to presenting test accuracy are presented in Section 13.3.7. You could consider using graphics to present test accuracy in the findings section of the main review.

13.3 Contents and structure of a plain language summary

We suggest including the following subheadings in the plain language summary and highlight key considerations for the content required under each subheading. We use the example of a review evaluating the accuracy of rapid swab tests for the diagnosis of strep sore throat in children (Cohen 2016), where the potential positive consequence of rapid swab tests would be to reduce unnecessary antibiotic use. This example is supplemented with alternative examples where needed to allow for different review and data formats, and the appendix contains a complete example.

13.3.1   Title

The main review question should be written in plain language. If the review title includes technical terms or jargon, consider re-writing it for the plain language summary. As a minimum, the review title should contain information about the following three key elements:

- The test or tests being studied (index tests). It is important to ensure that the type of test being studied is clear (e.g. a questionnaire, a blood test, a swab, a urine test or some form of medical imaging). Avoid using acronyms or characteristics of the index test, for example describing the index test as a 'rapid' test without including information about test type.
- The condition that the test (or tests) is designed to detect (the target condition).
- The people who will receive the test (for example adults, children, people with certain symptoms such as sore throat or low back pain). It may also be important to include any restrictions on the healthcare setting where the test will be applied; for example, if the test will only be used in hospital settings and not the community.

Examples of plain language summary title formats include:

> 'How accurate is index test for target condition in healthcare setting/population?'
>
> **Rapid swab tests for strep sore throat example**
> How accurate are rapid swab tests for strep sore throat in children?

13.3.2   Key messages

Use at least two and no more than three bullet points to summarize the main findings and implications of the review.

Start with a brief summary statement regarding whether the results of the review suggest that the index test has the potential to be useful to detect the target condition in the target population. This could be accompanied by a statement about the potential consequences of improved accuracy, no difference in accuracy or reduced accuracy, as indicated by the review findings. If the evidence reviewed is not sufficient to draw a conclusion, this should be stated here. For example, 'It is unclear whether [index test] can be used to detect [target condition] in [target population]'.

Important variation in test accuracy estimates, for example in different patient groups, due to different test thresholds, or with different versions of the test, can also be highlighted in this section. Where potential benefits from a reduction in test errors need to be balanced against other test attributes, such as cost, time to result, accessibility and acceptability, this can also be mentioned here. For example:

'The studies included in this review suggest that index test can/cannot identify population with target condition in setting. This may lead to consequences.

Estimates were similar for different versions of the index test.

Results suggest that index test is likely to be less useful in setting 1 than in setting 2.'

Rapid swab tests for strep sore throat example
- The studies in this review suggest that rapid swab tests can detect most bacterial infections (Strep A) in children with sore throats, leading to early and appropriate treatment with antibiotics.
- The number of children receiving unnecessary antibiotics following a rapid test is still likely to be lower than the number of children who would receive unnecessary antibiotics if the test is not used.
- Both types of rapid tests studied in the review had similar accuracy.

13.3.3 'Why is improving [. . .] diagnosis important?'

This section should include information about the target condition and a description of the potential consequences of false positive test errors and false negative test errors. It is helpful to introduce the concept of test errors in this section ahead of presenting results.

- What are the consequences of a false positive result (index test positive but target condition absent, i.e. incorrectly labelling individuals who actually do not have the condition as having the condition)?
- What are the consequences of a false negative result (index test negative but target condition present, i.e. missing the condition in individuals who actually have the condition)?

For example:

'[Describe target condition in terms of prevalence, morbidity, cost in the population of interest].

Not recognizing target condition when it is present (a false negative test result) may result in consequences of false negative.

An incorrect diagnosis of target condition (a false positive result) may result in consequences of false positive.'

Rapid swab tests for strep sore throat example
Why is improving the diagnosis of bacterial throat infection important?
Sore throat is very common in children. It can be caused by viruses or bacteria. Antibiotic treatment is only useful for sore throat caused by bacteria, most commonly group A streptococcus ('strep throat').

Not recognizing bacterial infection when it is present (a false negative test result) may result in delayed recovery and an increased risk of infecting others. It may also result in rare but serious complications such as abscesses in the throat, bacterial infection of the sinuses and ears, and rheumatic fever.

An incorrect diagnosis of bacterial infection (a false positive test result) may mean that children are given antibiotics when there is no benefit to be gained.

13.3.4 'What is the [...] test?'

This section should include a brief description of the index test and its proposed role in the diagnostic pathway (see Chapter 5).

- What was the index test(s) addressed in the review? Give enough information for readers to judge whether the test(s) being studied is relevant to them, for example where in the clinical pathway the test is likely to be applied (the community, hospital), who would conduct the test.
- Describe how use of the index test might benefit individuals suspected of having the target condition. For example, the index test may be more accurate, may provide quicker results, or may be more accessible (less costly, require less expertise) than tests currently in use.
- Describe potential negative effects of using the index test. For example, the index test may cause anxiety, pain, harms such as exposure to ionizing radiation, or be less accessible than tests currently in use.
- What is the role of the index test (e.g. triage, add-on, or replacement test; see Chapter 5, Section 5.3.1) (*Bossuyt 2006*)? Review authors should avoid using these technical terms and instead describe how the index test would be placed in the current testing pathway in relation to other tests.
- If there is more than one index test included in a review, the plain language summary should also explain how the tests differ. For example, one test may be quicker to give results or easier to perform, tests may be produced by a different manufacturer or require different processing techniques, one test may be a blood test and another a swab test.
- Describe the test result that indicates if the target condition is present (what is considered a positive test result) or absent (what is considered a negative test result).

Rapid swab tests for strep sore throat example
What are rapid swab tests for strep sore throat? Rapid swab tests require a simple throat swab taken by a nurse or doctor from the patient. This gives an immediate result allowing clinicians to decide whether to prescribe antibiotics. This is an advantage compared to conventional laboratory tests, which take 48 hours to give a result.   Two types of rapid swab tests were studied. These use different biochemical methods to identify the bacterial infection.

13.3.5 What did we want to find out?

State the aim of the review as concisely and simply as possible. If the review compares multiple index tests, then this should also be described.

> 'We wanted to find out how accurate index test(s) is in setting/population.'
>
> **Rapid swab tests for strep sore throat example**
> We wanted to find out how accurate rapid tests are for detecting bacterial infections in children with sore throat.
>
> **Different imaging tests for collapsed lung example**
> "We wanted to find out whether ultrasound imaging of the chest is better than an X-ray of the chest for diagnosing a collapsed lung in patients who have suffered a physical injury and present to the emergency department" (Chan 2020).

13.3.6   What did we do?

Briefly describe the review methods (for example, that the review searched for studies with specific characteristics, summarizing their results and evaluating the evidence). We suggest a sentence based on the following.

> 'We searched for studies that had investigated the accuracy of index tests for target condition in population and we combined the results across these studies.'
>
> **Rapid swab tests for strep sore throat example**
> We searched for studies that had investigated the accuracy of rapid swab tests for detecting bacterial infection in children and we combined the results across these studies.

13.3.7   What did we find?

This section should cover the number of included studies, the characteristics of the included studies, and the main results of the review.

13.3.7.1   Describing the included studies
This section should describe briefly the number of included studies and total number of participants. To clarify that the number of participants applies to the sum total of participants across included studies, it is helpful to structure this sentence as follows.

> 'The review included # relevant studies with a total of # participants.'
>
> **Rapid swab tests for strep sore throat example**
> The analysis included results from 98 studies that included 58,244 children with sore throat.

'The review included # relevant studies with a total of # participants. # studies (# participants) evaluated index test 1 and # studies (# participants) evaluated index test 2.'

Example where multiple index tests are evaluated
"The review included 34 studies with a total of 9339 participants. Thirty-one studies (8014 participants) evaluated chest CT; three studies evaluated chest X-rays (1243 participants) and one study evaluated lung ultrasound (100 participants)" (Islam 2021).

When describing included studies in reviews containing multiple tests, different versions of the same test or test accuracy in different subgroups, review authors should state the number of studies and number of participants contributing to each of the index test evaluations.

This section should also provide a brief summary of the characteristics of included studies as an indication of their applicability. The mean or median proportion of study participants with the target condition across studies should be included, provided this comes from single-group studies. Multi-group studies (also known as diagnostic case-control studies) should not be included in this summary, because the proportions with and without the target condition in such studies are determined by the researchers.

In addition, a brief summary of information on the applicability of the review findings should be presented. This information may include the organization of healthcare services that might have an impact on the accessibility of index tests and participant characteristics, such as symptoms, disease severity, age, sex and prior tests received. Details about how the index test is conducted, in terms of age or version of the technology, specific assays or expertise of the persons conducting the test, can also be mentioned.

For example:

'Studies were conducted in countries [comment on representativeness of geographical location]. The age range of participants/symptom severity/healthcare setting [comment on presentation and variation across studies]. Overall, an average of # out of every 100 (#%) participants were found to have target condition with this number ranging from # out of every 100 (#%) to # out of every 100 (#%).'

Rapid swab tests for strep sore throat example
Studies included in the review were carried out in 25 countries with almost half conducted in the USA. Tests produced by 42 different manufacturers were assessed. Children in included studies appeared to have more severe disease than typically seen in the community. The average age of children was 7 years. Overall, an average of 29 out of every 100 (29%) children were found to have a bacterial throat infection, with this number ranging from 10 out of every 100 (10%) to 67 out of every 100 (67%) across studies.

13.3.7.2   Presenting information on test accuracy
When it is considered appropriate to present numerical estimates of accuracy (single or summary estimates), the following are key points to consider.

- Natural frequencies are better understood than probabilities (*Gigerenzer* 2011). A natural frequency is a joint frequency of two events, such as the number of patients with the target condition and a positive test result. We suggest presenting accuracy based on a hypothetical group of individuals receiving the index test (e.g. 1000) with a proportion with the target condition that reflects the settings in which the index test is to be used.

- Presenting accuracy with reference to the index test result (predictive values) rather than actual disease status (sensitivity and specificity) may be preferred and more relevant to potential recipients of the test.
- Prominence should be given to test errors (false positives and false negatives) over true-positive and true-negative test results (*Whiting 2018a*).
- Keep numerical information to a minimum, while ensuring that the review objectives (as stated in Section 13.3.5) are addressed.

Chapter 11 illustrates how to derive natural frequencies from summary estimates of sensitivity and specificity from the systematic review and an estimate of the proportion with the target condition in those undergoing testing.

13.3.7.3 Presenting single estimates of accuracy
Where it is considered appropriate to present numerical results, based on the key points outlined we suggest the following template.

The results of these # studies indicate that if the index test were to be used in setting in a group of 1000 people where # (#%) have target condition then:

- An estimated [TP + FP] would have an index test result indicating target condition is present and of these [FP] would be incorrectly classified as having the [target condition].
- Of the [TN + FN] people with a result indicating that target condition is not present, FN would be incorrectly classified as not having target condition.

Rapid swab tests for strep sore throat example
The results of these studies indicate that if rapid swab tests were to be used in a group of 1000 children with sore throats, of whom 300 (30%) are actually caused by bacterial infection, then:

- An estimated 289 would have a rapid test result indicating that their sore throat is caused by a bacterial infection; of these, 32 (11%) would not have a bacterial infection.
- An estimated 711 children would have a rapid test result indicating that their sore throat is not caused by a bacterial infection; of these, 43 (6%) would actually have a bacterial infection.
- Both types of rapid test showed similar results.

To reduce numerical complexity, do not report confidence intervals in the plain language summary. Uncertainty in estimates of accuracy should be discussed as part of plain language summaries; see Section 13.3.8.

13.3.7.4   Presenting multiple estimates of accuracy: two index tests

A key objective of Cochrane Reviews of diagnostic test accuracy is comparison of test accuracy. Here we suggest how the user-tested template for presenting a single estimate of test accuracy might be modified for plain language summaries of reviews that compare two tests and for reviews that compare more than two tests.

When the accuracy of two index tests is compared, review authors can extend the basic template to report the accuracy of each test. For example:

Example where multiple index tests are evaluated

The results of these studies indicate that, in theory, if ultrasound of the chest was used on a group of 100 patients where 30 (30%) have a collapsed lung:

- An estimated 28 would have an ultrasound result indicating the presence of collapsed lung and of these one (3.6%) would be incorrectly classified as having a collapsed lung (FP).
- Of the 72 patients with a result indicating that they do not have a collapsed lung, three (4.2%) would actually have a collapsed lung (FN).

In contrast, if an X-ray of the chest was used on this same group of 100 patients where 30 (30%) have a collapsed lung:

- An estimated 14 would have a chest X-ray result indicating the presence of a collapsed lung and none of these would be incorrectly classified as having a collapsed lung (FP).
- Of the 86 patients with a result indicating that they do not have a collapsed lung, 16 (18.6%) would actually have a collapsed lung (FN).

Source: Based on Chan 2020.

Alternatively, absolute differences in sensitivity and specificity between the index tests could be illustrated in terms of the incremental change in the number of false positives and false negatives. For example:

Alternative example: Two index tests, incremental difference in accuracy

The results of these studies indicate that if Reflectance Confocal Microscopy (RCM) was used in 1000 lesions, of which 300 (30%) actually are melanoma:

- An estimated 396 would have an RCM result indicating that melanoma was present and, of these, 126 (32%) would not be melanoma (false positive results); in the same group of 1000 lesions, dermoscopy would indicate that 406 lesions were melanoma when they were not (false positive results). RCM would therefore avoid unnecessary surgery in an additional 280 lesions compared to dermoscopy.
- An estimated 604 lesions would have an RCM result indicating that melanoma was not present, of which 30 (5%) would actually be melanoma (false negatives); in the same group, dermoscopy would indicate that melanoma was not present in 324 lesions, of which 30 (9%) would actually be melanoma. The two tests would therefore miss the same number of lesions that are actually melanoma.

Source: Based on Dinnes 2018.

13.3.7.5   Presenting multiple estimates of accuracy: more than two index tests

Where more than two index tests are compared, the challenge is to balance complexity of numerical presentation with effective and non-selective reporting of results. Review authors may choose to report the accuracy of one test numerically, as outlined in the single-test example above, while making a narrative statement about the comparative accuracy of other included index tests. Review authors are advised to provide a statement about the accuracy of all included index tests to avoid the risk of selective reporting of results.

In the following plain language summary for rapid point-of-care molecular and antigen tests to diagnose COVID-19 infection, a total of 5 different antigen tests and 13 molecular tests were included. The review authors provided more detail on the larger volume of molecular test studies because they had less confidence in the smaller number of more heterogeneous antigen test studies. For example:

Example where multiple index tests are evaluated

There was considerable variation in the number of false negative test results (people in whom the test result indicated COVID-19 was absent when it was in fact present) across included antigen test studies. Antigen tests very rarely suggested that a person without COVID-19 actually had the disease (a small number of false positive results).

For the molecular tests, the results of these studies suggested that if the tests were to be used in a group of 1000 people of whom 100 actually have COVID-19:

- An estimated 105 people would have a test result indicating that they have COVID-19, and of these, 10 people (10%) would not have COVID-19 (false positive result).
- An estimated 895 people would test negative for COVID-19. Of these, 5 people (1%) would actually have COVID-19 (false negative result).

Source: Based on Dinnes 2020.

13.3.7.6   When presenting a numerical summary of test accuracy is not appropriate

Presentation of numerical estimates of test accuracy, even when accompanied by caveats about the volume of studies included, their risk of bias or applicability (Section 13.3.7), can misrepresent the trustworthiness of findings.

There may be valid reasons for not undertaking meta-analysis in a systematic review of test accuracy; for example, where data are sparse or when there is a substantial unexplained heterogeneity. Where meta-analysis is not possible because of sparse data, review authors may consider it appropriate to present the range of test accuracy estimates observed across included studies as an indication of index test performance. For example:

Example where numerical summaries are not presented

For detecting mild cognitive impairment, the results of these studies indicate that if the ACE-III or mini-ACE were to be used in a group of 1000 people with suspected mild cognitive impairment of whom 535 actually have mild cognitive impairment:

- An estimated 440 to 675 would have an ACE-III or mini-ACE result indicating the presence of mild cognitive impairment, and of these 98 to 167 (22% to 25%) would be incorrectly classified as having mild cognitive impairment (false positive).
- An estimated 325 to 560 people would have a result indicating the absence of mild cognitive impairment, and of these 27 to 193 (8% to 34%) would actually have mild cognitive impairment (false negative).

Source: Based on Beishon 2019.

Alternatively, in situations where a meta-analysis has not been conducted because to do so would be inappropriate (for example, methodologically flawed studies or substantial heterogeneity), review authors may not consider it appropriate to present any numerical estimates of test accuracy. For example:

Alternative example – no numerical estimate of test accuracy presented

Two studies evaluated the use of devices within the mouth (4938 tooth surfaces) and two studies (59 tooth surfaces) evaluated the use of devices on extracted teeth. Due to the small number of studies and differences between studies we could not provide an overall combined summary of the accuracy of the different tests.

Source: Based on Fee 2020.

13.3.7.7   Graphical illustration of test accuracy results

The use of graphics facilitates understanding of probabilistic information (Whiting 2015). An example of a test consequence graphic to complement the rapid swab tests for strep sore throat plain language summary example is provided in Figure 13.3.a and Figure 13.3.b (Whiting 2018b). A graphic could be included within the findings section of the main review or a link to a graphic could be provided in the online version of a Cochrane Review plain language summary (Macey 2020).

The graphic is populated using natural frequencies (see Chapter 11), combined with the information on the implications of positive (true positive and false positive) and negative (true negative and false negative) index test results.

A limitation of the structure of the test consequence graphic presented in Figure 13.3.a and Figure 13.3.b is that it rapidly becomes complicated when estimates of test accuracy for more than one index test are being presented.

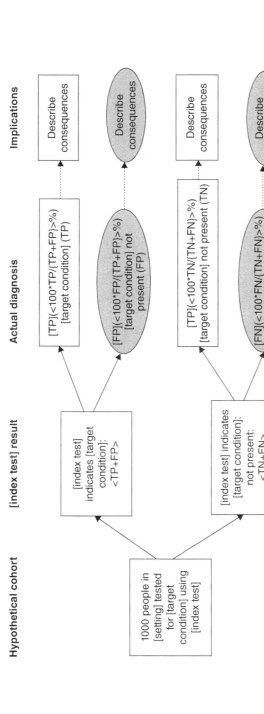

Hypothetical cohort

1000 people in [setting] tested for [target condition] using [index test]

[index test] result

[index test] indicates [target condition]: <TP+FP>

[index test] indicates [target condition]: not present: <TN+FN>

Actual diagnosis

[TP](<100*TP/{TP+FP}>%) [target condition] (TP)

[FP](<100*FP/{TP+FP}>%) [target condition] not present (FP)

[TP](<100*TN/{TN+FN}>%) [target condition] not present (TN)

[FN](<100*FN/{TN+FN}>%) [target condition] (FN)

Implications

Describe consequences

Describe consequences

Describe consequences

Describe consequences

TP: true positive – test is positive (indicates (target condition]) and patient has [target condition]
FP: false positive – test is positive (indicates [target condition]) but patient does not have [target condition]
TN: true negative – test is negative (indicates (target condition] not present) and patient does not have [target condition]
FN: false negative – test is negative (indicates [target condition] not present) but patient has [target condition]

Figure 13.3.a **Template for a test consequence graphic.** Text in square brackets, [], is replaced with text or numbers in the boxes in the final figure. Text in angle brackets, <>, indicates expressions to be calculated. Source: Whiting 2018.

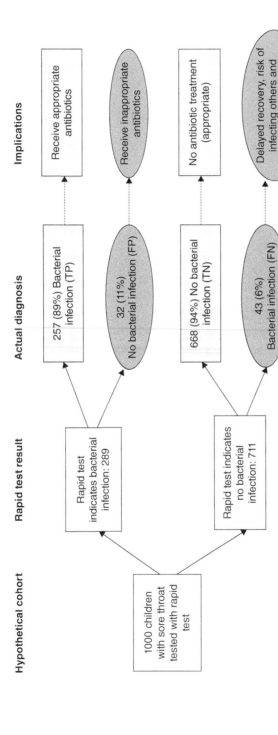

Hypothetical cohort

1000 children with sore throat tested with rapid test

Rapid test result

Rapid test indicates bacterial infection: 289

Rapid test indicates no bacterial infection: 711

Actual diagnosis

257 (89%) Bacterial infection (TP)

32 (11%) No bacterial infection (FP)

668 (94%) No bacterial infection (TN)

43 (6%) Bacterial infection (FN)

Implications

Receive appropriate antibiotics

Receive inappropriate antibiotics

No antibiotic treatment (appropriate)

Delayed recovery, risk of infecting others and possible severe complications

TP: true positive – test is positive (indicates (target condition]) and patient has [target condition]
FP: false positive – test is positive (indicates [target condition]) but patient does not have [target condition]
TN: true negative – test is negative (indicates (target condition] not present) and patient does not have [target condition]
FN: false negative – test is negative (indicates [target condition] not present) but patient has [target condition]

Figure 13.3.b **Application of the test consequence graphic.** *How accurate are rapid swab tests for bacterial infection in children with sore throat?*

13.3.8 What are the limitations of the evidence?

This section should describe the main limitations of the evidence. This should include a summary of the methodological quality of the studies included in the review and the potential impact of bias and uncertainty on estimates of accuracy. This section should also describe the reference standard used in the review and comment on the validity of the reference standard. For example:

'In the included studies, the diagnosis of target condition was made by assessing all patients with reference standard (the reference standard). This is likely to have been a reliable method for deciding whether patients really had target condition.'

Rapid swab tests for strep sore throat example
In the included studies, the diagnosis of bacterial infection was confirmed by the most accurate test available: seeing if bacteria could be grown in the laboratory from samples taken from children's throats (the reference standard).

If there was a potential for bias in the included studies, we suggest using a generic statement and then explaining how bias may have had an impact on estimates of test accuracy. We do not recommend going into detail about the type of bias that may have affected the included studies, such as verification bias or review bias. For example:

'However, there were some problems with how the studies were conducted. This may result in the index test appearing more accurate than it really is.'

Rapid swab tests for strep sore throat example
Although there were problems with the conduct of some studies, their results did not differ from the more reliable studies.

If there is heterogeneity in study results, this can be highlighted here. For example:

Limitations of the evidence – heterogeneity
'The test accuracy results presented are a summary based on studies in the review. However, as estimates from individual studies varied we cannot be sure that index test will always produce these results.'
    OR
'The test accuracy results presented are a summary based on studies in the review. However, as estimates from individual studies varied considerably, it is likely that use of index test in setting may give results that differ substantially from these estimates.'

Rapid swab tests for strep sore throat example
The numbers described above are a summary based on all studies. Because estimates of accuracy varied across individual studies, we cannot be sure that the summary accuracy estimates in this review could be replicated in practice.

Imprecision (wide confidence intervals around summary estimates) and/or small sample size can also be captured in this section. For example:

Limitations of the evidence – imprecision

'The test accuracy results presented in this review come from only # studies. It is likely that estimates of test accuracy will change as more studies become available.'

Where multiple index tests are evaluated, there may be different limitations in the evidence for the different tests evaluated. This should be captured in this section. For example:

Alternative example - limitations of the evidence – multiple index tests

'The test accuracy results presented in this review come from a small number of studies: four studies for the Care Start Malaria test and two studies for the Falcivax test. It is likely that estimates of test accuracy will change as more studies become available, particularly for the Falcivax test.'

Source: Based on Agarwal 2020.

13.3.9 How up to date is this evidence?

State the *month and year* review authors searched for the included studies, for instance by saying:

'The evidence is up to date to month and year of search.'

Rapid swab tests for strep sore throat example
The evidence is up to date to July 2015.

13.4 Chapter information

Authors: Penny Whiting (*Population Health Sciences, Bristol Medical School, University of Bristol, UK*) and Clare Davenport (*Institute of Applied Health Research, University of Birmingham, UK*).

Sources of support: The authors declare no sources of support for writing this chapter.

Declarations of interest: Penny Whiting and Clare Davenport led the development of the guidance on how to write a plain language summary for diagnostic test accuracy reviews. Clare Davenport is a member of Cochrane's Diagnostic Test Accuracy Editorial Team. The authors declare no other potential conflicts of interest relevant to the topic of this chapter.

Acknowledgements: This chapter prepared by Penny Whiting and Clare Davenport is based on the findings of research funded by the Cochrane Collaboration (in part by a Cochrane's Methods Innovation Fund Grant) and drawing on the plain language summary guidance for Cochrane Intervention Reviews. The authors thank Mariska Leeflang, Reem Mustafa, Nancy Santesso, Gowri Gopalakrishna, Geraldine Cooney, Emily Jesper and Joanne Thomas for their contributions to this project.

The authors would like to thank Denise Mitchell, Jenny Negus, Brian Duncan, Karen R. Steingart and Jacqueline Dinnes for helpful peer review comments.

13.5   References

Agarwal R, Choi L, Johnson S, Takwoingi Y. Rapid diagnostic tests for Plasmodium vivax malaria in endemic countries. *Cochrane Database of Systematic Reviews* 2020; **11**: CD013218.

Beishon LC, Batterham AP, Quinn TJ, Nelson CP, Panerai RB, Robinson T, Haunton VJ. Addenbrooke's Cognitive Examination III (ACE-III) and mini-ACE for the detection of dementia and mild cognitive impairment. *Cochrane Database of Systematic Reviews* 2019; **12**: CD013282.

Bossuyt PM, Irwig L, Craig J, Glasziou P. Comparative accuracy: assessing new tests against existing diagnostic pathways. *BMJ* 2006; **332**: 1089–1092.

Chan KK, Joo DA, McRae AD, Takwoingi Y, Premji ZA, Lang E, Wakai A. Chest ultrasonography versus supine chest radiography for diagnosis of pneumothorax in trauma patients in the emergency department. *Cochrane Database of Systematic Reviews* 2020; **7**: CD013031.

Cohen JF, Bertille N, Cohen R, Chalumeau M. Rapid antigen detection test for group A streptococcus in children with pharyngitis. *Cochrane Database of Systematic Reviews* 2016; **7**: CD010502.

Dinnes J, Deeks JJ, Saleh D, Chuchu N, Bayliss SE, Patel L, Davenport C, Takwoingi Y, Godfrey K, Matin RN, Patalay R, Williams HC. Reflectance confocal microscopy for diagnosing cutaneous melanoma in adults. *Cochrane Database of Systematic Reviews* 2018; **12**: CD013190.

Dinnes J, Deeks JJ, Adriano A, Berhane S, Davenport C, Dittrich S, Emperador D, Takwoingi Y, Cunningham J, Beese S, Dretzke J, Ferrante di Ruffano L, Harris IM, Price MJ, Taylor-Phillips S, Hooft L, Leeflang MM, Spijker R, Van den Bruel A. Rapid, point-of-care antigen and molecular-based tests for diagnosis of SARS-CoV-2 infection. *Cochrane Database of Systematic Reviews* 2020; **8**: CD013705.

Fee PA, Macey R, Walsh T, Clarkson JE, Ricketts D. Tests to detect and inform the diagnosis of root caries. *Cochrane Database of Systematic Reviews* 2020; **12**: CD013806.

Gigerenzer G. What are natural frequencies? *BMJ* 2011; **343**: d6386.

Islam N, Ebrahimzadeh S, Salameh JP, Kazi S, Fabiano N, Treanor L, Absi M, Hallgrimson Z, Leeflang MM, Hooft L, van der Pol CB, Prager R, Hare SS, Dennie C, Spijker R, Deeks JJ, Dinnes J, Jenniskens K, Korevaar DA, Cohen JF, Van den Bruel A, Takwoingi Y, van de Wijgert J, Damen JA, Wang J, McInnes MD. Thoracic imaging tests for the diagnosis of COVID-19. *Cochrane Database of Systematic Reviews* 2021; **3**: CD013639.

Leeflang MM, Deeks JJ, Gatsonis C, Bossuyt PM, Cochrane Diagnostic Test Accuracy Working Group. Systematic reviews of diagnostic test accuracy. *Annals of Internal Medicine* 2008; **149**: 889–897.

Macey R, Walsh T, Riley P, Glenny AM, Worthington HV, Fee PA, Clarkson JE, Ricketts D. Fluorescence devices for the detection of dental caries. *Cochrane Database of Systematic Reviews* 2020; **12**: CD013811.

Pitcher N, Mitchell D, Hughes C. Guidance for writing a Cochrane plain language summary Version 1, June 2021. community.cochrane.org/sites/default/files/uploads/inline-files/PLS%20guidance%20final%20draft%20%28v%2020%29.pdf.

Whiting P, Leeflang M, de Salis I, Mustafa RA, Santesso N, Gopalakrishna G, Cooney G, Jesper E, Thomas J, Davenport C. Guidance was developed on how to write a plain language summary for diagnostic test accuracy reviews. *Journal of Clinical Epidemiology* 2018a; **103**: 112–119.

Whiting P, Davenport C. Understanding test accuracy research: a test consequence graphic. *Diagnostic and Prognostic Research* 2018b; **2**: 2.

Whiting PF, Davenport C, Jameson C, Burke M, Sterne JA, Hyde C, Ben-Shlomo Y. How well do health professionals interpret diagnostic information? A systematic review. *BMJ Open* 2015; **5**: e008155.

Zhelev Z, Garside R, Hyde C. A qualitative study into the difficulties experienced by healthcare decision makers when reading a Cochrane diagnostic test accuracy review. *Systematic Reviews* 2013; **2**: 32.13.6

13.6 Appendix: Additional example plain language summary

How accurate is the Informant Questionnaire on Cognitive Decline in the Elderly (IQCODE) test for dementia in hospital?

Key messages

- The studies included in this review suggest the IQCODE can identify adults over 60 years in hospital who have dementia and require specialist assessment.
- The results suggest the IQCODE is likely to be less useful in specialist memory clinics and psychiatry wards than general hospital settings. The short version and different language versions of the IQCODE are as accurate as the standard English language long version.

Why is improving dementia diagnosis important?

Dementia is common and leads to memory problems. It also affects how you think, speak, feel and behave. It is important to diagnose dementia early so that treatment and support for patients and carers can have maximum effect and disease progression can be delayed. Not recognizing dementia when it is present (a false negative test result) results in lost opportunities for early help, including drug therapies or support for patients and carers. An incorrect diagnosis of dementia (a false positive test result) may result in anxiety, stress, wasted resources and unnecessary investigation and treatment.

What is the IQCODE test?

The IQCODE is a questionnaire that has been developed to help diagnose dementia. There are two versions of the IQCODE: a 'long' version (26 questions) and a 'short' version (16 questions). Each question asks if a person's ability to perform certain everyday tasks has changed. Both versions are completed based on information supplied by somebody close to the person being assessed for dementia. Questions are rated on a scale of 1 'has become much better' to 5 'has become much worse'. A diagnosis of dementia is more likely with higher scores.

What did we want to find out?

We wanted to find out how accurate the IQCODE questionnaire is for diagnosing dementia in hospital settings.

What did we do?

We searched for studies that had investigated the accuracy of the IQCODE test in hospital settings and we combined the results across these studies.

What did we find?

The review included 13 relevant studies with a total of 2745 participants. Studies included in the review were carried out in Europe, Australia, China, Singapore and Thailand. Some studies included patients because they had memory problems or other signs of dementia, other studies included general patients admitted to hospital. Average age ranged from 65 to 82 years. The percentage of people with a final diagnosis of dementia was between 11% and 87% across studies (an average of 51%).

The results of these studies indicate that in theory, if the IQCODE were to be used in hospital settings in a group of 1000 people, of whom 500 (50%) have dementia:

- An estimated 625 would have an IQCODE result indicating dementia and of these 170 (27%) would not have dementia.
- Of the 375 people with a result indicating that dementia is not present, 45 (12%) would actually have dementia.

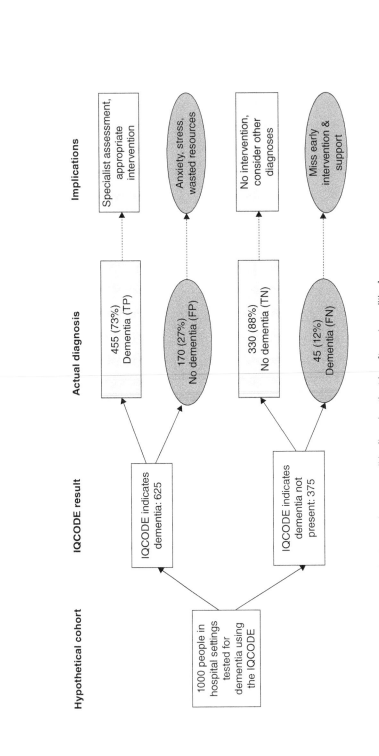

Hypothetical cohort

1000 people in hospital settings tested for dementia using the IQCODE

IQCODE result

IQCODE indicates dementia: 625

IQCODE indicates dementia not present: 375

Actual diagnosis

455 (73%) Dementia (TP)

170 (27%) No dementia (FP)

330 (88%) No dementia (TN)

45 (12%) Dementia (FN)

Implications

Specialist assessment, appropriate intervention

Anxiety, stress, wasted resources

No intervention, consider other diagnoses

Miss early intervention & support

TP: true positive – test is positive (indicates (target condition]) and patient has [target condition]
FP: false positive – test is positive (indicates [target condition]) but patient does not have [target condition]
TN: true negative – test is negative (indicates [target condition] not present) and patient does not have [target condition]
FN: false negative – test is negative (indicates [target condition] not present) but patient has [target condition]

The IQCODE produces more false positive and false negative results (more people in the red ovals in the diagram) in specialist memory clinics and psychiatry wards than in general hospital clinics and wards. There is no difference in results between long and short versions of the IQCODE or for languages other than English (similar numbers in each box in the diagram).

What are the limitations of the evidence?

In the included studies, the diagnosis of dementia was made by assessing all patients with an in-depth clinical interview (the reference standard). This is likely to have been a reliable method for deciding whether patients really had dementia. However, there were some problems with how the studies were conducted. This may result in the IQCODE appearing more accurate than it really is, increasing the number of correct IQCODE test results (green rectangles) in the diagram.

How up to date is this review?

The evidence is up to date to January 2013.

Source: Adapted from Harrison JK, Fearon P, Noel-Storr AH, McShane R, Stott DJ, Quinn TJ. Informant Questionnaire on Cognitive Decline in the Elderly (IQCODE) for the diagnosis of dementia within a secondary care setting. *Cochrane Database of Systematic Reviews* 2015; **3**:CD010772.

Index

Page locators in **bold** indicate tables. Page locators in *italics* indicate figures. This index uses letter-by-letter alphabetization.

2x2 tables
  data collection 134–135, 141–144, **142, 143, 145–146, 149–150**, 161
  measures of test accuracy 54, 56–57, **57**, 68, **69**
  meta-analysis 219, 236, 297, 316
  presenting findings 330
  study design 49

abstracts
  conference abstracts 132
  data collection 132, 144
  literature searches 98–100, 108, 112, 119–120
acceptability criteria 55–56
add-on tests 79
adverse events 151
advisory groups 12
Akaike's information criterion (AIC) 223
algorithmic search features 103, 119
allocation sequence 179
applicability *see* risk of bias and applicability assessment
area under the curve (AUC) 66, 113, 309
atypical data sets 296–305, *297–298, 302*, **303**, *305*
AUC *see* area under the curve
author contact 108, 134–135
Authors' conclusions 350, 369–374
author team
  criteria for authorship 12
  importance of the team 11

incorporating relevant perspectives and stakeholder involvement 12–13
planning a systematic review of test accuracy 11–13

bias *see individual bias types*; risk of bias and applicability assessment
bibliographic databases 101–104, 119, 121
binary data 54
BIOSIS Previews 103
bivariate model 215–219, *218*, **218**
  analysis with small numbers of studies 238–239
  Bayesian estimation in rjags 261–263, *263*, 287–291, *290–291*, 316–317, *318*
  comparing index tests 231–232, **233**, *233*, 237–238, **237**
  comparison of summary points 272–291
  estimation of a summary point 251–266
  fitting model using R 256–260, 284–287, 299–301
  fitting model using SAS 251–253, 274–280, *276*, 298–299
  fitting model using Stata 253–256, 280–284, *283*, 299
  generating an SROC plot 265, *276*
  imperfect reference standards 316–321, *318, 320*
  investigating heterogeneity 222–230, **225**, *226*
  monitoring convergence 263–264, *270*, 317, *318*

Cochrane Handbook for Systematic Reviews of Diagnostic Test Accuracy, First Edition. Edited by Jonathan J. Deeks, Patrick M. Bossuyt, Mariska M. Leeflang and Yemisi Takwoingi.
© 2023 The Cochrane Collaboration. Published 2023 by John Wiley & Sons Ltd.

bivariate model (*cont'd*)
  presenting findings 333, **334**
  sensitivity analysis 239–241, 266, 320–321
  sparse data and atypical data sets 297–303
  summary statistics 264–265, 289–291,
    317–320, *320*
  undertaking meta-analysis 250
blinding 176, 184
Boolean operators 112–113
Box-Cox transformations 222
broad questions 87–88

case-control studies
  risk of bias and applicability assessment
    177–178
  study design 39, *39*, 42
categorical data 151
Chi² statistic 223, 232
China National Knowledge Infrastructure
    (CNKI) 103
CINAHL 103–104, 115
clinical decisions 25
clinical pathway
  defining the clinical pathway 80–83, *81–82*
  unclear and multiple clinical pathways 83–84
clinical reference standard 45
clinical study reports (CSR) 133
Clopper–Pearson method 61
CNKI *see* China National Knowledge
    Infrastructure
CoCites 106
comparative studies
  drawing conclusions 359–362, 368
  evaluating medical tests 28
  measures of test accuracy 54, 68–71, **69**
  meta-analysis 206, 211, 216, 230–238,
    272–301
  presenting findings 330, 333–336, **334–335**
  risk of bias and applicability assessment 178–
    181, **180–181**, 188, **189**
  study design 45–47, *46–47*
composite reference standard 44, *302*
concealment of allocation 179
conclusions *see* drawing conclusions
conference abstracts 132
confidence intervals
  data collection 143–144
  drawing conclusions 355–356, 360, 361,
    364, 365
  measures of test accuracy 60–61, 68

meta-analysis 208, 210, 211, 216, 218, 226,
    237, *238*, **287**, 305, 311
  plain language summary 392
  presenting findings 334, 336, 337, 344–345,
    346
  risk of bias and applicability 171
conflicts of interest 14
confounders
  drawing conclusions 362, 368
  meta-analysis 231
  presenting findings 340
consecutive enrolment 176–177
consensus
  data collection 159
  drawing conclusions 367
consumer involvement 13
continuous data
  data collection 151
  measures of test accuracy 54
  review questions 91
controlled vocabulary 110–112
counts 54
coupled forest plots 208, *209, 267*
covariates
  data collection 151
  meta-analysis 215, 222–229
cross-classification
  measures of test accuracy 54, 56, **57**
  planning a systematic review of test
    accuracy 11
  study design 37
cross-referencing 133–134
cross-sectional studies
  review questions 88
  study design 37, *38–39*
CSR *see* clinical study reports
c-statistic *see* area under the curve

data collection 131–167
  2x2 contingency tables 134–135, 141–144,
    142, 143, 145–146, 149–150, 161
  checklist of data items 136, **136–137**
  concepts and definitions 132
  correspondence with investigators 134–135
  demographics 138
  extracting and converting study
    results 141–151
  extracting covariates 151
  extracting data from reports 157–160
  flow and timing 140–141

global measures 144
index test 139–140, **146**, *148*, **149–150**
individual patient data 133, 150
managing and sharing data and tools
    160–163, **161–163**
missing data and partial verification bias
    140, 148
multiple index tests from same study
    148–150, *149–150*
multiple reports and complex reviews
    158–159, 160–163, **161–163**
multiple thresholds and extracting data from
    ROC curves or graphics 147–148, *148*
other information to collect 151–152
participant characteristics and
    setting 138–139
sources of data 132–135
studies versus reports as unit of
    interest 133–134
study methods 137–138
subgroups of patients 150
target condition and reference
    standard 140, **145**
test failures 147
tools for data collection 152–157, **153–154**
what data to collect 135–137
data mining 120
decision analysis 24
deep learning 121
delayed verification 44
deviance information criterion (DIC) 223
diagnostic odds ratios (DOR)
    data collection 144
    drawing conclusions 360
    measures of test accuracy 63, *64*
    meta-analysis 219, 223, 228, 269
    presenting findings 330–332, *331*
    relative diagnostic odds ratio 228
    risk of bias and applicability assessment 192
Diagnostic Test Accuracy Editorial Team 5
DIC *see* deviance information criterion
Discussion section 350, 365–366
dissertations databases 104
DOR *see* diagnostic odds ratios
dot plots 147–148, *148*
drawing conclusions 349–376
  applicability of findings to review
    question 369
  assessing the strength of the evidence
    352–362
  Authors' conclusions 350, 369–374

Discussion section 350, 365–366
GRADE approach 362–365
heterogeneity 359–360, 364
implications for practice 370–373
implications for research 373–374
incomplete body of evidence 361–362
precision of summary estimates 360–361
risk of bias and applicability assessment 351,
    359, 363–364, 367
strengths and weaknesses of included
    studies 366–367
strengths and weaknesses of review 367–368
Summary of findings tables 350–352,
    353–358

ecological bias 340
eligibility/inclusion criteria
  data collection 133–134, 138
  drawing conclusions 369
  literature searches 120–121
  meta-analysis 205, 239
  plain language summary 384
  presenting findings 328
  review questions 77, 76, 88–93
  risk of bias and applicability assessment 178,
    193, **195**
  study design 36, 39–40
Embase 102–103, 105, 110–111, 115
errata
  data collection 132
  literature searches 114
explanatory studies 48–49

false negatives/false positives
  data collection 141–148
  drawing conclusions 351
  evaluating medical tests 23, 25
  measures of test accuracy 57, 68, 70
  meta-analysis 219, 297, 312, *315*
  plain language summary 381
  presenting findings 330–332, 341
  risk of bias and applicability assessment
    187, 192
  study design 43
field tags 111
fixed-effect meta-analysis 214, 302–303
flow and timing
  data collection 140–141
  presenting findings 340
  risk of bias and applicability assessment
    191–195, **194–195**

flow diagrams 174–175, *175*
forest plots
    coupled forest plots 208, *209, 267*
    data collection 151
    heterogeneity *338*
    meta-analysis 208, *209*, 210, *267, 297–298, 302, 338*
    reviews without meta-analysis 345
fraudulent studies 114, 159–160
full-text reports 120–121
fully paired design 179
funding 14
funnel plots 242

Gelman-Rubin statistic 264
global measures 144
gold standard 45, 187
Google Scholar 106–107
GRADE approach 352, 362–365
graphics/figures
    data collection 147–148, *148*
    plain language summary 388–390, *389, 390, 396*
    risk of bias and applicability assessment 196, *196*
    see also presenting findings
grey literature 100, 107
guidelines 105

heterogeneity
    drawing conclusions 359–360, 364
    meta-analysis 205, 214–215, 222–230, **225**, *226–227*, **229**, *230*, 299–302
    plain language summary 391
    presenting findings 333, 336–340, *338*, **339**, 344
    review questions 77
hierarchical summary receiver operating characteristic (HSROC) model 215–216, 219–220, *220*, **221**
    analysis with small numbers of studies 238–239
    Bayesian estimation of the model 268–272, *270, 272*, 294–296, *295*, 311–315, *315*
    comparing index tests 234–235, *235*
    comparison of summary curves 291–296
    estimation of a summary curve 266–272
    fitting model using R 306–311, *310–311*
    fitting model using SAS *267*, 268, 292
    imperfect reference standard 317–320
    investigating heterogeneity 222–230, 228–230, *227*, **229**, *230*

monitoring convergence 270–271
    multiple thresholds per study 221–222, 305–315, *310–311, 315*
    sensitivity analysis 239–241, 272
    sparse data and atypical data sets 299, 302
    specification of HSROC in rjags 268–272
    summary statistics 271, 295, 317–320, *320*
    undertaking meta-analysis 249–250
HSROC *see* hierarchical summary receiver operating characteristic model

I^2 statistic 214
incomplete reporting 108
inconclusive results 145–147
inconsistency *see* heterogeneity
indexing systems 99–100, 102, 108, 110–111
index test
    data collection 139–140, **146**, *148*, **149–150**
    drawing conclusions 351–352, 362, 372–373
    inconclusive index test results 55–56
    literature searches 100–101
    measures of test accuracy 53–56, **57**
    meta-analysis 230–238, **233**, *233, 234*, **237**, *238*
    plain language summary 380–383, 386–387, 391–392
    presenting findings 330, 345
    review questions 77, 82, 85, 90–91
    risk of bias and applicability assessment 182–186, **185–186**, 191
    study design 37–38, 48
individual participation data (IPD) 133, 150
information specialists 100–101, 108
intermediate results 55
interpretation bias 184, 188
IPD *see* individual participation data

joint classification 68, **69**
Jones multiple thresholds model 222, 305–315, *310–311*
journal articles 132

keyword searching 112–113, 119

language bias 113, 361
latent class analysis (LCA)
    meta-analysis 241, 316–321, *318, 320*
    study design 45
Latin American Caribbean Health Sciences Literature (LILACS) database 103, 115
LCA *see* latent class analysis

letters 132
likelihood ratios
  data collection 143
  drawing conclusions 352
  measures of test accuracy 61–63
  meta-analysis 216, 223, 229, 282
  presenting findings 332, **332**, 344
LILACS *see* Latin American Caribbean Health
    Sciences Literature
linear mixed-effects modelling 222
linked summary receiver operating characteristic
    plots 210
linking reports 134
literature searches 97–129
  co-citation searching 105–106, 115
  controlled vocabulary and text
      words 110–112
  designing search strategies 108–115
  documenting and reporting the search
      process 115–119, *118*
  drawing conclusions 367
  forward citation searching 105–106
  fraudulent studies, retracted publications,
      errata and comments 114
  future developments 121
  handsearching 105, 115
  information specialists 100–101, 108
  keyword searching 112–113, 119
  language, date and type of document
      restrictions 113
  minimizing risk-of-bias through search
      methods 114–115
  performance measures for search
      strategies 99
  review author roles 100–101
  search filters 113
  searching for studies 98–101
  selecting relevant studies 119–121
  sources to search 101–108
  structuring the search strategy 109–110,
      110, **111**
  text word or keyword searching 112–113
  working in partnership 100
logistic regression models 71

machine learning 120, 157
management studies 43
Markov chain Monte Carlo (MCMC)
    simulation 223, 250, 263, *263*, 270, *270*,
      295, 315, 317, *318*
measures of test accuracy 53–72

analysis of primary test accuracy study 56–64
comparative studies 68–71, **69**
concepts and definitions 53–54
confidence intervals 60–61
inconclusive index test results 55–56
interpretation 59–60
other measures 61–64, **62**, *64*
positivity thresholds 64–65, *65*
predictive values 58
pre-test and post-test probabilities 59
proportion with the target condition 58–59
receiver operating characteristic curves
    66–68, *67*
sensitivity and specificity 57–58, *64–65*, *67*
target condition 56
types of test data 54–55
medical test evaluation 21–33
  biomarker discovery/development 26–27
  clinical evaluations of test accuracy 28
  early evaluations of test accuracy 27
  how diagnostic tests affect patient
      outcomes 24–26
  purposes of medical testing 28–31, **28**
  test accuracy 23–24
  test development 26–28
  types of medical tests 22–23, **22**
MEDLINE 102–103, 105, 108, 112, 114, 121
meta-analysis 203–247, 249–325
  aims for reviews of test accuracy 204
  analysis with small numbers of
      studies 238–239
  Bayesian statistics 61, 221, 241, 250, 261–266,
      270, 268–272, *270*, *272*, 287–291, *290–291*,
      294–296, *295*, 311–320, *315*, *318*, 343
  comparing index tests 230–238, **233**, *233, 235*,
      237, *238*
  comparison of summary curves 291–296
  comparison of summary points 272–291
  data collection 150
  drawing conclusions 352, 366, 368, 369
  estimation of a summary curve 266–272
  estimation of a summary point 251–266
  facilitating convergence 297–301, *298*
  fitting hierarchical models 215–241
  fixed-effect meta-analysis 214, 302–303
  graphical and tabular presentation 208–211,
      209–210
  heterogeneity 205, 214–215, 222–230, **225**,
      226–227, **229**, *230*
  imperfect reference standard 241, 316–321,
      318, *320*

meta-analysis (*cont'd*)
  literature searches 105
  methodological developments 241
  monitoring convergence 263–264, *270,*
    270–271, 295, 317, *318*
  multiple thresholds per study 221–222,
    305–315, *310–311, 315*
  plain language summary 387
  planning a systematic review of test
    accuracy 15
  planning the analysis 207–208
  presenting findings 329–336, **334–335,**
    340–346, *342*
  publication bias 242–243
  regression analysis 223–224, 227–228
  reviews of test accuracy versus reviews of
    interventions 205–206
  sensitivity analysis 239–241, 266, 272,
    320–321
  simplifying hierarchical models 301–305, *302,*
    303, *305*
  sparse data and atypical data sets 296–305,
    297–298, 302, **303,** *305*
  special topics 241–243
  summary statistics 264–265, 271, 289–291,
    295, 317–320, *320*
  verification bias 241–242
  when not to use in a review 204–205
  see also bivariate model; hierarchical
    summary receiver operating
    characteristic model
meta-epidemiology 172
misclassification 187, 192
missing data
  data collection 134–135, 140, 144, 148
  drawing conclusions 361–362
  risk of bias and applicability assessment 194
multiple-group studies 39–42, *40*
multiple index tests
  data collection 148–150, *149–150*
  risk of bias and applicability assessment 184
multiple thresholds model
  data collection 147–148, *148*
  hierarchical summary receiver operating
    characteristic model 221–222, 305–315,
    310–311, 315
  Jones method 222, 305–315, *310–311*
  Steinhauser method 222, 305–315, *310–311*

narrative summary
  drawing conclusions 366

presenting findings 346, 347
  risk of bias and applicability assessment 197
  writing a plain language summary 377–397
narrow questions 87–88
national databases 103
network meta-analysis 236
non-randomized comparative accuracy
  studies 47

objectives 86, **87**
odds ratios *see* diagnostic odds ratios
online publications 132
ordinal data 54
overall accuracy 63

paired comparative accuracy studies 46, *46*
panel-based reference 44–45, *46*
partial verification bias 148, 192
participant selection *see* recruitment
patient outcomes
  altering clinical decisions and actions 25
  changes to time frames and
    populations 25–26
  direct test effects 25
  disease progression/recurrence 31
  drawing conclusions 372–373
  evaluating medical tests 24–26
  influencing patient and clinician
    perceptions 26
  study design 36
peer review
  data collection 132, 157
  literature searches 107, 117
PICO format 84
pilot testing 156–157
PIT format 84–86
plain language summary 377–397
  aims of review 382, 395
  audience and writing style 378–379
  case example 394–397, *396*
  concepts and definitions 377–378
  contents and structure 379–392
  description of index test 382, 394
  description of study benefits 381, 394–395
  how up to date the evidence is 392, 397
  included studies 383–384
  key messages 380–381, 394
  limitations of the evidence 391–392, 397
  multiple index tests 386–387, 392
  presenting findings 384–390, *389, 390,*
    395–397, *396*

review methods 382, 395–397
title 380
planning a systematic review of test
        accuracy 3–18
    author team 11–13
    Cochrane protocols 7–11
    conduct and reporting expectations 5–6
    data management and quality assurance 6
    Diagnostic Test Accuracy Editorial Team 5
    funding and conflicts of interest 14
    keeping review up to date 6
    proposing a new review 6–7, **8**
    rationale 7
    resources and support 13–15
    software tools 15
    specific features of Cochrane Reviews 5–6
    title formats 7, **8**
    training 14–15
point estimates
    drawing conclusions 359–360, 364
    measures of test accuracy 68
    meta-analysis 211, 225, 265, 284
    presenting findings 332, 333, 344, *346*
    review questions 77
point-of-care tests 79
populations
    data collection 138
    evaluating medical tests 25–26
    plain language summary 380
    review questions 77, 80–81, 84–85, 89
    study design 39–42, *40*
positivity thresholds
    data collection 147–148
    measures of test accuracy 64, *65*
    meta-analysis 212, 219, 222, 305–315, *310,*
        311, 315
    risk of bias and applicability assessment 183
post-test odds/probabilities 59, 345
pragmatic studies 48–49
precision
    drawing conclusions 360–361, 365
    literature searches 99, 108
    meta-analysis 270
    plain language summary 392
    risk of bias and applicability assessment 171
predictive tests 31
predictive value
    data collection 141–143, **142, 143**
    drawing conclusions 352, 366
    measures of test accuracy 58
    meta-analysis 217

positive/negative predictive value 58,
    141–143, **142, 143**
    presenting findings 334, 341–344, *342*
predisposition tests 29
preprints 132
presenting findings 327–348
    comparisons of test accuracy 333–336,
        334–335
    confidence intervals for differences in test
        accuracy 336–337
    description of included studies 328–329
    individual and summary estimates of
        test accuracy 329–333, *331,* **331–332**
    investigations of sources of heterogeneity
        336–340, *338,* **339**
    meta-analysis 208–211, *209–210,* 265, 308–
        311, *310–311,* 317–320, *320, 338*
    methodological quality of included
        studies 329
    narrative summary 197
    plain language summary 377–397
    re-expressing summary estimates
        numerically 340–344, *342*
    results of the search 328
    Summary of findings tables 211, 345,
        350–352, **353–358**
    summary points 211–214, 333–334, **334**
    uncertainty and heterogeneity in summary
        statistics 332
    when meta-analysis cannot be
        performed 344–346
    see also forest plots; summary receiver
        operating characteristic plots
pre-test odds/probabilities 59, 345
prevalence 341–344, *342*
prior distribution function 261, 269–270,
    287, 294
PRISMA-S/PRISMA-DTA 5, 116–119, *118*
probability 59, 70–71, 345
prognostic tests 30
proof-of-concept studies
    evaluating medical tests 27
    study design 41
prospective studies 48
PsycINFO 103–104
publication bias
    drawing conclusions 361–362, 365
    funnel plots 242
    literature searches 98, 107
    meta-analysis 242
PubMed 102–103, 106, 111

QUADAS-2/QUADAS-C *see* risk of bias and
applicability assessment
quality assurance 6

random-effects meta-analysis 214, 226, 303
randomization
    comparative accuracy studies 46–47, *47*
    enrolment 176–177
    review questions 77
    sampling 192
    study design 179
RDOR *see* relative diagnostic odds ratio
receiver operating characteristic (ROC) plots
    data collection 144, 147–148
    measures of test accuracy 54, 66–68, *67*
    risk of bias and applicability assessment 183
    see also hierarchical summary receiver
        operating characteristic model; summary
        receiver operating characteristic plots
recruitment
    data collection 133, 137–138
    risk of bias and applicability assessment
        176–182, **180–181**
reference lists 100, 105, 115, 119
reference management software 119
reference standard
    clinical reference standard 45
    composite reference standard 44
    data collection 140–145, **145**
    delayed verification 44
    evaluating medical tests 23
    gold standard 45, 187
    latent class analysis 45, 241, 316–321, *318, 320*
    literature searches 99, 120
    measures of test accuracy 54, **57**
    meta-analysis 241, *302*, 316–321, *318, 320*
    multiple reference standards 42–43, *43*
    panel-based reference 44–45
    plain language summary 391
    presenting findings 340, 345
    review questions 81, 92–93
    risk of bias and applicability assessment 182,
        187–190, **189–190**
    study design 37–38, 42–45, *43*
regional databases 103
regression analysis 223–224, 227–228
regulatory reviews 133
relative diagnostic odds ratio (RDOR) 228
relative risks 71
reliability 159
replacement tests 78

reporting bias
    drawing conclusions 361
    literature searches 113
reports 158–159
representativeness 177
requests for information 108
retracted publications 114
retrospective studies 48
review bias 391
review questions 75–95
    add-on tests 79
    aims of systematic reviews of test
        accuracy 76–77
    broad versus narrow questions 87–88
    concepts and definitions 75–76
    defining the clinical pathway 80–83, *81–82*
    defining the review question 84–88
    drawing conclusions 369
    eligibility criteria 77, 80, 88–93
    identifying the clinical problem 77–84
    index test 77, 82, 85, 90–91
    investigations of heterogeneity 77
    objectives 86, **87**
    plain language summary 380–381
    populations 77, 80–81, 84–85, 89
    reference standard 81, 92–93
    replacement tests 78
    risk of bias and applicability
        assessment 169–172
    role of a new test 77–80
    target condition 57–58, 84–86, 91–92
    triage tests 78, 82
    unclear and multiple clinical pathways 83–84
RevMan
    data collection 142–143
    meta-analysis 215–216, 221, 253, 265
    planning a systematic review of test
        accuracy 15
risk of bias and applicability
        assessment 169–201
    bias and imprecision 171
    biases in test accuracy studies: empirical
        evidence 172
    bias versus applicability 171–172
    concepts and definitions 170
    drawing conclusions 351, 359, 363, 367–368
    literature searches 114–115
    narrative summary of assessment 197
    presenting findings 196, *196*, 327–328, 345
    QUADAS-2
        applicability assessment 174

background 173
flow and timing 191–195, **194–195**
flow diagrams 174–175, *175*
index test 182–186, **185–186**
participant selection 176–182, **194–195**
performing the QUADAS-2
   assessment 175–176
reference standard 182, 187–190,
   189–190
risk of bias assessment 173–174
using and tailoring QUADAS-2 174
QUADAS-C
   background 173
   flow and timing 193–195, **195**
   index test 182–186, **185–186**
   participant selection 178–181, **180–181**
   reference standard 188–189, **189–190**
study design 43
risk stratification 29
ROC *see* receiver operating characteristic
Rutter and Gatsonis HSROC model *see*
      hierarchical summary receiver operating
      characteristic model

sample size 141, **142, 143**
sampling methods 137–138
scientific misconduct 159–160
screening tests 29
search filters 113
search recall 99, 108
sensitivity/specificity
   data collection 141–144, **142**, *148*
   drawing conclusions 350–352, 360, 361, 366
   evaluating medical tests 23, 27
   literature searches 99, 115
   measures of test accuracy 57–58, *64–65, 67*
   meta-analysis 205–241, *218*, **218**, *220*, **221**,
      238, 252, 261–273, 276, 282, **287**,
      297–311, *305, 310–311*, 320–321
   presenting findings 330–336, **331–332, 334,**
      335, 337, 341–346, *342, 346*
   risk of bias and applicability assessment
      181, 192
setting
   data collection 138–139
   plain language summary 391
   review questions 80–81
software tools 15
sparse data sets
   meta-analysis 296–305, *297–298, 302*, **303**, *305*
   plain language summary 387

SROC *see* summary receiver operating
      characteristic
staging tests 29–30
stakeholder involvement 12–13
standard error
   data collection 144
   meta-analysis 224, 239
Steinhauser multiple thresholds model 222,
      305–315, *310–311*
study design 35–51
   basic design for test accuracy study 36–39,
      38–39
   clinical reference standard 45
   comparative studies 45–47, *46–47*
   composite reference standard 44
   concepts and definitions 35
   delayed verification 44
   gold standard 45
   latent class analysis 45
   multiple groups of participants 39–42, *40*
   multiple reference standards 42–43, *43*
   panel-based reference 44–45, *46*
   pragmatic versus explanatory studies 48–49
   prospective versus retrospective studies 48
   risk of bias and applicability assessment 178
study methods 137–138
subgroups of patients 150
subject headings 112
subject-specific databases 103–104
Summary of findings tables
   drawing conclusions 350–352, **353–358**
   meta-analysis 211
   presenting findings 345
summary receiver operating characteristic
      (SROC) plots
   comparisons of test accuracy 334–336, **335**
   drawing conclusions 351, 360
   individual and summary estimates of test
      accuracy 330–332, *331*
   meta-analysis 208–210, *210*, 265, *276*
   planning a systematic review of test
      accuracy 15
   reviews without meta-analysis 345, *346*
   see also hierarchical summary receiver
      operating characteristic model
surveillance 31
systematic reviews of interventions 24

tables of findings *see* Summary of findings tables
target condition
   data collection 140–145

target condition (*cont'd*)
  drawing conclusions 360
  evaluating medical tests 23, 27
  literature searches 100, 120
  measures of test accuracy 53–72
  plain language summary 380–381, 391
  planning a systematic review of test accuracy
        6–7
  presenting findings 340–346, *342*
  review questions 57–58, 84–86, 91–92
  risk of bias and applicability assessment
        187–190
  study design 35–39, 42–43, 48
test failures 147
test positives/test negatives
  data collection 141–144
  evaluating medical tests 23, 30
  measures of test accuracy 54, 56, 64–65, *65*
  meta-analysis 219
  presenting findings 330–331
  review questions 82–83, 91
  risk of bias and applicability assessment 192
  study design 42–43
text words 110–112
therapeutic monitoring 31
theses databases 104
time frames 25–26
timing *see* flow and timing
title
  plain language summary 380

planning a systematic review of test accuracy 7, **8**
  title searches 119
training 14–15
treatment efficacy 31
treatment selection 30
triage tests 78, 82
trial registries
  data collection 133
  literature searches 107–108, 115
two-group/two-gate studies 40–41, *40*

uncertainty
  drawing conclusions 351, 363, 373
  measures of test accuracy 60
  plain language summary 391
  presenting findings 332
unexpected findings 151
univariate tests 214
unverified participants 192

validity 359
variance–covariance matrix 255, 256, 260, 261,
        287, 292, 297, 301, 303, **303**
verification bias 241–242, 391
  see also partial verification bias

web searching 106–107
Wilson score interval 61

Youden's index 63–64, 308–311, *310–311*